W9-DIY-495

in China manipulating animal viruses to study their potential to infect humans. Dr. Fauci has publicly denied any responsibility, but Senator Rand Paul has methodically exposed Fauci's obfuscation, denial, and cover-up. In *Deception*, Paul gives a riveting account of how these and other lapses in oversight and skirting of regulation to carry out gain-of-function experiments could have catalyzed the pandemic. Paul demands action to reform out-of-control scientists and their enablers, who may have caused the worst peacetime public health catastrophe in history."

—Jay Bhattacharya, M.D., Ph.D., professor of health policy, Stanford University

"It happens from time to time in history that one person is the right person for the time and place, without whom everything would have been different, and much more dreadful. That is the case with Senator Rand Paul, who has earned for himself a heroic place. Imagine: without Rand Paul, Anthony Fauci, who preferred hiding behind friendly reporters during the ruination of American liberty from 2020 to 2022, might never have encountered a critic. This is the accounting that we so desperately need."

—Jeffrey A. Tucker, president and founder, the Brownstone Institute

"Senator Rand Paul has written an eye-opening account countering many of America's public health leaders and government officials who fail to fully explore facts about the origins of the SARS-CoV-2 pandemic. Adding to revelations about gross incompetence, censorship of disagreement, and dishonest distortions by public health leaders to unethically manipulate the public, Senator Paul refutes the effort by leading scientists, prestigious medical journals, the WHO, and the NIH itself to thwart discovery of the truth. If their systemic effort was intended to conceal malfeasance by America's

NIH, led by Drs. Collins and Fauci, who sent American tax dollars to fund dangerous gain-of-function research in Wuhan and circumvent Obama-era restrictions, then we are witnessing perhaps the deadliest cover-up scandal in history."

—Scott W. Atlas, M.D., Robert Wesson Senior Fellow in Health Policy, Hoover Institution, Stanford University, and former advisor to the President of the United States and member of the White House Coronavirus Task Force

"Rand Paul has been the rare political leader who relentlessly interrogated our deeply misguided pandemic policies. This true public servant worked tirelessly to expose the corruption and conflicts of interest driving our public health apparatus down this destructive path. Here he gives us the insider's view from the front lines of the political battle for the health of our nation. *Deception* is essential reading for Americans who do not want to live permanently under a biomedical security state."

—Aaron Kheriaty, M.D., director of the Bioethics and American Democracy Program, Ethics and Public Policy Center

"I can count on one hand the number of elected officials who dared to question the approved narrative crafted by Dr. Fauci & Co. during the COVID pandemic. Senator Rand Paul was one of those officials. *Deception* is the pinnacle of his tireless efforts to shed light on the malfeasance that led to the worst public policy decisions of our lifetime. The truths he exposes will hopefully lead to the dismantling of the most corrupt class of professionals to lead our once-trusted government institutions. Let it be so—and quickly!"

—Justin Hart, author of *Gone Viral: How Covid Drove the World Insane*

DECEPTION

ALSO BY RAND PAUL

The Case Against Socialism

Our Presidents and Their Prayers

Taking a Stand

Government Bullies

The Tea Party Goes to Washington

DECEPTION
The Great COVID Cover-Up

RAND PAUL
WITH KELLEY ASHBY PAUL

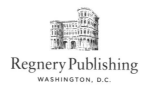

Regnery Publishing
WASHINGTON, D.C.

Regnery® is a registered trademark and its colophon is a trademark of Salem Communications Holding Corporation

Cataloging-in-Publication data on file with the Library of Congress

ISBN: 978-1-68451-513-4
eISBN: 978-1-68451-514-1

Library of Congress Control Number: 2023941988

Published in the United States by
Regnery Publishing
A Division of Salem Media Group
Washington, D.C.
www.Regnery.com

Manufactured in the United States of America

10 9 8 7 6 5 4 3 2 1

Books are available in quantity for promotional or premium use. For information on discounts and terms, please visit our website: www.Regnery.com.

For Kelley:

When my hair begins to thin
We will be lodged and snuggled
Safe from the north-eastern winds
The drafty caulking
The aging woodwork
Lofty ceilings and unadorned timbers
Threaten cold
But we will be protected by woolen blankets
And perhaps a sip of wine by the fire
And the heat of bodies so close

Happiness deferred if you can call it that
The so long suffering
Mourned about
But immediately missed
The long day
The daily doing
The stuff of living will be followed
By the glow of picking through the photographs
The memories of children laughing
And mothers weeping
And stoic dads who solemnly
Stand erect at the changing of the guard
All of us bystanders
But finally having the time to appreciate
The splendor
The time to wait and sit
To move the bishop without
Concern that the queen may be in danger
Or that the pawns might rebel
There will be time
When no intrusion will obscure
The butterfly or deter her flight
A time for reflection
Before the coming of goodnight

Contents

Preface

For a contrarian like me, it's hard not to idolize Li Wenliang. He was a young ophthalmologist, just as I once was. Full of youth, unapologetic, and a force for truth even living in the midst of Communist China, where citizens are serenaded by drones hovering outside the balconies of their high-rise apartments singing the true state anthem: "Control your soul's desire for freedom."[1]

Li Wenliang gave his life taking care of COVID patients and trying to warn the world of the impending pandemic. Meanwhile American government scientists essentially spit on his grave as they buried the truth to cover their asses. At every turn, Anthony Fauci has worked to obscure any connections between the NIH-funded Wuhan lab and COVID-19. Did Li know that his postings on Weibo chat about an unknown SARS-like virus that was killing people in Wuhan would essentially be his last words?

How was this hero, this truth-teller, treated by the Communist Chinese? He was summoned and reprimanded for "spreading rumors" and "severely disturbing the social order." Li was forced to sign a confession.[2]

Realize that he was accused of spreading "misinformation"—the same sort of accusations that would soon be leveled in the land of the free. I should know. They made the same accusations against me. Major media platforms such as Facebook labeled anyone suggesting that COVID could have originated in the Wuhan lab a purveyor of this so-called misinformation.[3] The term would become the watchword of the American left, desperate to control the narrative by silencing those who questioned it.

According to the official Chinese narrative, Li died from COVID.

He was only thirty-three years old. The death rate from COVID or with COVID in the United States for adults between the ages of thirty and thirty-nine is about 0.04 percent, quite rare.[4] Likely, that rate is even lower if patients with significant comorbidities are excluded. Li's death was a great loss but also a rare occurrence in his age bracket.

Extraordinarily rare.

In an authoritarian society, such deaths linger and lead to whispers regarding the veracity of official causes of death...

When his death was posted online sometime after midnight, the comments on Weibo quickly came in: "I knew you would post this in the middle of the night.... You think we've all gone to sleep? No. We haven't."

Another commenter posted that "countless young people will mature overnight after today: the world is not as beautiful as we imagined. Are you angry? If any of us here is fortunate enough to speak up for the public in the future, please make sure you remember tonight's anger."[5]

The wistful responses of China's youth to the loss of one of their own generation remind me of the Parveen Shakir poem:

They insist upon catching the firefly in the daylight
The children of our age, have grown wiser.[6]

It is yet to be determined whether a new generation of Chinese youth will rise up, remembering the hope that came when Deng Xiaoping dismantled Mao's brutal shackles. Will a new generation channel the despair of Tiananmen Square to forge a new China? A China whose government does not threaten to one day unleash upon the world, either by accident or by intent, a biological scourge that civilization might struggle to survive?

With Li's untimely passing, even China's National Supervisory Commission, an anti-corruption department of government, chimed in, saying they would investigate Li's death "in response to issues raised by the masses." As CNN reported, "The short statement did not elaborate on the nature of the 'issues' raised."[7]

Li Wenliang was a hero, and I dedicate this book to Li and all others who resist censorship in the hope that the DNA of resistance and independent thought will never be stamped out by government censors.[8]

Introduction

Once upon a Nightmare...

A s news of the mysterious and deadly virus spread, one can only imagine the flop sweat that must have soaked through Shi Zhengli's clothing as she paced her office in the Wuhan Institute of Virology (WIV). Known worldwide as the "bat scientist," Dr. Shi trembled at the thought that a worldwide pandemic may have originated in her lab.[1] News that three of her colleagues were seriously ill with a pneumonia of unknown origin sent shock waves throughout the WIV. Yet in Communist China, one's first worry isn't always about the truth, but how the party reacts to the truth. Shi had to act quickly if she were to survive.

She knew there was no tolerance for criticism. She'd seen what happened to colleagues, such as Huang Yanling, who didn't toe the party line. She didn't know yet that Huang would ultimately go missing, but Shi wasn't naïve. Shi hadn't reached this pinnacle of success in the Chinese research world without understanding the Communist Party roadblocks that could stymie anyone's ascent to leadership. Any misstep might be her last.

Dr. Shi's accomplishments were legion. From her field expeditions to remote caves to her collection and identification of over a hundred new coronaviruses to her collaboration with famous American scientists, Shi knew she was a star in government circles. But Shi also understood that no one in China is ever truly safe. Everyone is ultimately expendable, and the trick was staying ahead of the curve, avoiding the hangman's ax.

Her lab was now under direct military control—not that her lab had ever *not* been under the military's watchful eye. It might help her survive if the new military command understood that she had just been following orders. It might help her survive if she reminded everyone that she listened to and obeyed the direct orders of military scientist General Zhou Yusen.

Shi simply provided him with samples of the mutant virus. He promised a general vaccine for all coronaviruses. General Zhou insisted that the virus must have significant ability to infect humans; the coronavirus needed to have a special site to allow it to enter human cells. Shi could do that. Shi had even submitted an application for a U.S. defense agency grant to do precisely that. Shi didn't yet know the virus from her lab would kill millions, but she did hope that the world would one day judge her based on her desire to save lives.

As for her personal survival, Shi pinned her hopes on the "I was just following orders" defense. General Zhou was really the one in charge. He was official military, for goodness' sake. Surely, he would either absorb the blame or take the fall. Dr. Shi would not know until the spring that General Zhou would not survive the year.

Was he killed because the leaked virus killed millions of Chinese? Or did he commit suicide because the vaccine he developed was not really that effective? Dr. Shi didn't know General Zhou's fate yet. All Dr. Shi knew at the time was that mistakes were not tolerated, that errors of this magnitude were terminal, and Shi knew that survival depended not only on demonstrating her usefulness but also showing her party loyalty by expertly covering up all traces of the virus's true origin.

But now it was a race against time. All evidence of the virus so carefully cultivated in her lab must be eliminated, not just to destroy the evidence but to protect any other lab workers from dying. Once the danger abated enough for her to think, Shi knew the next step was to prevent the world from knowing that the virus originated in her lab.

So late one night in September on a muggy day with midday temperatures exceeding ninety degrees, Dr. Shi destroyed the online coronavirus database she had so painstakingly compiled over the years. Much of that research was financed by the U.S. taxpayer.

The cover-up had begun.*

And it was only September 2019. The rest of the world would have to wait until January 2020 to learn of the COVID pandemic. And even then, the Chinese government would begin by swearing that the virus did not transmit from human to human…

So many lies.

Not just the lies of the Chinese government—even our own government lied. And lied even more as it tried to hide every bit of evidence of U.S. government funding of dangerous coronavirus gain-of-function experiments in Wuhan.

---

* This opening is based on facts but fictionalizes Shi Zhengli's feelings and thoughts about the origins of COVID. Obviously, this revery is conjecture, and the character does not purport to be an objective portrait of any real person living or dead.

PART I

The Cover-Up

CHAPTER I

The COVID Cover-Up Begins in a Whirlwind

In early January 2020, there were reports from Wuhan of a mysterious pneumonia. At first Chinese officials reported that it did not appear to be passed from human to human,[1] but within days they couldn't contain the lie. Not only was it found to be quite contagious, it also was quickly shown to kill.

The cover-up likely began even before Anthony Fauci knew for certain how dangerous the pandemic would become. Previous lab leaks had never killed more than a few thousand people. Fauci would not be fully aware of how readily this virus was adapted to humans for several more weeks. What Fauci did know was that he had—for several years now—personally approved gain-of-function research in Wuhan.[2]

He knew that his reputation and the billion-dollar "business of science" depended on distancing himself, the NIH (National Institutes of

Health), and the NIAID (National Institute of Allergy and Infectious Diseases) from any research in Wuhan.

In a remarkable display of scientific prowess, Professor Yong-Zhen Zhang of Fudan University obtained a sample from a pneumonia patient and sequenced the virus in an astonishing forty-hour sprint.[3] Zhang completed the analysis at 2:00 a.m. on January 6. The Chinese government told him "in no uncertain terms not to publish anything."[4]

Throughout this period, the Chinese were not forthcoming with the truth about the pneumonia-causing virus from Wuhan. For weeks the Chinese government maintained that there was no evidence of human-to-human transmission.

The Chinese government also withheld the RNA sequence from the public for several weeks and only revealed it after Zhang and Eddie Holmes, a virologist from the University of Sydney, revealed the sequence in January on virological.org. That same day, China reported its first death from COVID-19. Only when these scientists finally revealed the sequence online did the Chinese government release their own sequencing analysis—an analysis likely completed at least by late December 2019.[5]

Redfield Catches the Scent

In the next weeks, virologists around the world would scramble to analyze the new virus's genome. One virologist, Robert Redfield, head of the CDC, voiced his concern early on that the virus might have originated in the Wuhan Institute of Virology.[6]

Redfield had been an Army physician and a professor at the University of Maryland. While in the military, Redfield founded the Department of Retroviral Research. His prestigious career also included serving as Chief of Infectious Diseases at the University of Maryland School of Medicine. As a virologist and cofounder of the University of

Maryland's Institute of Human Virology, he was uniquely qualified to delve into the origin of COVID-19.

As such, Redfield was sounding the alarm worldwide by mid-January of 2020, calling Tedros Adhanom Ghebreyesus, director general of the World Health Organization (WHO), Jeremy Farrar, head of Wellcome Trust in the United Kingdom, and of course, Anthony Fauci. He contacted each scientist separately with the same urgent message: "We had to take the lab-leak hypothesis with extreme seriousness."[7]

Instead of answers, shockingly, Redfield was excluded from Fauci-led meetings concerning COVID-19. Why would a virologist *who is also head of the CDC* not be included in discussions concerning the origins of COVID-19?

According to Redfield, Fauci excluded him from meetings of the inner circle from the get-go because Redfield was open to the possibility that COVID-19 could have leaked from the Wuhan lab. Redfield didn't learn the full extent of his exclusion until he read the emails that a federal judge forced Fauci to reveal under the Freedom of Information Act.[8]

Redfield remembers getting his first situation report on "a new unspecified pneumonia on January 1st," and he immediately doubted the veracity of the reports coming from China's government.[9]

George Gao, the head of China's CDC, told Redfield that there was "no evidence of human-to-human transmission, no hospital transmission," and that the infected were only people who had been to the wet market.

But only a few days later, Gao called back and said, "Bob, the epidemic is out of control with cases everywhere and it has nothing to do with the wet market."[10]

To Redfield, the origin of the virus—that is, whether it arose naturally from an animal host or leaked from a lab—was an extremely important piece of information. What alarmed Redfield from the beginning was the ease of COVID-19's transmission from human to human. Previous coronaviruses that came from animals never adapted to transmit easily from human to human. But COVID-19 was exploding in growth, showing no difficulty transmitting between humans.[11]

Indeed, the previous outbreaks of the coronaviruses SARS and MERS could be contained because the virus never evolved to become very contagious among humans. Crucially, a virus that was pressured in the lab to adapt to survive in human cells could leak from a lab fully able to easily infect humans and then be transmitted human to human.

Clearly, whether the virus came from nature or from a lab leak *mattered*, not only in assessing culpability but in preparing for how widespread the epidemic would become. Fauci's dismissal of the lab leak likely centered on his wanting to escape blame, but it also erroneously suggested that COVID-19 might behave like SARS and MERS and not be so contagious.[12]

The true nature of COVID-19's contagiousness would become apparent within the next several weeks. And Redfield was not shy about bringing his concerns to each and every meeting with Fauci and others.

Within the first weeks of January, Redfield and Fauci were already at odds. Redfield describes it: "Fauci and I kind of got into it.... I'm a virologist and Tony is an immunologist. I told Fauci that I'm very concerned that he was championing this theory that it came from animals, but there is another theory: that it came from a laboratory."[13]

This was not the first time Redfield and Fauci had tangled. About ten years before, Redfield had sided with those who believed it was dangerous to perform gain-of-function studies to mutate bird flu so it could be aerosolized. Redfield argued against publishing these studies, explaining that the information would become a road map for potential terrorists. Fauci argued that the scientific knowledge obtained was worth the risk.[14]

Americans were deliberately kept ignorant of the raging debate in the scientific community over gain-of-function research. Fauci was deeply invested in having people believe there was overwhelming scientific consensus concerning the great value of gain-of-function research as a method to identify threats and prevent future pandemics. In reality, there is rarely overwhelming consensus in science—that is, except in modern times when billions in grant money is dangled, as we will see was the case here. In fact, many prominent scientists argued that the creation of new pathogens not found in nature had deadly risks for humankind.[15]

When I cross-examined Fauci as he testified before the Senate HELP (Health, Education, Labor and Pensions) Committee, he flatly and angrily denied that he ever funded gain-of-function research. Redfield was aghast. Redfield said, "Tony may have overplayed his hand when he was so aggressive with Congress, saying that he was never involved in funding gain of function research. There's too much evidence that's just not true."[16]

Paul Thacker, a former Senate investigator, put it this way: "When Fauci testified before Congress and denied funding gain of function research, because he has his own definition of gain of function, I immediately thought, 'This guy just lied before Congress.'"[17]

The Smoke Screen Takes Shape

Even Peter Daszak, who coauthored the findings on the research with Shi in Wuhan, explicitly referred to his research as "gain of function." According to emails obtained by FOIA, Daszak responded to NIH officials who approved the resumption of his funding with: "We are very happy to hear that our Gain of Function research funding pause has been lifted."[18]

Disturbingly, most of these insights into the timeline of the cover-up come from documents held by Fauci and the NIH and were only released when demanded by a federal judge through the Freedom of Information Act.

As Columbia economist Jeffrey Sachs puts it, "The most interesting things that I got as chair of the *Lancet* commission came from Freedom of Information Act (FOIA) lawsuits and whistleblower leaks from inside the U.S. government. Isn't that terrible? NIH was actually asked at one point: give us your research program on SARS-like viruses. And you know what they did? They released the cover page and redacted 290 pages. They gave us a cover page and 290 blank pages! That's NIH, for heaven's sake. That's not some corporation. That is the U.S. government charged with keeping us healthy."[19]

About this time, Jeremy Farrar of Wellcome Trust, perhaps the largest private provider of research dollars, remembers seeing email exchanges among respected scientists suggesting the virus had characteristics that appeared to be manipulated or even engineered to infect human cells.[20]

Farrar is a British M.D./Ph.D. who identified the re-emergence of bird flu, H5N1, in humans in 2004. If you searched a "Who's Who" of infectious diseases and vaccines, you'd find his name. He's also a former editor of the *New England Journal of Medicine*. Farrar might be considered as powerful, or more so, than Anthony Fauci.

In his book *Spike*, Farrar recounts that "by the second week in January [2020], I was beginning to realize the scale of what was happening."[21] Farrar writes, "During that period, I would do things I had never done before: acquire a burner phone, hold clandestine meetings, keep difficult secrets."[22]

Farrar does not make clear who he was afraid of. The Chinese government? The public? Were the burner phone and the secret meeting necessary to hide from the public the possibility that the virus had leaked from the Wuhan Institute of Virology? He reveals that he got advice from Wellcome chair Eliza Manningham-Buller, who, curiously, was also previously the head of Britain's intelligence agency—MI5.

It is revealing that, in trying to unravel the cover-up of COVID-19's origins, one finds a recurring intersection between spies and infectious diseases.

Why? Because even though the government scientists have circled the wagons to deny COVID-19 leaked from a lab, they know that it is a real possibility that spies across the world are constantly searching for dangerous bioweapons research or unintentional leaks of what they euphemistically refer to as "dual-use research." In other words, they are on the alert for viruses that might be intentionally designed to kill an enemy or viruses ostensibly just created "for study"—that might be just as dangerous.

It's not hard to see where problems might arise in this murky gray area between weapons and research.

As the rumors swirled that the virus might have leaked from the Wuhan Institute of Virology, Farrar's wife, Christiane, insists that he ring "people close to us, so they would understand what was going on in case anything happened to [you]." Farrar told his brother that "a few scientists, including me, were beginning to suspect this might be a lab accident...." Farrar also told his brother that the British and American intelligence agencies were in the loop.[23]

Whatever his reason for doing so, Farrar painted a dangerous scenario: "'If anything happens to me in the next few weeks,' I told them nervously, 'this is what you need to know.'"[24]

Why was Farrar so alarmed? He admits that his "starting bias was that it was odd for a spillover event, from animals to humans, to take off in people so immediately and spectacularly—in a city with a bio lab."[25]

The Furin Site Telltale

Furin is one of the enzymes that activates the genetic code that initiates protein synthesis in cells. A cleavage site is a spot for the enzyme to attach to genetic material and serve as a key to activate the making of specific proteins, the building blocks of life. Farrar was alarmed that this coronavirus was the first of its kind to have a furin cleavage site that "enhances infectivity" and "seemed almost designed to infect human cells."[26]

Likewise, when Redfield first learned that COVID-19 had a furin cleavage site, he said, "This isn't natural."[27] Redfield, like others, noted that the genetic code that creates COVID-19's furin cleavage site is the code most often found in *humans*, not in bats. Bizarrely, the cleavage site was so adapted to humans that it no longer allowed the virus to enter a bat cell at all.[28]

If anyone doubts that Fauci and his yes-men knew that a lab leak would boomerang and direct blame back on them, the emails obtained by Freedom of Information court orders make this point explicitly.

The compressed timeline of phone calls, Zoom conferences, and midnight emails provides a sense of the panic building in the last days of January 2020. These emails show that by January 27, the level of alarm had risen to a fever pitch. At 6:24 p.m., one of Fauci's deputies, Greg Folkers, emailed talking points for Fauci for that evening's White House press conference. The email reminded Fauci that he had approved NIAID funding for coronavirus research, including research in Wuhan. Folkers goes on to remind Fauci of the main players in the joint research with Wuhan: EcoHealth's Peter Daszak, UNC's Ralph Baric, Ian Lipkin, and Shi Zhengli of Wuhan. Folkers even lists the NIAID identifying number for a gain-of-function research grant to Baric and Shi. Fauci's own assistant labels the grant "gain of function,"[29] though Fauci himself would later vehemently assert to the American people that "the NIH has not ever and does not now fund gain-of-function research in the Wuhan Institute of Virology."[30]

That same day across the Atlantic, Farrar sends an email to Fauci: "We should use different phones: avoid putting things in emails; and ditch our normal email addresses and phone contacts." In his memoir, *Spike*, Farrar recounts, "I didn't know the term then but I now had a burner phone, which I could use only for this purpose and then get rid of."[31]

How can anyone read that and not conclude that the pursuit of the truth was taking a back seat to the secrecy of covering up?

A day later, January 28, Farrar called Eddie Holmes, the British evolutionary biologist and virologist. Farrar was worried about internet discussion that the virus may have leaked from the Wuhan lab. Farrar wanted to discuss with Holmes a preprint journal article from a few days before that had reported that the COVID-19 RNA sequence was 96 percent similar to another Wuhan virus known as RaTG13.[32]

On January 29, Kristian Andersen, professor of immunology and microbiology at Scripps Research, shared a journal article that describes a technique to modify the spike protein of the original SARS that caused the pneumonia outbreak and deaths in 2003. According to Farrar, Andersen said this study "looked like a how-to-manual for building the Wuhan coronavirus in a laboratory." Farrar describes Andersen as alarmed that this journal article suggests that researchers could have created COVID-19 in the Wuhan lab.[33]

That same day, Andersen emailed Eddie Holmes: ". . . can we talk? I need to be pulled off the ledge here." (This is Holmes's recollection.) Holmes remembers Andersen saying that ". . . there's this furin cleavage site between the S1 and S2 junctions." Additionally, "There are two restriction sites, BamHI, around it. And that section, between the restriction sites, looks like it has reduced variation."[34]

Restriction sites are areas of genetic sequences recognized by restriction enzymes. They allow scientists to insert new DNA. Andersen is saying it looks like the nucleotide sequence between the restriction sites is *not of natural origin and likely inserted by scientists.*

Holmes's response holds nothing back: "Fuck, this is bad."[35]

A few days later on January 31, the back-and-forth between the virologists concerned that COVID-19 came from a lab reached a fever pitch.

A Sickening Realization Dawns on Fauci's Yes-Men

At 5:23 p.m., on January 31, 2020, Jeremy Farrar emailed Fauci requesting a phone call. Farrar says he "contacted Tony Fauci about the rumours over the origins of the virus and asked him to speak to Kristian Andersen at Scripps."[36] The phone number is redacted from the email, but one might reasonably assume it's Farrar's burner phone. Realize it's after 10:00 p.m. in England. Something big is afoot.[37] Farrar describes his feelings at the time: "I remember becoming a little nervous about my own personal safety around this time. I don't really know what I was scared of."[38]

Farrar was in a frenzied twenty-four-hour-a-day back-and-forth with international virologists. His wife reports seventeen calls in just one night, all of which were over concerns that COVID-19 might have originated in a lab in Wuhan[39]—and now he can't explain what he was afraid of? This beggars belief.

What might be the state of a scientist in such a condition of horrified epiphany?

Might he fear retribution from the Chinese government if he is complicit in revealing that the virus might have come from a Wuhan lab? Or might he fear that the billion-dollar "business of science" could be damaged if the public becomes aware that the pandemic may have originated in a lab?

Perhaps both?

Farrar told Fauci the names of the scientists already "involved"—Kristian Andersen, Bob Garry, and Eddie Holmes—provided their contact information, and told Fauci to call Andersen.[40]

That same day, *Science* magazine released an article: "Mining Coronavirus Genomes for Clues to the Outbreak's Origins," by Jon Cohen. The article is written with the intent to dispel any possibility of a lab leak. Cohen even refers to any such hypothesis as a "conspiracy" theory.

Cohen favorably quotes Trevor Bedford, who argues that COVID-19 is "at least" twenty-five years distant evolutionarily from RaTG13. Cohen does quote a longtime critic of gain-of-function research, Professor Richard Ebright, who expresses worry about the safety protocol at the Wuhan Institute of Virology. But Cohen depicts Ebright as an outlier or gadfly of the consensus.[41] The intent is to diminish any critique from him.

The truth is that Ebright is a thirty-year-tenured molecular chemist with 175 peer-reviewed papers to his name. Ebright was also an editor of the *Journal of Biochemistry* for sixteen years. And since 2004, Ebright had been the most prominent scientist to argue for more controls on gain-of-function research.[42]

A few hours later, still on January 31, at 8:43 p.m., Fauci emailed the article indicating that gain-of-function research was going on in Wuhan (and funded by his NIAID) but its products were safely contained to Farrar and Andersen.[43] At some point, Fauci presumably called Andersen. The contents of that call are unknown.

At 10:32 p.m. on January 31, 2020, the COVID cover-up began to take shape.

The RNA genome of the Wuhan virus had only been released by Chinese scientists a few weeks earlier. But it didn't take long for virologists to notice that something was amiss. The RNA sequence showed anomalies suggestive of laboratory manipulation.

On the evening of January 31, a mad scramble of the nation's elite virologists contacted Tony Fauci to alert him of what he already should have suspected—the Wuhan virus appeared to have been manipulated in a lab to make it more infectious in humans. One of these virologists, a confidant of Fauci, Kristian Andersen, at 10:32 p.m. sent this harried email to Fauci:

> One has to look really closely at all the sequences to see that some of the features (potentially) look engineered....Eddie, Bob, Mike, and myself all find the genome inconsistent with expectations from evolutionary theory.[44]

The other three virologists are Eddie Holmes, Bob Garry, and presumably Mike Farzan. That Andersen doesn't list their last names indicates how well Fauci must have known each of them.[45]

Garry, a researcher at the University of Tulane, echoed Andersen's conclusion. Garry had looked at COVID's RNA sequence and was troubled by anomalies in this genetic sequence not normally found in nature.

In an email obtained by federal order, Garry describes in sheer wonderment the genetic sequence of COVID-19:

> Before I left the office for the ball, I aligned nCoV with the 96% bat CoV sequenced at WIV. Except for the RBD the S proteins are essentially identical at the amino acid level—well all but the perfect insertion of 12 nucleotides that adds the furin site. S2 is over its whole length essentially identical. I really can't think of a plausible natural scenario where you get from the bat virus or one very similar to it to nCoV where you insert exactly 4 amino acids 12 nucleotide that all have to be added at the exact same time to gain this function—that and you don't change any other amino acid in S2? I just can't figure out how this gets accomplished in nature. Do the alignment of the spikes at

the amino acid level—it's stunning. Of course, in the lab it would be easy to generate the perfect 12 base insert that you wanted. Another scenario is that the progenitor of nCoV was a bat virus with the perfect furin cleavage site generated over evolutionary times. In this scenario RaTG13 the WIV virus was generated by a perfect deletion of 12 nucleotides while essentially not changing any other S2 amino acid. Even more implausible IMO.[46]

Two years later, when interviewed by Megyn Kelly, Garry attempted to laugh off his early support for the lab-leak theory by saying scientists often play devil's advocate, as if he never really believed in the lab-leak theory, despite flatly saying otherwise and calling a natural origin implausible in private correspondence. His actual emails from the time tell the true story.[47]

On January 31, all of those we might label Fauci's "yes-men" were frantically worried that COVID-19 came from a lab—worried because they all knew Fauci's NIAID had been funding the Wuhan lab for years. They all were independently reaching the same conclusions: COVID did not appear to be a product of nature. COVID appeared to be manipulated by scientists.

On the evening of January 31, 2020, all four of these virologists agreed that the RNA genome of this new virus appeared "inconsistent with expectations from evolutionary theory." They were confident enough to directly contact the ultimate dispenser of research grant money in the Free World—Anthony Fauci.

These scientists didn't quibble, they didn't equivocate. These scientists presented succinctly and definitively that they didn't "find" the new virus's genome consistent with having arisen from nature. It doesn't take a crystal ball to imagine the worried look that might have furrowed Fauci's brow.

Less than two hours later, at 12:29 a.m. that same night, Fauci emailed his second-in-command, Dr. Hugh Auchincloss. As Congressman Jim Jordan explains at The Federalist, "In the email, Dr. Fauci attached a paper written by Dr. Ralph Baric and Dr. Zhengli-Li Shi—the so-called 'bat woman' from Wuhan Institute of Virology (WIV). The paper highlighted taxpayer-funded gain-of-function research on coronaviruses conducted by the WIV. Dr. Fauci told Dr. Auchincloss: '*It is essential that we speak this [morning]. Keep your cell phone on…read this paper…you will have tasks today that must be done.*'"[48]

I don't know about you, but I've never emailed an employee after midnight, nor have I ever shown such fierce and forceful language to indicate in the wee hours of the night that there will be "tasks today that must be done."

It's hard not to read those words and surmise that fear was gripping Tony Fauci's heart. But Fauci wasn't done for the night. He must have lain awake worrying.

Just before 3:00 a.m., Dr. Fauci sent another email, this one to Dr. Robert Kadlec, Trump's Assistant Secretary for Preparedness and Response at Health and Human Services. Fauci attached an article that argued against a lab leak and for a natural or evolutionary origin to COVID-19. Keeping his own worry under wraps, Fauci began covering up any suggestion that the virus could have leaked from the Wuhan lab.

His email to Kadlec read, "*Bob: This came out today. Gives a balanced view.*"[49]

When I first learned of this 3:00 a.m. email, I wondered what the rest of the story must be. Why email Bob Kadlec at 3:00 a.m.? I was perplexed until I learned that one of Kadlec's duties was to chair the P3CO Committee, the group that is supposed to screen gain-of-function proposals and disapprove experiments it deems too dangerous.

So, the source of Fauci's restless night is the worry that Kadlec might soon discover that the gain-of-function research in Wuhan never came before his committee, that Fauci was allowing gain-of-function research to bypass scrutiny by never referring it for scrutiny.

So, in the middle of the night, just four hours after he was informed by four trusted and, importantly, *loyal* scientists, that the pandemic virus from Wuhan appeared to be manipulated in the lab, Anthony Fauci made the audacious decision to cover up any information or hypothesis that might link the virus to a leak from the lab.

The Mad Scramble of Deceit

In those fateful hours, Fauci struck out on a dangerous path of deceit, the scale of which has likely never before been undertaken. We know of these email exchanges only because a federal judge forced Fauci to reveal them.

It's likely, though, that even before the first email at 10:32 p.m., Fauci had an inkling that the virus might have come from the lab. Fauci knew, as did many of his colleagues, that dangerous gain-of-function research was going on in Wuhan at both civilian and military installations. Fauci knew that both labs were involved in making lethal viruses more contagious in humans.

In fact, when Fauci's assistant Auchincloss responded at about noon to Fauci's midnight email, he revealed, to some extent, the reason for Fauci's alarm:

> *The paper you sent me says the experiments were performed before the gain-of-function pause but have since been reviewed and approved by NIH.* **Not sure what this means since [we are] sure that no coronavirus work has**

gone through the P3 framework. [We] will try to determine
if we have any distant ties to this work abroad.[50]

In this email, Auchincloss expresses hope that the research in question did not occur during the "pause" when NIH had decided to pause gain-of-function research. Hope is necessary because Auchincloss comes to the same conclusion that any objective observer would: the research that NIH funded in Wuhan was unquestionably gain-of-function research.

Hope was the main theme of the email from Auchincloss because that outcome would be necessary to absolve Fauci and the NIH of blame. Further, Dr. Auchincloss seems to take solace in the fact that "no coronavirus" research has been approved by the Pandemic Committee, a committee commissioned to review dangerous gain-of-function research.[51]

What Auchincloss doesn't reveal, or may not know yet, is that NIH was indeed funding coronavirus gain-of-function research but purposefully not sending it for review to the Pandemic, or P3CO, Committee.

While Auchincloss was busy trying to cover the tracks of Fauci and the NIH funding of gain-of-function research, he still had time to do a little day trading. Auchincloss's insider knowledge told him that this was no run-of-the-mill flu bug. He already suspected it leaked from a lab, thus making it pre-adapted to spread from human to human and much more dangerous than previous outbreaks that came from animals. As a consequence, Auchincloss quickly unloaded between $111,000 and $350,000 of stocks to protect his bottom line.[52]

Just hours later, on February 1 at 11:48 a.m., NIH head Francis Collins sent Fauci a preprint by Dr. Shi. The paper by Shi revealed RaTG13, the closest relative to COVID-19. Interestingly, Collins didn't discuss Shi's discovery. Instead, Collins seemed more interested in distancing the NIH from Shi. Collins told Fauci, "No evidence this work was supported by NIH."[53]

By no evidence, what he really meant was there was no NIH number attached by Dr. Shi to the paper. Of course, what went unspoken were the millions of dollars Fauci and Collins had funneled to Dr. Shi over the past decade via EcoHealth Alliance and various U.S. universities.[54]

Within days, though, after further discussions with Fauci, Kristian Andersen, the author of the 10:32 p.m. email, along with his colleagues, suddenly and inexplicably reversed all of the group's previous conclusions and came to a completely different one.

They had "evolved" from finding the genome inconsistent with a natural origin to aggressively writing and lobbying to suppress any voices that argued that COVID was the product of a lab leak.

By February 4, Andersen had completely flipped his previous argument. Instead of arguing as he had five days previously that COVID-19 was "inconsistent" with natural evolution, he now emailed Daszak. "If one of the main purposes of this document is to counter those fringe theories, I think it's very important that we do so strongly and in plain language ('consistent with' [natural evolution] is a favorite of mine when talking to scientists, but not when talking to the public—especially conspiracy theorists)," he wrote.[55]

Typically, scientists don't speak of political purposes in doing research; presumably, the purpose is seeking the truth. But in this email, Andersen tips his hat—his purpose is entirely political, to dispel "fringe theories" and silence "conspiracy theorists."

Andersen's language reveals how polemical he's willing to get. In the same email, he writes, "The main crackpot theories going around at the moment relate to this virus being engineered with intent and that is demonstrably not the case."[56]

By extension, Andersen was describing some of the world's most distinguished virologists who were open to the possibility that

COVID-19 leaked from a lab (a position he himself held just days earlier) as crackpots.

Can any objective reader fail to conclude that Andersen is engaging in partisan political posturing to cover up the possibility that the virus may have leaked from a Chinese lab supported by U.S. tax dollars?

My guess is the many scientists, including Nobel laureate David Baltimore, who sought an honest debate over the origins of COVID-19, would not be pleased to be scornfully labeled "conspiracy theorists."

It is worth noting that, while Fauci's men dispelled even the possibility of a lab leak as "conspiracy theory," few if any of these supposedly conspiracy-minded scientists arguing that COVID might have come from the lab deny that it could have possibly come from animals.

Conflicts of Interest Abound

Virtually every virologist who has written, studied, or come forward with evidence suggesting a lab leak has couched his conclusion with the caveat that, so far, the evidence is not conclusive for either theory.

But I've seen exactly zero evidence of proponents of the lab leak using language such as "crackpot," "conspiracy," or "fringe" to describe fellow scientists advancing the opposite theory, that of an animal origin.

So, the zealotry and closed-mindedness come almost entirely from one side. And it's not hard to conclude why.

Fauci and his men had a conflict of interest.

They knew they had approved the funding for the Wuhan lab.[57] They knew they had deceitfully hidden it from review by the Pandemic Committee.[58] They knew the research was gain of function and controversial.[59] And they knew if COVID-19 came from the Wuhan lab, they would all bear responsibility for the pandemic.

Coincidently or not, Andersen and Daszak, by pliantly doing Fauci's dirty work, would ultimately be rewarded with millions of dollars in

NIH grants just months after they led the public battle to discredit any notion that the virus might have originated in a lab.[60]

Finally, two years later, after previously running headlines calling me a "sniveling moron" for daring to question Fauci, *Vanity Fair*, of all publications, would run a piece encapsulating what happened in these early days: "As for transparency-minded scientists in the U.S., Daszak early on set about covertly organizing a letter in the *Lancet* medical journal that sought to present the lab-leak hypothesis as a groundless and destructive conspiracy theory. And Fauci and a small group of scientists, including Andersen and Garry, worked to enshrine the natural-origin theory during confidential discussions in early February 2020, even though several of them privately expressed that they felt a lab-related incident was likelier."[61]

Contrary to all notions of justice, Daszak would continue to get large NIH grants throughout the pandemic.

It's hard to establish quid pro quo in any relationship, but it certainly seems that it pays to do Anthony Fauci's bidding.[62]

How quickly did Kristian Andersen, Eddie Holmes, and Bob Garry flip their positions on the origins of COVID? Well, at 10:32 p.m. on January 31, they seemed unanimous in "finding" the COVID genome inconsistent with natural evolution.

The next evening, February 1, in a teleconference with Anthony Fauci, Andersen and Holmes reiterated their belief that COVID looked to have been manipulated in a lab. Also on the call were several other international virologists.

During the February 1, 2020, teleconference, Andersen was still "60 to 70 per cent convinced" COVID-19 came from a laboratory, while Edward Holmes was still putting the odds that this was a lab leak at "80 per cent." According to Farrar, "Andrew [Rambaut] and Bob [Garry] were not far behind" in their assessment of the odds. Farrar himself admits that he would "have to be persuaded that things were not as sinister as they seemed."[63]

The next day Farrar emails Fauci: "On a spectrum if 0 is nature and 100 is release—I am honestly at 50! My guess is that this will remain grey, unless there is access to the Wuhan lab—and I suspect that is unlikely!"[64]

And yet…these very same scientists who privately were still leaning toward a lab origin publicly set about busily condemning anyone with the temerity to make the lab-origin argument.[65]

Professor Mike Farzan—like his colleague at Scripps Research in La Jolla, California, Kristian Andersen—was also privately vocal at this time about his conclusion that COVID must have leaked from a lab. Farzan's expertise included discovering how COVID attaches to human cells utilizing a furin cleavage site. (This furin cleavage site had never before been identified in this family of coronaviruses). Farrar indicates in an email that Farzan thought it quite unlikely that the furin cleavage site that allows COVID to enter human cells developed naturally.

Farzan tells Andersen that he's "struggling to figure out how the new coronavirus could have acquired its features in a natural way."[66]

Farzan participates in the February 1 phone call with Fauci, Collins, Farrar, and the rest. According to reporter Caroline Downey, Farzan voiced his conclusion that "SARS-CoV-2 had the marking of laboratory experimentation that resulted in a virus that immediately proved highly infectious to humans."

Looking at the COVID-19 sequence, Farzan concluded that "a likely explanation [for the virus's origin] could be something as simple as passage SARS-live CoVs in tissue culture on human cell lines (under BSL-2) for an extended period of time, accidentally creating a virus that would be primed for rapid transmission between humans via gain of furin site (from tissue culture) and adaptation to human ACE2 receptor via repeated passage."[67]

So, Farzan argues that the COVID-19 genetic sequence could be explained by serial passage in culture as has been previously accomplished with human coronaviruses. Farzan believes that serial passage could account for the furin cleavage site. He acknowledges that a furin cleavage site could occur in nature but is "highly unlikely."

With regard to "accidental release or natural event," Farzan concludes, "I am 70:30 or 60:40."[68]

Many of the emails concerning the February 1 teleconference are redacted. An accurate account of this teleconference likely holds the key to revealing the organization of the cover-up.

While Andersen, Holmes, Garry, Rambaut, Farzan, and Farrar *all* leaned heavily in favor of a lab leak initially, there were others who from the beginning lobbied against the lab leak.

Not surprisingly, the loudest lobbyists against the lab leak were gain-of-function researchers such as Ron Fouchier.

Fauci and Farrar chose to include Ron Fouchier and Marion Koopmans, his colleague from Erasmus University, in their secret discussions.[69] No stranger to controversy, Fouchier was "a longtime advocate, and practitioner, of gain-of-function studies."[70] COVID-19 was not the first big scare involving a laboratory-created virus. Fauci had also been intimately involved in the furor over Ron Fouchier's gain-of-function influenza research, which exploded on the scene in 2011.[71]

Fouchier genetically altered the virus H5N1, an avian influenza strain, to make it more transmissible, or infectious. According to Martin Enserink at *Science*, "Scientists believe it's likely that the pathogen [created by Fouchier], if it emerged in nature or were released, would trigger an influenza pandemic, quite possibly with many millions of deaths."[72]

The debate over whether or not publication of this research would become a how-to manual for creating lethal viruses was heated. Ebright, Redfield, and others argued against publication and for additional regulations on gain-of-function research.[73] Fauci sided with Fouchier and pushed for publication of the method used to create this killer virus.

Fauci responded at the time, "I think the benefits that will come out of the Fouchier paper in stimulating thought and pursuing ways to understand better the transmissibility, adaptation, pathogenicity [of H5N1] in my mind far outweigh the risk of nefarious use of this information."[74]

David A. Relman, M.D., of Stanford University, disagreed with Fauci and argued that the Fouchier study should never have been allowed, or published. "Basically, I was and still am opposed to this particular work, because the risks outweighed the benefits, from the start, and still do," Relman stated. "I don't believe that the benefits, even if they (e.g., early detection in birds and animals) could be realized in the near term, are worth the significant risks. Accidental release is a major concern, as well as malignant disregard for public safety."[75]

Gain-of-Function Research Rears Its Ugly Head

One would think that enhancing an aerosolized influenza virus that could kill millions is reason enough to prohibit or, at the very least, greatly scrutinize such research. As Enserink reports, "The virus could escape from the lab, or bioterrorists or rogue nations could use the published results to fashion a bioweapon with the potential for mass destruction." According to Richard Ebright, a molecular biologist at Rutgers, "This work should never have been done."[76]

Fauci was intimately aware of this debate. Fouchier's research was funded by the NIH.[77] Fauci, with his signature hubris, was unfazed by the danger of the research. On the contrary, he weighed in to support gain-of-function research in a 2012 paper.

Fauci wrote, "In an unlikely but conceivable turn of events, what if that scientist becomes infected with the virus, which leads to an outbreak and ultimately triggers a pandemic.... Scientists working in this field might say—as indeed I have said—that the benefits of such experiments and the resulting knowledge outweigh the risks."[78]

Fauci's past would predict his future. To him, the benefits of gain-of-function research outweighed the risks. I wonder if the six million people who died from COVID-19 would agree.

As with every debate concerning the billions of dollars controlled by the NIH, Fauci was right in the middle of the debate over Fouchier's dangerous juicing up of the influenza virus.

Fauci fought hard for the continuance of gain-of-function research, but he ultimately acceded to a pause of this dangerous research for three years and the establishment of a committee to assess the risks of individual gain-of-function research proposals on one condition: that he be given the exclusive right to grant exemptions.[79]

Like so many "reforms" in government, this reform was more whitewash than real improvement. During the so-called pause in gain-of-function research, Fauci granted exemption after exemption to the pause and, in the case of the Wuhan gain-of-function research, simply exempted the research from any scrutiny at all by the Pandemic Safety Committee.[80]

Jeffrey Sachs, an economist at Columbia University, describes the so-called pause in gain-of-function research: "And there was actually a moratorium in 2014. But the champions of this kind of research pushed on, they applied for waivers, which they got, and finally the moratorium came off in 2017. And they said how important it is to do this dangerous kind of research, because they claimed, 'Well, there are lots of viruses out there. And we don't know when they're going to become highly pathogenic, and we need to develop drugs and vaccines against a wide spectrum of them. So we have to test all these viruses that we can find, to see whether they have high spillover potential.'"

"But," as Sachs explains,

they weren't actually aiming to just test viruses that they were collecting in nature. They were aiming to *modify* those viruses. Because the scientists knew that a SARS-like virus without a furin cleavage site wouldn't be that dangerous. But they wanted to test their drugs and vaccines and theories against dangerous viruses. Their proposal was to take hundreds, by the way—or [at] least they talked about in one proposal more than 180 previously unreported strains—and test them for their so-called 'spillover potential.' How effective would they be? And to look: do they have a furin cleavage site, or technically what's called a proteolytic cleavage site? And if not, *put them in.* For heaven's sake. My God! Are you kidding?[81]

When I cross-examined Fauci in committee about this dangerous research being approved by him, he argued that his experts all informed him that the research was not gain-of-function or dangerous.[82] But one wonders how he was informed of this opinion since the research in question had never been examined by the very committee expressly set up to evaluate the risk of creating pandemic viruses.

If a Fauci-commissioned group of scientists determined that the Shi-Baric experiments inserting S proteins from unknown coronavirus on SARS1 backbones were not gain of function, let us see the reports.

If such reports don't exist, then it is difficult to avoid the conclusion that Fauci was lying to me under oath in a Senate committee hearing.

The "Proximal Origin" Propaganda Piece

Despite privately expressing the opinion that COVID-19 appeared to be inconsistent with natural evolution, Bob Garry and Kristian Andersen assisted Fauci in covering up any possible evidence that COVID came from a lab. Garry and Andersen agreed to get a journal article out as soon as possible arguing that the evidence was overwhelmingly in favor of a natural origin for COVID.

So, the very day they were privately 60–80 percent sure the virus came from a lab leak, they completed the first draft of a paper entitled "Proximal Origin," which argued against a lab leak and became, as Jeff Carlson and Hans Mahncke put it, "the media's and the public health establishment's go-to evidence of a natural origin for the virus."[83]

According to Representative Jim Jordan, just four days after this teleconference, "Dr. Andersen, the virologist who sent the original 10:32 p.m. email on January 31, went public with this statement: 'The main crackpot theories going around at the moment relate to this virus being somehow engineered...*and that is demonstrably false.*'"[84]

Fauci must have made some powerful inducements to convince Andersen and the other scientists in four days that they were wrong to think COVID-19 was inconsistent with natural evolution.

Emails between Fauci and Francis Collins, the head of NIH, reveal the line of self-serving reasoning that likely won over the doubting scientists.

The day after the teleconference, Fouchier emailed Farrar and the team: "It is my opinion that a non-natural origin of 2019-nCoV is highly unlikely at present. Any conspiracy theory can be approached with factual information."[85]

Already the pejorative "conspiracy theory" was being bandied about.

Fouchier also emails, "It is good that this possibility was discussed in detail with a team of experts. However, further debate about such accusations would unnecessarily distract top researchers from their active duties and do unnecessary harm to science in general and science in China in particular."[86]

Fouchier is here floating the idea that there is a greater good, greater than the truth, a need to defend "science"—or, to be more accurate, a desire to defend the "funding of science."

Investigative journalist Katherine Eban ponders, "Could it have been to protect science from the ravings of conspiracy theorists? Or to protect against a revelation that could prove fatal to certain risky research that they deem indispensable? Or to protect vast streams of grant money from political interference or government regulation?"[87]

In like manner, Farrar, Collins, and Fauci were floating the idea that there was a good greater than the truth. In an email from Jeremy Farrar, director of Wellcome Trust, sent to Fauci and Collins, Farrar argues that it is entirely possible that COVID came from a lab leak.

Collins didn't attempt to dispute the details of the analysis but rather responded that such debate would open a Pandora's box that might damage "international harmony."[88] Collins echoed Fouchier's caution that "further debate would…do unnecessary harm to science in general and science in China in particular."[89]

To paraphrase: *Sure the virus looks manipulated in a lab, but to admit it won't be good for our relations with China and might harm "science."*

My interpretation of what Collins really meant by harming science was that if the pandemic were discovered to have sprung from the Wuhan lab, that knowledge might harm the *business* of science and presumably the funders of science, namely himself and his always-present colleague, Anthony Fauci.[90]

Redfield disagreed. He argued that such maneuvers were "the antithesis [of science], that they were harming science. The way to protect science is approach this scientifically."[91] To this day, he remains convinced "that consciously or subconsciously—some of both—[Collins and Fauci are] trying to protect science. Fauci knows that he's funded this research. He also knows that he misled Congress." Redfield describes Fauci and Collins as being in "protection mode."[92]

Collins further concluded to Farrar, "I share your view that a swift convening of experts in a confidence-inspiring framework...is needed, or the voices of conspiracy will quickly dominate, doing great potential harm to science and international harmony."[93]

Redfield remembers the whole response as "orchestrated." "Fauci and Collins...used their political power within the scientific community to set the narrative. And Jeremy Farrar, if you will, was sort of the front person."[94]

Later these scientists, particularly Andersen, would claim that they changed their views slowly as new evidence accumulated. But the truth is that the cover-up began with Fauci's flurry of emails on January 31 and the coup d'état was essentially complete after the teleconference on February 1.

The Cover-Up Show Hits the Road

By February 3, 2020, Fauci had taken the cover-up show on the road. He gave a presentation at the National Academies of Sciences, Engineering, and Medicine pushing as accepted fact that COVID had come from nature, even though his most trusted virologists were still arguing privately that a lab leak was more probable.[95]

It is telling that by February 6, 2020, mainstream media organs were already parroting Fauci's talking points in their reports and incorporating his assumptions into the very questions they asked him. In an interview with Fauci, ABC News's chief medical correspondent, Dr. Jennifer Ashton, asked him whether he had any "concerns that stem from misinformation online that the novel coronavirus could have been engineered or deliberately released."[96] This wasn't a question but an affirmation of Fauci's assertions. So much for investigative journalism.

As Fauci busily proceeded to cover up the laboratory origin of the Wuhan virus, he may not have known yet how contagious or how adapted to humans the COVID virus would be, but he was hearing reports of hundreds if not thousands of people in Wuhan with pneumonia.

He knew one thing for certain. He had funded those labs.[97] He had publicly supported gain-of-function research,[98] and he had purposely allowed that research to avoid the scrutiny of the Pandemic Pathogen Committee.[99]

He must have understood that if it became known that the virus originated in a lab that he funded, he would bear some responsibility for the pandemic.[100] And one can only conclude that he weighed the odds and decided that cover-up was his best option.

CHAPTER 2

Fauci Organizes a Formal Cover-Up

D esperate times call for desperate measures. As Jeremy Farrar recounts in *Spike*, "Just a few of us—Eddie, Kristian, Tony and I—were now privy to sensitive information that, if proved to be true, might set off a whole series of events that would be far bigger than any of us. It felt as if a storm was gathering...."[1]

While we still don't know what Fauci said to so convincingly enlist scientists—otherwise privately still concerned that COVID-19 might have come from a lab—to immediately begin writing a conclusion-laden defense stating that the virus couldn't possibly have come from a lab, we do know that they quickly adapted to the task to provide a statement that was 180 degrees opposite to their private conclusions.

Robert Redfield, the former head of the CDC, describes this so-called epiphany: "You have to question why someone flips his position within 72 hours and then gets a huge grant later.... I don't think they flipped their position without someone influencing them.... I think they flipped because it was in their personal interest."[2]

The Origins of Deceit

The product was "Proximal Origin" by Andersen, Garry, Holmes, Lipkin, and Rambaut. It was written up within days and published on March 17, 2020, in *Nature*. Already by February 4, 2020, the authors were showing Fauci advanced copies of the paper. Fauci responds by email to the authors: "Very thoughtful summary and analysis."[3]

These authors, all virologists, were an international team, hand-picked by Fauci. Andersen was from Scripps Research, Holmes from the University of Sydney, Garry from Tulane, Rambaut from the University of Edinburgh, and Lipkin from Columbia.

"Proximal Origin" was commissioned and pre-approved by Fauci and Farrar. The paper was urgently needed, according to Fauci and others, to clamp down on any insinuation that COVID-19 might have come from the Wuhan lab.[4]

Publication of this paper came days after these same scientists in private were still expressing grave doubt about the virus coming from nature. Andersen was still harboring misgivings even as they rushed the paper into publication: "I was battling with the idea that, having raised the alarm, I might end up being the person who proved this new virus came from a lab.... And I didn't necessarily want to be that person...."[5]

Why didn't he want to be "that person?" Perhaps deep down he knew that, if COVID-19 came from a lab, it might disrupt the so-called business of science, the multimillion-dollar grants and the international scientific meetings conveniently held at Swiss ski resorts. Andersen, no doubt, wanted to keep his membership in the club.

Andersen and his coauthors make an unequivocal pronouncement in the "Proximal Origin" paper's headline. For readers that don't dive into the details, the bold conclusion is presented up front: "Our analyses clearly show that SARS-CoV-2 is NOT a laboratory construct or a purposefully manipulated virus" [emphasis added].[6]

Seems to be an overly certain conclusion when elsewhere in the paper they admit that their conclusion is based on the fact that COVID-19 binding to ACE2 is "not ideal" and "different" from the binding of SARS 1. From this argument, the authors conclude, that it "most likely" has a natural origin. But instead of going with the conclusion, right there in the paper, that they only consider this prospect "most likely," they begin and end with the declaration in absolute tones that SARS-CoV-2 "is not" a laboratory construct.

Throughout the body of the paper, the authors couch their analysis in terms of probability: "It is improbable that SARS-CoV-2 emerged through laboratory manipulation of a related SARS-CoV-like coronavirus."[7] Yet, they leave no room for likelihoods and chances in their rigidly categorical headline stating that SARS-CoV-2 "is not a laboratory construct."

The authors argue, "Although no animal coronavirus has been identified that is sufficiently similar to have served as the direct progenitor of SARS-CoV-2, the diversity of coronaviruses in bats and other species is massively undersampled."[8] The exact same disingenuous argument could be made that a laboratory coronavirus may exist that is sufficiently similar to be a direct progenitor of SARS-CoV-2 but just hasn't been reported. And were this really the case, it would likely *never* be reported, at least not by the Wuhan Institute of Virology. Such a revelation would immediately attach culpability to the lab for the pandemic.

The authors do admit, however, that, "In theory, it is possible that SARS-CoV-2 acquired RBD mutations (Fig. 1a) during adaptation to passage in cell culture, as has been observed in studies of SARS-CoV."[9]

But they conclude, "The finding of SARS-CoV-like coronaviruses from pangolins with nearly identical RBDs, however, provides a much stronger and more parsimonious explanation of how SARS-CoV-2 acquired these via recombination or mutation."[10] So, the authors hang their hat on Occam's razor—an argument, to be sure, but not sufficient or proportionate to their declaratory conclusion that COVID-19 "is not a laboratory construct."

In contrast to Fauci's yes-men, many scientists were looking at the origins question with an open mind. Dr. Alina Chan is a postdoctoral researcher at the Broad Institute of MIT. She and science writer Matt Ridley point out in their book *Viral* that research first submitted in the spring of 2020 cataloged animals sold in the Wuhan wet market and determined "that no pangolin or bat had been found among the animals for sale...." The authors of that research concluded, "Our comprehensive survey data corroborates that pangolins are unlikely implicated as spill-over hosts in the COVID-19 outbreak."[11]

The "Proximal Origin" authors admit that no animal host for COVID-19 has been discovered. They don't mention that eighty thousand animals from the Wuhan wet market were tested and *none* of them were positive for COVID-19. They don't mention that no animal handlers have been found to have COVID-19 antibodies. This is at the very least suggestive that interaction with animals was not the source. They don't mention that in nine thousand blood samples from Wuhan patients from 2019, *none* showed antibodies to COVID.[12] Antibodies are typically formed when we are infected by a virus, and they are specific to that virus. A test for antibodies is a test for whether or not that virus was present in the body and the body created defenses against it. The fact that no stored blood from 2019 in Wuhan had antibodies to COVID argues for a sudden exposure, such as a lab leak. If the origin had been from an animal source, almost assuredly blood samples would show antibodies beginning in 2019. Typically, when a virus infecting humans comes from animals, it is successful only after many tries. Statistically, some of the viral pneumonia cases in 2019 in Wuhan should have been COVID. Instead, zero patients from a sample of over nine thousand had antibodies to COVID.

Contradictions and Holes in Logic from the Start

"Proximal Origin" adamantly stated that COVID-19 was not a product of a lab leak, but its authors did not discuss the lack of genetic diversity in the initial virus genetic sequences. Typically, when a virus comes from animals, such as the original SARS in 2003–2004, the genetic sequence shows many different lineages until the virus finally mutates to become more transmissible in humans. Genetically engineered viruses lack diversity.

In *Viral*, Alina Chan recounts how she and her team at MIT noticed that "there were no signs that the new virus was evolving and accumulating useful mutations to infect human beings more efficiently—as the SARS virus had done at the beginning of the 2003 epidemic."[13] COVID-19 seemed to show up in Wuhan instantly pre-adapted to transmit easily in humans.

In contrast, Redfield describes that the previous encounters with SARS and MERS "weren't really great threats because they never really learned how to transmit effectively human to human."[14]

As Chan explains it, COVID-19 "more closely resembled SARS in the late phase of the 2003 epidemic after the virus had already picked up numerous advantageous adaptations for human infection and transmission.... The early genomes of the 2003 SARS virus diversified like a tall tree.... The early genomes of [COVID-19]... were all highly similar...."[15]

WHO came to the same conclusion. "Current findings show that the virus has been remarkably stable since it was first reported in

Wuhan, with sequences well conserved in different countries, suggesting that the virus was well adapted to human transmission from the moment of first detection."[16]

While Fauci's men would diligently try to find evidence that the virus originated in the Wuhan wet market, Chan points out that environmental samples taken from the market "were more than 99.9% identical to the human virus isolates.... This suggested *human* contamination of the market rather than the presence of infected animals... at the market...." In other words, one would expect the samples from surfaces in the Wuhan wet market to be genetically different from later viral sequences found in humans, if the market were the original source.[17]

By May, the head of China's CDC came to the same conclusion: "The virus had existed long before the market."[18] So, genetic analysis strongly suggested the Wuhan wet market was *not* the source of the virus but rather had served as a super-spreading site for the virus after it appeared.[19]

But the authors of "Proximal Origin" were adamant. COVID-19 could not have come from a lab, they claimed.

Yet despite the overly certain headline conclusion that COVID-19 "is not a laboratory construct," the conclusion in the body of the paper is more nuanced: "We do not believe that any type of laboratory-based scenario is plausible."[20]

It is clear that they were counting on the lazy American press simply to repeat the headline with no scrutiny or understanding of the paper itself. The bias and utter stupidity of our major media outlets are dangerous features of our current time. We need a press that will uncover truth, question falsehood, and be skeptical. Unfortunately, we have only lapdogs for the powerful.

Now that we have access to the private emails the "Proximal Origin" authors sent during this same time, it is an extraordinary contrast to compare what they say privately with the adamant categorical pronouncements of "Proximal Origin."

Coauthor Bob Garry admits in an email, "Seeing that [the furin cleavage site] in the new SARS-CoV-2 when those sequences came out for the first time actually kept me up all night."[21] Despite that admission of profound worry, Garry, an assistant professor of microbiology and immunology at Tulane University School of Medicine, flipped from an attitude of initial skepticism and even fear to coauthoring a *Nature* paper that emphatically declared that the virus did not originate in a lab.[22]

It seems that after worrying all night, he became abruptly worry-free and certain within days—confident enough to declare that the virus "is not a laboratory construct."

Likewise, another coauthor of "Proximal Origin," Andrew Rambaut, had only days before in a February 2 email indicated his own doubts that COVID-19 came from nature: "From a (natural) evolutionary point of view the only thing here that strikes me as unusual is the furin cleavage site." Rambaut explained that the furin cleavage site was not found in nature in this particular family of coronaviruses and its presence "resulted in an extremely fit virus in humans," making COVID-19 much more transmissible.[23]

Nevertheless, all of these authors came forward in public to argue that the sequence of COVID-19 is not a sequence most researchers would choose, so therefore the virus *must* have come from nature. "You couldn't predict that [sequence] with any computer program," Garry still argues today. "Nature usually is better at doing things than we can figure out with a computer these days. That's pretty good evidence that this virus did evolve to bind to human ACE-2 on its own. Nobody helped it. If somebody had designed it, they would have used a different solution."[24]

And the journalists of today followed right along. Shayla Love of *Vice* presents Garry's argument as so much received truth: "It's an indication that the alterations in the binding were selected for through natural selection, not genetic engineering."[25]

For the first several months of the pandemic, I was not overly intrigued by the virus's origin. I read news reports of scientists that concluded COVID-19 came from animals just like SARS and MERS had. I didn't give it a second thought, that is, until I came across Nicholas Wade's amazing article on the subject, self-published on Medium.com.[26]

One Real Journalist Examines the Evidence and Sounds a Warning

As a former *New York Times* science writer, Nicholas Wade was an accomplished investigative reporter and could translate scientific jargon into English. Wade and others argued that by using serial passage, repeatedly passing a virus through culture or humanized animals, natural selection could be accelerated and leave no trace that the virus has been manipulated in a lab. A virus can be quickly pushed to evolve and to adapt and grow in human cells without ever using genetic splicing.

Wade's analysis is brilliant and worth examining. It is hard not to worry about the state of free speech when you learn that no mainstream media outlet would publish this extensive piece by a long-established writer, especially now that much of the scientific community is coming forward to admit that his argument was valid.

Wade begins by analyzing the arguments that Fauci's men make in the "Proximal Origin" paper. He explains that the lack of overt evidence of laboratory manipulation is not as simple as the authors contend.

Wade writes, "True, some older methods of cutting and pasting viral genomes retain tell-tale signs of manipulation. But newer methods, called 'no-see-um' or 'seamless' approaches, leave no defining marks. Nor do other methods for manipulating viruses such as serial passage, the repeated transfer of viruses from one culture of cells to another. If a virus has been manipulated, whether with a seamless method or by serial passage, there is no way of knowing that this is the case. Andersen and his colleagues were assuring their readers of something they could not know."

Wade dissects the argument that if scientists created a virus, they would never have chosen to design it the way COVID-19 is sequenced. The authors of "Proximal Origin" argue that the COVID-19 sequence is not consistent with their calculations of how best to create a binding site for the virus to attach.

Wade writes, "If this argument seems hard to grasp, it's because it's so strained. The authors' basic assumption, not spelled out, is that anyone trying to make a bat virus bind to human cells could do so in only one way. First they would calculate the strongest possible fit between the human ACE2 receptor and the spike protein with which the virus latches onto it. They would then design the spike protein accordingly (by selecting the right string of amino acid units that compose it). Since the SARS2 spike protein is not of this calculated best design, the Andersen paper says, therefore it can't have been manipulated."[27]

Two Pentagon scientists, Jean-Paul Chretien, at the Defense Advanced Research Projects Agency, and Robert Cutlip, a research scientist at the Defense Intelligence Agency looked carefully at the arguments from "Proximal Origin." Chretien and Cutlip disputed the argument "that if someone wanted to design a coronavirus with high affinity to human ACE2, they would not have designed SARS-COV-2, since the computational analysis they would have undertaken in the planning stage would have predicted lower affinity...."[28]

Chretien and Cutlip respond, "This is not a scientific argument but rather an assumption of intent or methodology for a hypothesized scientist." They point out that the literature is replete with scientists testing the effects of "one or more receptor binding domain variants" to study infectivity or binding empirically, not necessarily only to create maximal affinity.

Chretien and Cutlip cite dozens of coronavirus experiments, many in Wuhan, who argue against only one mindset being logical for scientists to utilize.[29]

Why didn't we learn of this devastating critique when it was written only weeks after the "Proximal Origin" paper was published? Because as with virtually every important piece of information about the origin of COVID, the paper by Chretien and Cutlip was hidden by the powers that be.

For years, any discussion of the possibility of a lab leak was censored or ridiculed as conspiracy, while this important paper remained hidden. It came to light only because the internet group DRASTIC (Decentralized Radical Autonomous Search Team Investigating COVID-19) revealed it to the public in May of 2023. Without this whistleblower leak, Fauci's cover-up would never have been brought to the light of day.

In the spring of 2020, though, with the ink barely dried on "Proximal Origin," Fauci took to the White House podium to declare that the virus must have come from nature because this important paper in *Nature* said so.[30]

Fauci apparently did not feel compelled to reveal that he had in principle commissioned and edited the paper for the express purpose of quelling any inconvenient facts indicating the possibility of a lab origin.

Wade's analysis agrees that researchers do not choose only one pathway to research:

> This ignores the way that virologists do in fact get spike proteins to bind to chosen targets, which is not by calculation but by splicing in spike protein genes from other viruses or by serial passage. With serial passage, each time the virus's

progeny are transferred to new cell cultures or animals, the more successful are selected until one emerges that makes a really tight bind to human cells. Natural selection has done all the heavy lifting. The Andersen paper's speculation about designing a viral spike protein through calculation has no bearing on whether or not the virus was manipulated by one of the other two methods.[31]

Through serial passage, scientists obtain a sort of forced or accelerated natural selection. A virus is grown in human cells or mice created with humanized lungs and passed repeatedly to select for the viruses that demonstrate a fitness to thrive. It's a process just like evolution but accelerated greatly in time and forced in the direction of better ability to grow in human cells.

Fauci's yes-men, the coauthors of "Proximal Origin," make another argument against COVID-19 being the product of manipulation. They argue that COVID-19 does not have a genetic "backbone" previously used by scientists. As Wade summarizes it, "Only a certain number of these DNA backbones have been described in the scientific literature. Anyone manipulating the SARS2 virus 'would probably' have used one of these known backbones...."[32]

The authors of "Proximal Origin" argue that since COVID-19 does not use a known genetic backbone, this proves it was not manipulated in a lab. But, as Wade points out, "the argument is conspicuously inconclusive. DNA backbones are quite easy to make, so it's obviously possible that SARS2 was manipulated using an unpublished DNA backbone."[33]

In the final analysis, Fauci's yes-men therefore hang their hat on two arguments: one, that if COVID-19 was designed in a lab the designers would have done it more perfectly, and two, they would have used a known genetic backbone. As Wade describes it, "this conclusion, grounded in nothing but two inconclusive speculations, convinced the world's press that SARS2 could not have escaped from a lab."[34]

Fauci-whisperers Kristian Andersen and Bob Garry, in essence, argue that COVID-19 couldn't have been manipulated by scientists in the lab because the viral RNA sequence doesn't appear to use techniques, inserts, or known viral backbones to reach the final product of COVID-19. "Proximal Origin" coauthor Eddie Holmes writes that scientists "wouldn't use some random bat virus in their own lab. They'd use a familiar strain that they knew could infect cells," while Marion Koopmans argued that the virus must have come from nature because "there was just no close genetic backbone in the literature...."[35]

One might add: Sure—unless the backbone is a virus that the Chinese have never released to the public...

What's more, a private Bob Garry email obtained by court order makes the complete opposite argument that if "[y]ou were doing gain of function research you would NOT use an existing close [clone] of SARS or MERSv. These viruses are already human pathogens. What you would do is [choose] a bat virus th[at] had not yet emerged."[36]

The Deep Flaws of "Proximal Origin"

Virologist Jesse Bloom discovered several coronavirus sequences from Wuhan that had been *removed* from the NIH gene database by Wuhan scientists. None of them was a progenitor of COVID-19, but his analysis indicated that COVID-19 had been circulating in Wuhan "preceding the Huanan seafood market" super-spreading event.[37]

Is it possible the Chinese have other coronavirus sequences that have not yet or maybe never will be released? We know that the closest coronavirus relative to COVID-19, "RaTG13," was found in a bat cave in Southern China and associated with the deaths of three miners. We also know that Dr. Shi mislabeled and obscured the origins of this close relative of COVID-19 until investigative scientists discovered the truth.[38]

In December 2019, Daszak bragged that he and the Wuhan Institute of Virology had discovered "over a hundred new SARS-related coronaviruses." As Chan and Ridley point out, however, "an up-to-date catalogue of viruses sampled by the WIV has not been shared publicly."[39]

So, yes, it's quite possible there are many coronaviruses the Chinese have not been forthcoming about.

With "Proximal Origin" Fauci's yes-men produced what became one of the most cited journal articles of all time, referenced over two thousand times. The paper was used as justification by the mainstream media to either ignore or dismiss anyone arguing that COVID-19 might have come from the Wuhan lab.

For the next year and a half, it would appear to the world that these scientists were united and had no doubt that the virus came from nature. Only a Freedom of Information Act lawsuit would finally reveal that all five of the authors of "Proximal Origin" had initially concluded, after reviewing the genetic sequence of COVID-19, that the virus was not consistent with natural evolution.

One of the five, Ian Lipkin, also failed to disclose his association with EcoHealth Alliance, one of the principal intermediaries in delivering NIH funds to Wuhan.[40]

As Elaine Dewar reports in her book *On the Origin of the Deadliest Pandemic in 100 Years*, Lipkin's Mailman School of Public Health received over $4 million in the years leading up to the pandemic. This might have been a conflict of interest worth noting, but it was never voluntarily revealed.[41]

Interestingly, about a year after the appearance of "Proximal Origin," in May 2021, coauthor Lipkin come to a different conclusion. He commented on the fact that the Shi gain-of-function experiments were not performed in the appropriate BSL-4 biosafety level environment: "That's screwed up. It shouldn't have happened.... My view has changed."[42]

In an article on Lipkin, U.S. Right to Know reporter Emily Kopp quotes David Relman, a Stanford University microbiologist who warns of the danger of not disclosing conflicts of interest. "For any major, controversial issue, I believe that all of us have an even greater responsibility to reveal those conflicts upfront—and let others have an opportunity to judge what effect those conflicts might have had."[43]

Relman also disputes the main argument of "Proximal Origin." The viral backbone could simply have been one of the many unreported viruses held at the Wuhan Institute of Virology.

As Kopp describes, Relman believes that "the disappearance of the lab's coronavirus sequence database in 2019 and the lab's history of gain-of-function experiments also weaken the claims of Lipkin and his coauthors."

According to Relman, "The Proximal Origins paper is flawed in its assumptions, logic and the soundness of its conclusions. I was very surprised that it passed review at *Nature Medicine*."[44]

Chapter 3

The Politicization of *The Lancet*

Early in 2020, Fauci's men had the "Proximal Origin" paper in the hopper, but it wouldn't be published until March. They wanted something immediately. They needed to preempt any discussion of a possible lab leak. So on February 19, Daszak and his merry band took to the pages of the once prestigious medical journal *The Lancet* in another attempt to stifle debate. Daszak organized the composition and official coauthors for the letter. Jeremy Farrar signed on. They used language rarely, if ever, found in a scientific journal, such as, "We stand together to strongly condemn conspiracy theories suggesting that COVID-19 does not have a natural origin."[1]

The language sounded like it had been appropriated from the daily polemics of a CNN or MSNBC. Instead of arguing the merits of their case, the Fauci yes-men chose ad hominem attacks.

Daszak and the rest had jumped into the fray without even an iota of humility. As science writer Nicholas Wade puts it, they spoke out definitively "when it was really far too soon for anyone to be sure what had happened. Scientists 'overwhelmingly conclude that this coronavirus originated in wildlife,' they said, with a stirring rallying call...to stand with Chinese colleagues on the frontline of fighting the disease." Wade continues, "The Daszak and Andersen letters were really political, not scientific statements, yet were amazingly effective. Articles in the mainstream press repeatedly stated that a consensus of experts had ruled lab escape out of the question or extremely unlikely."[2]

That *The Lancet*, one of the world's premier journals, had allowed itself to be used as a propaganda tool by printing the Daszak letter without acknowledging that Daszak and several of the signatories of the piece were economically intertwined with the Wuhan lab is appalling.

Freedom of Information court orders forced emails into the public sphere that revealed that not only had the principal funder of Wuhan research, Daszak, organized the letter, but he privately collaborated with Ralph Baric, the principal scientific collaborator with EcoHealth Alliance and Wuhan's Dr. Shi.

Daszak emails Baric, "[You] should not sign this statement, so it has some distance from us and therefore doesn't work in a counterproductive way.... We'll put it out in a way that doesn't link it back to our collaboration so we maximize an independent voice."

Baric responds, "I also think this is a good decision. Otherwise it looks self-serving and we lose impact."[3]

Research professor Billy Bostickson remembers *The Lancet* letter as being a motivating factor in the formation of his organization DRASTIC (Decentralized Radical Autonomous Search Team Investigating COVID-19). Bostickson in an interview put it this way: "The Lancet letter looked to us very much like fake moral outrage parading as science."[4]

Major Science Magazines Go All-In on the Fauci Propaganda

Some might argue that the official organs of the scientific establishment had become subservient to Chinese overlords. *Nature*, which published "Proximal Origin," was embarrassingly compromised as well. The embarrassment was compounded when it was discovered that the conglomerate that publishes it "voluntarily" censored more than a thousand articles in two political journals on subjects the Chinese government did not want its citizens to see, including articles on "Taiwan, Tibet, and the Cultural Revolution."[5]

A group of professors from Heidelberg University chose to disassociate themselves from *Nature* after learning of the censorship. They wrote, "For a scholarly publisher, this is an unacceptable breach of trust both with the authors and the international scholarly community."

The publisher of *Nature* argued that, on balance, it was better to accept Chinese Communist censorship than to be precluded from publishing in China. The Heidelberg University professors point out, though, that "there is no 'law' in China that bans treatment of these topics but only an informal unpublished directive from the Communist Party's Propaganda Department...."[6]

The publisher of *Nature* further argued that they were only censoring about 1 percent of their international content for the Chinese censors. The Heidelberg professors were unimpressed. They responded that "once this door of accepting censorship orders is opened, nothing stands in the way of China (or any other state) expanding its list of banned subjects." The bad example set by the publisher of *Nature* will guarantee that other authoritarian states will, likewise, "ban the scholarly discussion of topics they find objectionable for religious, ideological, political, race or other reasons."[7]

Eventually, *The Lancet* would indirectly admit its culpability as a pawn for misdirection by forming *The Lancet* Commission to investigate the origins of COVID-19 and by amending the original Daszak letter to note his monetary conflicts of interest.[8]

The money question speaks to whether the Daszak and Andersen letters were simply political statements or actually covert attempts to hide the truth, to hide culpability. Either could be argued. Or both. As Dr. Alina Chan and Matt Ridley point out in their exposé *Viral*, Daszak, a long-time collaborator of a scientist at the center of the investigation, "has a personal stake in ensuring current Chinese practices continue."[9]

Allowing Daszak to be a part of the initial WHO investigation was absurd. Clearly any indication that the pandemic began in a lab he funded would be devastating for his reputation and career. In fact, Tony Fauci stood to lose even more. His long career was coming to a close, and he surely feared that his decision to fund dangerous research in China may have led to a worldwide pandemic threatened to become his legacy.

One signatory of *The Lancet* letter calling the lab-leak theory a "conspiracy theory" was Dr. Bernard Roizman, who, like Lipkin, eventually changed his mind. In May 2021, he wrote, "I'm convinced that what happened is that the virus was brought to a lab, they started to work with it…and some sloppy individual brought it out…they can't admit they did something so stupid."[10]

Shilling for China

Nicholas Wade recounts an interview Daszak gave December 9, 2019, where "he talked in glowing terms of how researchers at the Wuhan Institute of Virology had been reprogramming the spike protein and generating chimeric coronaviruses capable of infecting humanized mice."[11]

Just three weeks later, though, Daszak was no longer gushing over his collaboration on these gain-of-function experiments. Instead,

Daszak was busy shilling for China and fawning over them for their transparency.

Upon returning from the WHO investigation, Daszak had nothing but praise for China. According to the Associated Press, Daszak claimed China extended "a level of openness that even he hadn't expected." Daszak could barely contain his enthusiasm for his Chinese government handlers: "We were asked where we wanted to go. We gave our hosts a list…and you can see from where we've been, we've been to all the key places." If you weren't paying close attention to the time and place, you might be forgiven for wondering if Daszak had traveled back in time and was reporting from a Potemkin village.[12]

From day one, Daszak was adamant that the virus did not leak from the Wuhan lab. He wasn't just arguing that natural spillover was more plausible. He actively derided anyone who dared mention the lab-leak hypothesis. By April he would declare, "The idea that this virus escaped from a lab is just pure baloney. It's simply not true."[13]

Yet modern history is replete with lab leaks.

Deadly viruses have escaped from research laboratories nearly every year since the fatal smallpox leaks from British labs in the 1960s and '70s. In three separate lab leaks, at least eighty smallpox cases and three deaths were reported. And more recently, the SARS1 virus has leaked out of research labs in both Taiwan and Singapore—and a staggering four times from China's National Institute of Virology in Beijing.[14]

And the lab leaks are not limited to Asia. Alison Young looked at reported accidental exposures or leaks from 2006 to 2013 and found over fifteen hundred incidents just in the United States.[15] Even though Ralph Baric is described as carefully applying the best of safety standards, mice infected with SARS viruses have escaped UNC labs.[16]

The authors of "Proximal Origin" also have to overcome the incredible coincidence of COVID-19 beginning in a city hundreds of miles away from the bats that carry SARS-like viruses. As Nicholas

Wade puts it, "Start with geography. The two closest known relatives of the SARS2 virus were collected from bats living in caves in Yunnan, a province of southern China. If the SARS2 virus had first infected people living around the Yunnan caves, that would strongly support the idea that the virus had spilled over to people naturally. But this isn't what happened. The pandemic broke out 1,500 kilometers away, in Wuhan."[17]

Even Ralph Baric, world-famous gain-of-function researcher and collaborator with Wuhan's Dr. Shi, admitted, "So they [the Wuhan Institute of Virology] have a very large collection of viruses in their laboratory. And so it's—you know—proximity is a problem. It's a problem."[18]

The Wuhan Lab and the Wet-Market Smoke Screen

Dr. Shi herself would describe lying awake at night worried that COVID-19 might somehow be associated with her lab. Ultimately, she concluded that it wasn't. But her initial response was a genuine fear that it might have even originated in her lab.[19]

According to her narrative, though, a review of all her viruses confirmed to her, at least, that her lab was not culpable. In fact, as the evidence began to accumulate that the virus likely did come from a lab, Shi became increasingly and emotionally charged in her denunciations demanding "those who believe and spread malicious media rumors to close their stinky mouths."[20]

Steven Quay, M.D., Ph.D., and CEO of Atossa Therapeutics, presents evidence that COVID came from Wuhan but didn't originate in the market. He notes,

> The Chinese first told the world that the COVID pandemic began in the Huanan Seafood Market because approximately one-half of early cases had been associated with that

location. This would have been reminiscent of the two previous coronavirus epidemics as both SARS1 and MERS began in live animal markets. However, after 18 months of investigation, we now know it did not begin in a market in Wuhan for three reasons.

First, none of the 11 patients from the Huanan market or another market were infected with the earliest virus, meaning they came into the market already infected. The four patients with the earliest version of the virus all had one thing in common: none had any exposure to the Huanan Market.[21]

Even WHO finally admitted in 2021 that "the first family cluster of infections in Wuhan had no exposure to the Huanan seafood market."[22] Indeed, the first man diagnosed in early December 2019 had not visited the wet market.[23]

A U.S. Defense Intelligence Agency (DIA) report also determined that "about 33 percent of the original 41 identified [COVID-19] cases did not have direct exposure" to the market.[24]

As Chan and Ridley note, "Damningly, one of the early lineages of SARS-CoV-2 was not detected at or associated with the cases from the market—pointing to the more likely scenario that a person had brought one of the early variants of the virus into the market where a superspreading event occurred in a poorly ventilated and crowded venue."[25]

Former Stanford School of Medicine professor and biomedical startup founder Steven Quay agrees: "We knew in January 2020 from public scientific databases that the patient with the earliest first complete virus sequence was a 39-year-old man treated at the General Hospital of Central Theater Command of the People's Liberation Army of China, located on Wuluo Road in the Wuchang District of Wuhan, about 3 km from the Wuhan Institute of Virology. After 18 months and almost 3 million viruses sequenced worldwide his virus remains the earliest."[26]

Quay analyzed the public databases and determined that of the market specimens, zero showed infection with the earliest form of the virus, which indicates that the virus had already evolved before it made its way to the market. Some Chinese scientists claimed that COVID was introduced to the market via frozen foods. But "environmental specimens from the market" included well over a thousand "samples of frozen food," and all were negative test results for COVID-19.

Quay's arguments against a natural origin of COVID are also based on the extensive testing of the 457 Huanan market animals, all of which tested negative. In addition, Quay reported that 616 animals that were brought into the market from other providers all tested negative. Another 1,864 wild animals of similar type from the same region in Southern China also all tested negative.

There is no doubt that a preponderance of public data published by the WHO establishes, as Quay concludes, "that it did not begin in the Huanan Market or any other market in Wuhan."[27]

Indeed, the Chinese went beyond testing in the Wuhan wet market to test across China. The Chinese government tested approximately eighty thousand samples of animals, including 209 unique species, not only market and farm animals but wild animals as well. Given that the virus was not discovered in "a single specimen," Quay estimates that "the probability of this for a community-acquired infection is about one in a million. This is what you expect for a lab-acquired infection."[28]

In the spring of 2020, the head of the Chinese CDC, George Gao, acknowledged that the wet market was not the original site for COVID.[29] Nevertheless, the American press still, to this day, writes that COVID likely originated in the wet market.[30]

Even Baric understood the damning nature of a coronavirus pandemic occurring during the winter when bats hibernate, particularly since the pandemic began hundreds of miles from the known cave sources of SARS-like viruses.

Yet he steadfastly joined with the Fauci yes-men in attacking anyone who dared to argue that COVID-19 came from a lab. Baric communicated with Daszak on organizing *The Lancet* letter. He was intimately aware of *The Lancet* letter language calling lab-leak proponents "conspiracy theorists." Daszak directed him not to sign the letter to make the effort appear less coordinated. But a year into the discussion, Baric seems to have become more agnostic and signed a letter with Alina Chan, David Relman, Jesse Bloom, and others "calling for a proper investigation of a possible leak...."[31]

That Baric would now call for a more even-keeled investigation might indicate that he is not concealing data that might implicate the Wuhan Institute of Virology and, as the pandemic raged, never once admitted to this proposed research. He deserves to be given the chance to cooperate in the investigation. We do know, however, that he coauthored a 2018 DARPA grant proposal with EcoHealth Alliance and Dr. Shi to insert furin cleavage sites into coronaviruses—a proposal that could create what we now know as COVID-19.[32] Even the U.S. government, not always known for diligence in screening dangerous experiments, turned this proposal down. That Baric would propose and not voluntarily reveal such experiments concerns anyone inclined to give him the benefit of the doubt.[33]

Jesse Bloom, an evolutionary virologist at Fred Hutch Cancer Center, was initially agnostic about COVID's origins. Bloom, in a phone call, explained to me that seeing Dr. Shi's DARPA grant proposal from 2018 to insert human furin cleavage sites into SARS-like viruses further convinced him to consider that COVID-19 could have originated from a lab.[34]

That Baric would not ever volunteer that the 2018 DEFUSE grant existed is also troubling. When Baric learned that COVID-19 was the first SARS-like coronavirus to have a furin cleavage site, would alarm bells have gone off in his head? Wouldn't he immediately ask himself the obvious question: Did Shi actually perform the experiments proposed in the DEFUSE grant? Did Shi actually insert a furin cleavage site into a coronavirus and then an accident happened?

We will likely never know Baric's true thoughts at the time, but we do know he did not breathe a word of how similar the DEFUSE grant, which he proposed with Shi, was to the actual structure of what became known as COVID-19.

We also know that Fauci, under oath, would seek to distance himself from Baric.

Fauci's integrity would be tested when he was deposed by the attorneys general of Louisiana and Missouri. When questioned about Ralph Baric, the gain-of-function guru at UNC, Fauci acknowledged that he knew of him and that NIH had funded Baric, but Fauci couldn't "recall" if he'd ever met Baric.

In the deposition, he was asked, "But you don't remember ever meeting him in person?" Fauci: "I don't recall. I could have met him. I run into several thousands of scientists that we refer to, but I don't recall, certainly, having a relationship with him."[35]

But as Zachary Stieber of *Epoch Times* reports, "Fauci's official calendar lists a one-on-one meeting with Baric on Feb. 11, 2020." In an email, one of Baric's colleagues, Matt Frieman, a professor at University of Maryland recalls a phone call with Baric after Baric's meeting with Fauci. Baric told Frieman that the meeting was in person and included extensive discussion of "the outbreak and chimeras."[36]

Is it possible the Fauci could have forgotten a one-on-one meeting with one of the world's premier virologists, a specialist in coronaviruses, just as the pandemic was beginning to spread worldwide?

But it wasn't just this one meeting that Fauci now cannot recall. In 2013, Fauci kicked off a six-hour symposium on coronaviruses. The speaker who immediately followed him to the podium? None other than Ralph Baric. Fauci then seats himself in the first row and is visible for at least the first hour and a half of the six-hour conference.[37]

Fauci, also in the deposition, doesn't seem familiar with the renowned Baric collaborator, Dr. Shi Zhengli. Fauci lets the lawyers know that he's not good with "Asian names."[38]

Why would Fauci pretend not to know Ralph Baric? Why would his memory be foggy when questioned about Dr. Shi? Perhaps, Fauci fears that when all is said and done and the historical record is complete, culpability will attach to anyone having anything to do with gain-of-function research at the Wuhan lab.

The Wet–Market Fairy Tale Unravels

Is "Proximal Origin" coauthor Dr. Baric an honest broker of the truth? Well, just as the pandemic began, Baric testified before Congress on February 26, 2020. His talk was meant to inform Congress in general about coronaviruses. He mentioned that the Chinese commonly eat bats and that likely bats were for sale at the Wuhan wet market. (Both of these insights are now largely debunked.[39])

What Baric *failed* to mention was his extensive partnership with the Wuhan Institute of Virology and his decade-long collaboration with its lead bat scientist—Dr. Shi. He somehow never got around to letting us know that the Wuhan lab hosts the largest collection of coronaviruses in the world.[40] Meanwhile, Baric had worked behind the scenes with Peter Daszak to brand anyone with the temerity to question the possibility of a lab leak as a "conspiracy theorist."[41]

During this time, I sent letters to the Democrat chairmen Gary Peters of Homeland Security and Patty Murray of HELP (Health, Education, Labor and Pensions) seeking investigative hearings. For the most part, the answers were a steadfast no. My recollection is that at one point they offered to let me have a witness in a hearing that would touch on bioterrorism but not directly discuss COVID's origin.

My calls for a series of hearings on the danger of gain-of-function research, my entreaties to investigate the origins of the virus, my pleas for a major investigation of a virus that killed at least six million people worldwide were met only with resistance from the Democrats in charge. On my own, I was able to, under considerable duress, get the CIA, DOE, and FBI to give me briefings, but not one Democrat senator attended.

In addition to having to overcome the "coincidence" that COVID-19 began in the city that just happened to house the world's largest collection of coronaviruses, Fauci's yes-men had to explain why COVID-19 appeared to show up pre-adapted to transmit easily among humans. Redfield and others had noted this anomaly early on. The original SARS1 never really evolved to be readily transmissible among humans. SARS1 did have human-to-human transmission that evolved over time, but it never reached the level of transmissibility that COVID-19 had from the beginning.

As Nicholas Wade explains, "Viruses don't just make one time jumps from one species to another. The coronavirus spike protein, adapted to attack bat cells, needs repeated jumps to another species, most of which fail, before it gains a lucky mutation."

When the first SARS epidemic occurred in 2003–2004, researchers discovered that its initial genetic sequence evolved over time to become better adapted to infect human cells. As Wade describes it, "successive changes" occurred in the SARS1 "spike protein as the virus evolved step by step into a dangerous pathogen. After it had gotten from bats into civets, there were six further changes in its spike protein before it became a mild pathogen in people. After a further 14 changes, the virus was much better adapted to humans, and with a further 4, the epidemic took off."

COVID-19 was a much different story. As Wade says, "When you look for the fingerprints of a similar transition in [COVID-19], a strange surprise awaits. The virus has changed hardly at all, at least until recently. From its very first appearance, it was well adapted to human cells."[42]

While many scientists have now confirmed that COVID-19 appeared to arrive "pre-adapted" to infect humans, Dr. Alina Chan of the Broad Institute at MIT noticed in March of 2020 that the COVID-19 genome had changed very little in the first several months.[43]

It was this dramatic lack of evolutionary changes in COVID-19 that prompted further study from Dr. Alina Chan. She discovered that COVID-19 "more closely resembled" SARS1 toward the end of that epidemic after it had "picked up numerous advantageous adaptations for human infection and transmission."[44] What intrigued Chan was that COVID-19 in the first weeks of the pandemic had already evolved to be more transmissible than SARS1 was even after evolving in humans.

In other words, COVID-19 did not appear to have made multiple leaps from animals to humans, and COVID-19 did not appear to evolve in humans to become more infective. COVID-19 showed up day one ready-made for human transmission.

Even Dr. Baric admits that "early strains identified in Wuhan, China, showed limited genetic diversity, which suggests that the virus may have been introduced from a single source."[45]

Fauci's yes-men argued in "Proximal Origin" that natural spillover was the least complicated answer. But as Wade points out, "Proponents of lab leak have a simpler explanation. SARS2 was adapted to human cells from the start because it was grown in humanized mice or in lab cultures of human cells, just as described in Dr. Daszak's grant proposal. Its genome shows little diversity because the hallmark of lab cultures is uniformity."[46]

Trevor Bedford, a professor of biostatistics at the Fred Hutch Cancer Center, also commented on COVID-19's genetic sequence showing up already pre-adapted for human transmissibility. COVID-19, according to Bedford, "had acquired only seven nucleotide changes since the pandemic burst on the scene, a very slow rate of change."[47]

That COVID-19's genetic sequence from the very beginning was pre-adapted for human transmissibility goes against the Occam's razor argument of "Proximal Origin" that the simplest explanation is that of a natural spillover from the animal kingdom. Perhaps the simplest argument is that, given the lack of genetic diversity, the lack of animal carriers, the lack of antibodies in animal caretakers, the evidence for a single source of entry, *and* the world's largest repository of coronaviruses nearby…

Perhaps the simplest explanation was, after all, really a lab leak.

The Obvious Alternative

The Fauci yes-men argued that all of the genetic sequences needed for COVID-19 to evolve naturally exist in other coronaviruses. One problem with this hypothesis is that the genetic sequences necessary are not found in close relatives of COVID-19. The fact that researchers have located a distant coronavirus with a furin cleavage site is unlikely to be relevant. As Wade notes, "Beta-coronaviruses will only combine with other beta-coronaviruses but can acquire, by [laboratory] recombination, almost any genetic element present in the collective genomic pool."[48]

Rossana Segreto, Ph.D., of the Department of Microbiology at the University of Innsbruck, published a review of the scientific literature with several other scientists. This group concluded that "there is also no indication of recombination between the subgenus *Sarbecovirus* [sic] and other *Betacoronavirus* subgena [sic] or species of the *Alpha*,

Gamma or *Deltacoronavirus* genera. Indeed, in the subgenera of *Betacoronaviruses*: *Embecovirus*, *Merbecovirus* and *Sarbecovirus*, gene exchange is restricted to members of the same subgroup."[49]

Quay also points out that "since 1992, in Gain-of-Function experiments, the WIV and other laboratories around the world have inserted furin sites into viruses repeatedly. It is the only sure method that always works and makes viruses more infectious."[50] We know that experiments involving the deliberate insertion or deletion of furin cleavage sites have been conducted for over a decade.

According to Quay, the particular codon sequence found in the furin cleavage site of COVID-19—CGG-CGG—"is commonly used in laboratories around the world, including the WIV. You can literally order it from a supply company on the internet."[51]

Fauci's yes-men argue that furin sites and CGG-CGG codon sequences occur in other groups of coronaviruses and can be explained by recombination within the coronavirus family.

Quay responds, "This is wrong for three reasons based on well-known, fundamental biology. Because coronaviruses **do** exchange genetic material so easily the very existence and stability of the five distinct groups is evidence from nature that there must be barriers to the exchange of genetic material" between the different families of coronaviruses.[52]

For example, the *sarbecovirus* family of coronaviruses has been stable for a thousand years. If recombination between separate families were common, the families would have likely consolidated and not stayed separate for such a long period of time.

Dr. Quay explains why recombination is unlikely between groups: "First, recombination happens when one poor bat is infected with two different viruses and during that co-infection genetic material is exchanged. Here, the groups of viruses that have furin sites or CGG dimers don't infect the same bat species as the COVID-like viruses that don't have these features. The COVID virus can only exchange genetic material within its own group; a group that has not had a furin site or a CGG-CGG dimer for a thousand years."[53]

A second impediment to distantly related coronaviruses exchanging genetic information is, as Quay explains, that "unique gene sequences are required for genetic exchange or recombination to occur. The 'hot spots,' where exchange can occur are different for each group [of coronaviruses] and incompatible between different groups."[54]

Given that SARS-related beta-coronaviruses do not need furin cleavage sites in order to infect bat cells, there is no evolutionary pressure for bats to obtain one. To date, none has been found. And incidentally, when a coronavirus appeared with a furin cleavage site, it turned out that virus, COVID-19, didn't infect bat cells very well at all.

COVID-19 transmission from animals was not meeting the Occam's razor test of being the simplest explanation, to say the least.

CHAPTER 4

The Case for the Lab-Leak Theory

Proponents of the natural-spillover theory, which hypothesizes that COVID-19 was naturally transmitted from bats to some intermediate animal and then to humans, point to the SARS1 epidemic in 2003–2004. Within months, researchers discovered that civets carried SARS1. The human handlers of civets more frequently had antibodies to SARS1 than the general public, and when the civets were slaughtered, the epidemic petered out. The epidemic also dwindled because, as former CDC director Robert Redfield mentioned, SARS1 never adapted to become easily transmitted among humans, especially when compared to COVID-19.

Likewise, MERS or Middle Eastern Respiratory Syndrome—another SARS-like virus—was soon traced to camels.

Probably the strongest argument against COVID-19 originating from natural spillover is that eighty thousand animals have been tested from the Wuhan wet market, and indeed across China, and no animal host has been found.[1] In addition, animal handlers in China have been checked for an increased prevalence of antibodies to COVID-19, and that testing has been negative. While the Chinese government's investigation cannot be accepted at face value, they certainly have no incentive to obscure a wet-market origin. Evidence that COVID came from the market would certainly lessen the possibility that the virus originated in a Wuhan lab.

Preserved blood drawn from Wuhan patients with flu-like symptoms in 2019 would be expected to have antibodies to COVID-19, and no such evidence has been found.

As Dr. Quay summarizes, "After testing 9,952 stored human blood specimens from hospitals in Wuhan from before December 2019, there was not a single case of COVID in any specimen. It was expected that between 100 and 400 would be positive. The probability of this for a community-acquired infection is also about one in a million. This is what you expect for a lab-acquired infection."[2]

If COVID-19 came from animals, you would expect multiple, different animal-to-human infections. In fact, animal-to-human infections, at first, are typically clumsy and unsuccessful until the virus mutates enough to readily infect humans.

This was true of SARS1. Initially, it was poorly transmitted among humans, but as it evolved it became more transmissible. But you can look at the genetic sequence of early cases and see multiple, individual, and separate infections from animals to humans.

With COVID-19, Dr. Quay points out, "There is no evidence of multiple animal-to-human transmissions. With two prior coronavirus outbreaks, SARS1 and MERS, 50–90% of early cases were from various animal-to-human infections. For SARS-CoV-2, 249 early cases of COVID-19 were examined genetically, and they were all human-to-human transmissions. For a community-acquired zoonosis, the probability of this occurring is the same as flipping a coin 249 times and getting heads every single time. This **is** however what you expect for a lab-acquired infection."[3]

Another point that persuades scientists that the furin cleavage site may have been added to COVID-19 is the fact that the RNA codons in COVID-19 that code for the furin cleavage site use an unusual code. Of the thirty-six different possible codes, COVID-19 uses the CGG-CGG code, a code often used by scientists intent on deliberately adding a furin cleavage site to a virus.

The uniqueness, according to Quay, is that not only is the CGG-CGG code distinctive in the SARS-like viruses, but "an MIT group shows that there has never been a furin site or the CGG-CGG letter code in this group of coronaviruses for at least one thousand years—since William won the Battle of Hastings in 1066 to become monarch of England."[4]

Nicholas Wade explains this point as well: "There are several curious features about this insert but the oddest is that of the two side-by-side CGG codons, only 5% of SARS2's arginine codons are CGG, and the double codon CGG-CGG has not been found in any other beta-coronavirus. So how did SARS2 acquire a pair of arginine codons that are favored by human cells but not by coronaviruses?"[5]

Quay reminds us that nearly a dozen gain-of-function experiments adding furin cleavage sites in the lab have used the CGG-CGG genetic codon sequence, including experiments published by Dr. Shi of the Wuhan Institute of Virology.[6] As Nicholas Wade writes, "For the lab escape scenario, the double CGG codon is no surprise. The human-preferred codon is routinely used in labs. So anyone who wanted to insert a furin cleavage site into the virus's genome would synthesize the [genes for the furin cleavage site] in the lab and would be likely to use CGG codons to do so."[7]

Nobel laureate David Baltimore, a famous virologist and president emeritus of CalTech, remarked, "When I first saw the furin cleavage site in the viral sequence, with its arginine codons, I said to my wife it was the smoking gun for the origin of the virus." It must have greatly distressed Fauci's yes-men when they arrived at the same obvious conclusion as Baltimore: "These features make a powerful challenge to the idea of a natural origin for SARS2."[8]

Why is the furin site so important to COVID-19? As we've seen, the one tried-and-true way to make a virus more transmissible is for scientists to add a furin cleavage site. Furin sites are found in deadly transmissible viruses like yellow fever, Ebola, Zika, and HIV.[9]

However, Kristian Andersen, the Fauci apparatchik, still claims in a *New York Times* interview that "furin cleavage sites are found all across the coronavirus family, including in the betacoronavirus genus that SARS-CoV-2 belongs to."[10] What Andersen fails to divulge is that in the closely related subgenus of *sarbecoviruses*, zero have furin cleavage sites.[11]

The aspect of COVID-19 that brought so many scientists together to suspect the lab leak is that COVID-19 was, as Quay describes it, "pre-adapted for human-to-human transmission from the first patient. Specifically, the part of the virus that interacts with human cells was 99.5% optimized. When SARS1 first jumped to humans it had only 17% of the changes needed to cause an epidemic. As evidence of the relevance of this work, the UK strain that emerged in the fall of 2020 that was more infective was a change in one of the few spots that was not optimized at the beginning."[12]

Virologists who argue that COVID-19 was not pre-adapted state that COVID-19 shows evidence of mutation from the beginning in the various strains that have developed, such as the Delta and Omicron variants. Quay argues that "the details tell another story. COVID does randomly make, on average, about one genetic mistake every two weeks. So, after a year of circling the globe, it will naturally have on average about 26 changes somewhere in its gene code compared to when it started. But the vast majority of those mistakes are either neutral, having no effect on the deadliness of the virus, or actually detrimental, making the virus weaker. Less than 1% actually improve the virus."[13]

How did COVID-19 become pre-adapted to be virtually perfectly transmissible among humans? One possibility is the use of a lab technique called serial passage. Mice with "humanized" lungs are infected with a virus. These mice have been genetically programmed to grow lungs that have all of the cell-surface markers of humans. After a week, the virus is recovered from the mice with the most severe symptoms of infection. The process is repeated until scientists have created a more deadly virus that will kill every humanized mouse. This is called "directed evolution," or gain of function. Creating the hybridized mice is technically difficult—but not when you already have an outside supply. Fortunately for the Wuhan Institute of Virology (and unfortunately for the human race), Ralph Baric of UNC allowed Dr. Shi access to the humanized mice that he had created.[14]

Animals Don't Become Infected

To this day, Fauci's yes-men continue to argue that it is more probable that COVID-19 came from an animal as natural spillover. Another near-insuperable problem with their theory is that COVID-19, even the earliest strains, doesn't infect any animal very well. If COVID came from bats, it should still easily infect bats—yet it doesn't.

In a publication in the March 2021 issue of *Environmental Chemistry Letters*, Rossana Segreto and her coauthors show that, even though bats are considered to be the natural reservoirs for COVID-19, they are "poorly infected by SARS-CoV-2, and they are therefore unlikely to be the direct source for human infection."[15]

Segreto cites studies showing COVID-19 does not grow in the kidneys or lung cells of common bat species *R. sinicus*, and binds poorly to *R. sinicus* ACE2 receptors. Furthermore, modeling predicts for thirty-seven bat species a very low or low "binding affinity." Which, according to Segreto and her coauthors "indicates a significant and unexplained evolutionary distance between SARS-CoV-2 and bats."

The paper points out that COVID-19's "combination of high human adaptation and poor bat susceptibility" contrasts "greatly [with] the evolution of MERS-CoV and SARS-CoV."[16] Observers are right to question why a virus that "jumped" from bats would no longer show much ability to infect bats.

To add fuel to the fire, apparently labs in Wuhan were already inserting furin cleavage sites in coronaviruses in 2015. Huazhong Agricultural University in Wuhan inserted a furin cleavage site into a live coronavirus and showed that the virus gained functional infectiousness. The Key Laboratory of Animal Epidemiology of the Ministry of Agriculture in Beijing also experimentally inserted a furin cleavage site into a chicken coronavirus and found that the virus was made more lethal and could cross the blood/brain barrier to damage the central nervous system.[17]

The evidence for a lab leak is withering and relentless. No animals in the wet market had COVID-19. No stored blood had antibodies to COVID-19. COVID-19 didn't struggle to infect humans as previous coronaviruses had. And the pandemic coincidentally started just steps away from the largest collection of coronaviruses in the world? Perhaps the simplest answer is the most accurate—that the virus was indeed a leak from one of the many experimental coronavirus labs in Wuhan.[18]

The Furin Cleavage Site Is Essential Evidence

Virtually every scientist reacted the same way to the discovery that COVID-19 had a furin cleavage site—the internet abbreviation sums it up best—WTF!

Initially, this finding led even Fauci's yes-men to pause in late January 2020, before the cover-up was in full swing. During a Zoom call between Andersen and *This Week in Virology* podcast host Eddie Holmes discussing the furin cleavage site, Andersen confides, "I need to be pulled back from a ledge here."[19]

Andersen was bothered by the presence of the furin cleavage site. According to Holmes, Andersen said, "There's... this furin cleavage site between the S1 and S2 junctions. There are two restriction sites, BamHI, around it. And that section, between the restriction sites... looks like it's got reduced variation."[20]

Andersen's conclusion, before he was conveniently convinced otherwise, was that the furin cleavage site appeared to be the result of lab manipulation or genetic engineering. As U.S. Right to Know health reporter Emily Kopp explains in her excellent timeline, "Restriction sites are snippets of the genome recognized by restriction enzymes that cleave at or near that site. And the portion of the genome between these sites did not at first appear natural."[21]

Holmes, who would within days call the lab leak a "conspiracy theory," responded much more directly and with no obfuscation: "Fuck, this is bad!"[22]

The Disturbing Findings of DRASTIC

Charles Rixey is a member of DRASTIC, a loose group of internet mavens and sleuths who chased the lab-leak theory around the world and down a thousand rabbit holes. Rixey served as a WMD professional in the U.S. Marines and calls attention to the so-called gain-of-function pause to ask, "In 2014, who served as the final approval authority for Baric's pending research, which ultimately allowed it to be grandfathered under the impending GOF ban?"[23] Why were the Baric-Shi experiments not reviewed by the P3CO Committee?

When I met Bob Kadlec, who chaired the P3CO Committee, I asked him the same question. He responded that his committee was never given the opportunity to review the Baric/Shi experiments.

He told me it seemed strange to him that one of his duties as preparedness undersecretary would be to vet gain-of-function experiments for degree of danger and for approval. First, it seemed to him too big a job to be assigned to one person, especially someone with many other tasks. Second, he observed that the head of the Pandemic Review Committee would be assigned that task and little else, and they were not. He was also distressed that the Pandemic Committee, P3CO, had no power to compel grants to be sent to them for review and no power to defund or stop dangerous research.

Kadlec acknowledged that the system failed. He had no control over choosing which grants to review and had no binding decision-making authority to grant or deny funds in any case.[24] This should outrage every American.

If we can ever get Democrats to consider regulating gain-of-function research, the reforms must give the Oversight Committee the power to decide which grants it scrutinizes and the power to block grants deemed to be dangerous.

CHAPTER 5

The Lancet Commission

It was too little, too late, but *The Lancet* editor Richard Horton finally came clean a year and a half after Daszak used the pages of the once non-political journal to facilitate a cover-up of COVID-19's origins. After being utterly humiliated and used by Peter Daszak, *The Lancet* finally recognized Daszak's many, many conflicts of interest. As the *Washington Times*' Rowan Scarborough put it, "The Lancet has had a breakup with Peter Daszak, the scientist whose public letter hosted by the British medical journal protected China's spooky Wuhan laboratory at a pivotal time as the coronavirus began contaminating the world."[1]

Editor Richard Horton wrote in a December 2021 edition of *The Lancet*, "[Daszak and his coauthors] argued that the overwhelming majority of scientific opinion supported the view that SARS-CoV-2 'originated in wildlife.' And they signed off their letter, 'We declare no competing interests.' But what fast became clear is that one author of that *Lancet* letter did indeed have an interest to declare, and an incendiary one at that—a direct link to the Wuhan Institute of Virology, including experiments on viral spillover events and recombinant bat coronaviruses."[2]

Called before a British Parliament committee, Horton admitted, "In this particular case, regrettably, the authors claim that they have no competing interests, and of course...there were indeed competing interests that were significant, particularly in relation to Peter Daszak."[3]

Peter Daszak had crossed the line that had always united dispassionate scientists: conflict of interest. Science is a big business with billions of dollars changing hands. The bare minimum expected of all scientists is to reveal the source of their funding. When Daszak wrote a letter condemning anyone who questioned the origin of COVID-19 and didn't reveal that he was the leading U.S. funder of the Wuhan lab, he crossed a line that should have forever banished him from further scientific discourse.[4]

The Lancet understood this breach of ethics and tried to make amends. The NIH, on the other hand, was still actively funding Daszak's EcoHealth Alliance into the summer of 2023.[5] This begs the question of whether there was ultimately more to discover concerning Fauci's own culpability regarding NIH funding of Wuhan gain-of-function research.

A Non-Partisan Approach...

To *The Lancet*'s credit, they not only admitted to being duped by Daszak but went a step further to appoint a blue-ribbon commission to investigate the origins of COVID-19.[6]

They picked Columbia economist Jeffrey Sachs to head the commission. To anyone who might suspect that *The Lancet* allowed "right-wingers" to run this commission, Professor Sachs has a thoroughly progressive resume and, more importantly, a reputation for honesty. Sachs has been a special advisor to several UN secretaries general, led WHO commissions, and is currently the director of the Center for Sustainable Development at Columbia University.

In fact, when I mentioned to Senator Susan Collins how impressed I was with Sachs, she remarked in a light-hearted way, "You know he's Bernie Sanders's favorite economist."[7] When I spoke with Sachs on the phone, he mentioned that he went to undergrad at Harvard with Senator Chuck Schumer.[8] I saw Schumer later on the Senate floor and couldn't resist needling him a bit. "I spoke to one of your Harvard classmates today."

"Yah, who?"

"Jeffery Sachs."

Schumer got a twinkle in his eye as he responded, "Yah, he complains that I'm too conservative."

I tried to explain to Schumer that Sachs had led a year-long investigation into the origin of COVID-19 and concluded that it likely originated in a lab. Schumer's eyes suddenly darted around the room as if looking for someone else to rescue him from the topic. He did offer to read Sachs's report, and I sent it to him.[9] No report back on whether he actually ever read it.

I also sent a copy of Alina Chan and Matt Ridley's *Viral* to the Chairman of the Homeland Security Committee, Gary Peters (D-MI), and the Chairman of the Health Committee, Bernie Sanders (I-VT), hoping that one day someone on the Left would read the eye-opening evidence that COVID-19 likely leaked from a lab. Perhaps they might even become concerned enough, or curious enough, to support investigation into the source of the virus.

A few days later, I ran into Bernie Sanders on the floor. "I think you know Jeffrey Sachs?"

"Sure," Bernie mumbled from behind his mask. I recounted that Sachs had started out accepting, like everyone else, the so-called consensus opinion that COVID spilled over from nature and couldn't have leaked from the Wuhan lab. Bernie listened offhandedly and said, "Now you're not saying it's some kind of weapon?"

I replied, "No, no. Not at all."

As Sanders walked away, he offered, "Because I'm not interested in just beating up on China."[10]

To get Democrats to examine the case for a lab leak, I had to somehow break through a resistance to even investigate. It wasn't that they had concluded the evidence of a lab leak was insufficient; they had essentially decided against even examining the question.

For me to uncover the full extent of the cover-up and ultimately craft legislative reform, I would have to first break down the barriers of resistance that had hardened since the pandemic began.

When Sachs began *The Lancet* investigation, he initially leaned toward the Daszak narrative. He even appointed Daszak to lead the origins division of the investigation. As Sachs describes it, "Well, more than that: I appointed him—this was Peter Daszak—I appointed him to chair the task force of the pandemic commission that I was running for the *Lancet*. And he headed a task force on the origins. I thought, naively at the beginning, 'Well, here's a guy who is so connected, he would know.' And then I realized he was not telling me the truth. And it took me some months, but the more I saw it, the more I resented it."[11]

By the summer of 2022, Sachs had seen Daszak's true stripes. Sachs "recused" Daszak in June of 2022 without a public explanation, but later he would say that Daszak had not been forthright about his conflicts of interest.[12]

Sachs describes Daszak's dishonesty and obstructionism: "Well, he could have explained to me right from the beginning that there was a big research program and that they were manipulating the viruses, and here's how."[13]

Not only did Daszak not offer to describe the gain-of-function research he was funding, he also refused, when asked, to reveal any of the research information. As Sachs recalls, "When I asked him for one of the research proposals, he said, 'No, my lawyer says I can't give it to you.' I said, 'What? You're heading a commission. We're a transparent commission. You're telling me your *lawyer* says you can't give me your project proposal.' I said, 'Well, then you can't be on this commission. This is not even a close call.'"[14]

Sachs goes on to say that it wasn't just information Daszak refused to divulge; he engaged in an active and deceptive "misdirection."[15]

In December of 2022, Sachs did a Zoom presentation from Austria for me and Senators Collins, Johnson, Marshall, and Tuberville. He was quite explicit that his investigation was as much about the future as it was about the past. Sachs warned that COVID-19 was not a one-off fluke, but that risky gain-of-function research was ongoing, funded by the U.S. government, and presented a risk of leading to future pandemics.[16]

Sachs concluded after two years of investigation that he was "pretty convinced" that COVID "came out of U.S. lab biotechnology, not out of nature." Sachs went on to state that COVID-19 is "a blunder, in my view, of biotech, not an accident of a natural spillover.... And it's not being investigated, not in the United States, not anywhere. And I think for real reasons they don't want to look under the rug...."[17]

Sachs Raises Worldwide Concerns

The Jeffrey Sachs interview by Nathan Robinson in the August 2022 edition of *Current Affairs* gives an excellent glimpse into Sachs's experience leading *The Lancet* Commission.

According to Robinson, Sachs concludes "that there is clear proof that the National Institutes of Health and many members of the scientific community have been impeding a serious investigation of the origins of COVID-19 and deflecting attention away from the hypothesis that risky U.S.-supported research may have led to millions of deaths." Robinson explains the disturbing ramifications of Sachs's statement: "If that hypothesis is true, the implications would be earth-shaking, because it might mean that esteemed members of the scientific community bore responsibility for a global calamity."[18]

This is precisely what I told an incredulous and sputtering Anthony Fauci to his face during one of our committee exchanges. It was gratifying to finally see others who had extensively investigated the origins of COVID-19 coming to the same conclusion.

Sachs explains what he believes likely happened:

The alternative hypothesis is quite straightforward. And that is that there was a lot of research underway in the United States and China on taking SARS-like viruses, manipulating them in the laboratory, and creating potentially far more dangerous viruses. And the particular virus that causes COVID-19, called SARS-Cov-2, is notable because it has a piece of its genetic makeup that makes the virus more dangerous. And that piece of the genome is called the "furin cleavage site." Now, what's interesting, and concerning if I may say so, is that the research that was underway very actively and being promoted, was to insert furin cleavage sites into SARS-like viruses to see what would happen. Oops![19]

Instead of, at least, exploring this alternative hypothesis, Fauci and his yes-men, according to Sachs, kept "telling us, 'Look at the market, look at the market, look at the market!' But they don't address this alternative. They don't even look at the data. They don't even ask questions. And the truth is from the beginning, they haven't asked the real questions."[20]

Perhaps nothing is more antithetical to science and more dangerous to humankind than a climate of fear that chills the asking of real questions.

Sachs was disturbed by the chicanery that occurred behind the scenes in late January and early February 2020. Sachs recounts that

> at the beginning, which we could date from the first phone call of the National Institutes of Health (NIH) with a group of virologists on February 1, 2020, the virologists basically said "Oh my god, that is strange, that could well be a laboratory creation. What is that furin cleavage site doing in there?" Because scientists knew that was part of an active ongoing research program. And yet, by February 3, the same group is saying "No, no, it's natural, it's natural." By February 4, they start to draft the papers that are telling the public, "Don't worry, it's natural." By March, they write a paper—totally spurious, in my view—called the proximal origins paper that is the most cited bio paper in 2020. It said: it is absolutely natural. [Note: the paper's conclusion is "we do not believe that any type of laboratory-based scenario is plausible."][21]

Sachs expresses shock at the lack of scientific inquiry by

> the scientists like those that talk about the Huanan market, they don't even discuss that [gain-of-function] research that was underway. That is just misdirection, to my mind. It's like sleight of hand art. Don't look over there. Look over here. But we know that there was a tremendous amount of this research underway. We have interviews by the lead

scientists. We have these research proposals. I know the intention of doing this research from discussions. I've read so many studies of the importance of this research claimed by the scientists. And yet I see NIH with its head in the ground. "Oh, no, nothing here to look at." And then I see the scientists. "Oh, nothing here to look at. We know it's the market. Did we find an animal? No. Do we have an explanation of where that furin cleavage site came in? No. We don't have an explanation of the timing, which doesn't quite look right. Oh, but *don't look over there,* because there's nothing there," they keep telling us. Well, that's a little silly.[22]

When Robinson asked Sachs why Fauci and his colleagues would try to cover up the origins of COVID, Sachs responded, "There are at least two reasons why they might be doing what they're doing. One is, as you say, the implications are huge. Imagine if this came out of a lab. And we have, by some estimates, about 18 million dead worldwide from this. That's not the official count. But that's the estimated excess mortality from COVID. Well, the implications of that—the ethical, the moral, the geopolitical—everything is enormous."[23]

Viral author Alina Chan's take is similar when asked about the possibility that the pandemic originated as a lab leak: "It would be terrifying to be blamed for millions of cases of COVID-19...."[24]

Sachs went on to indicate that the "business" of research may also explain the cover-up.

There's a second matter that is really important, too. One thing that is rather clear to me is that there is so much dangerous research underway right now under the umbrella of biodefense or other things that we don't know about, that is not being properly controlled. This is for sure. And that's happening around the world. And governments say "don't poke your nose into that." That's our business, not your business. But it's actually our business. It's our business to understand what is going on with this. This is not to be kept secret. We don't trust you.

Let me put it this way: I don't trust them right now. I want to know. Because even what we know of the dangerous research is enough to raise a lot of questions of responsibility for the future. And to pose the question: "Hey, what other viruses are you guys working on? What should we know?" Because no matter what the truth is on SARS-Cov-2, what is pretty clear is we've got so much technological capacity to engineer dangerous pathogens right now. And a lot of that is being done. And it's classified. It's secret, and we don't know what it is. And I don't like that feeling at all. I don't recommend it for us and for the world.[25]

Sachs went on to compare the risks of gain-of-function research to nuclear weapons: "We've kind of understood the nuclear risk—even that, of course, is in a lot of ways hidden from view. But this is a clear and present risk. And there's reason to believe we're actually in the midst of it, not just hypothetically. So come on: it's time to open the books everywhere. It's time to find out. Maybe it was the marketplace. Maybe it wasn't a lab. But we need to get real answers, now."[26]

Growing Cover-Up Concerns and Revelations

In May of 2022, Sachs and Columbia pharmacology professor Neil Harrison published a significant paper in *Proceedings of the National Academy of Sciences.*

The paper described how Daszak's EcoHealth Alliance (EHA) and others refused to cooperate in *The Lancet* Commission's investigation.

"EHA, UNC, NIH, USAID, and other research partners have failed to disclose their activities to the US scientific community and the US public, instead declaring that they were not involved in any experiments that could have resulted in the emergence of SARS-CoV-2," wrote Sachs and Harrison.[27]

The NIH argues that COVID-19 "could not have resulted" from research that it sponsored because of the differences between SARS-CoV-2 and "the published viral sequences."[28]

But this is a misdirection argument. Arguments for a lab leak do not posit that COVID-19 came from any published precursor but from a precursor that has *not* been divulged. This is China, after all, not exactly known for transparent institutional governance.

Records gathered so far via federal court order (FOIA) show that the collaboration between EcoHealth Alliance and the Wuhan Institute of Virology and Dr. Baric's UNC lab involved many SARS-like viruses yet to be published.[29]

Sachs and Harrison point out that the NIH argument is entirely dependent on the very limited data that is available. We would need access to the unpublished viral sequences currently stored in Chinese and U.S. databases in order to verify such claims.

Even NIH director Lawrence Tabak admitted in congressional testimony that genetic sequences for several viruses have been hidden from public view at the behest of researchers in China and the United States.[30]

If gain-of-function researchers, like Daszak, are not cooperating or revealing and updating the NIH on their experiments, surely their NIH funds should be stopped. Instead, even though they have missed deadline after deadline and refused to divulge lab data to the NIH and independent investigators, the NIH continues to grant EcoHealth millions more in taxpayer money. Hard to fathom. It makes one question if the additional money is perhaps intended to encourage EcoHealth's continued silence and obstruction.

As recently as May 2023, the NIH was initiating new grants to EcoHealth Alliance.[31] As writer Jocelyn Kaiser reported in a May 2023 article in *Science*, "Three years after then-President Donald Trump pressured the National Institutes of Health (NIH) to suspend a research grant to a U.S. group studying bat coronaviruses with partners in China, the agency has restarted the award." She quotes Richard Ebright calling the new four-year grant "'an outrage' because EcoHealth 'flagrantly and repeatedly' violated the terms of the grant" and a "pleased" Peter Daszak saying, "Now we have the ability to finally get back to work."[32] Daszak's words are especially galling considering that after his grant was retracted in April of 2020, he wrote in an email, "My plan is to continue this work, unfunded for now."[33]

This man's intellectual hubris knows no bounds. Not only are U.S. government grant funders oblivious that tax dollars may have funded the pandemic, they are supremely arrogant to keep funneling tax dollars out the door with little or no oversight.

In the midst of revelations concerning NIH's ongoing funding of research in Wuhan via EcoHealth Alliance, I introduced an amendment to stop all U.S. government funding of research in Wuhan. Senate Democrats allowed my amendment go in but then quietly worked with Nancy Pelosi to strip the language out of the bill that ultimately passed. Such arrogance and sleight of hand should disturb every American, regardless of political party.

A Tsunami of Gain-of-Function Evidence Builds

Many observers have posited various ways that COVID-19 could have occurred by accident during gain-of-function research. A worker digging bat guano in South China could have been infected and returned to Wuhan beginning the pandemic.[34] A lab worker could have been bitten by a laboratory animal or infected by aerosol.[35] A gain-of-function coronavirus could have infected a lab worker. All of these possibilities were discounted by Daszak and other Fauci yes-men as fantasies.

As time wore on, Fauci would advance the absurd argument that a lab worker being bitten and infected by a bat was *not* a lab leak, but an example of "natural spillover."[36]

Sachs and Harrison also make the novel argument that the genetic sequence for COVID-19's furin cleavage site of COVID is actually identical to an epithelial sodium channel called ENaC that just coincidentally has been "extensively characterized at UNC."[37] UNC, of course, being the home also to Dr. Baric, the longtime collaborator with Dr. Shi's Wuhan Institute.

In an interview with The Intercept, Rutgers molecular biologist Richard Ebright elaborated that the discovery of identical amino acid sequences in COVID-19's furin cleavage site and human EnaC at first did not seem "particularly suspicious." He continues, "I had known for more than a year that there was a perfect match to an eight-amino acid sequence present in human ENaC. What I had not known was that the sequence was known to be a functional furin cleavage site and that it was a sequence extensively studied at UNC."

For Ebright, the coincidence of finding a furin cleavage site in COVID-19 that was identical to a furin cleavage site being studied at UNC deserved more scrutiny.[38]

A team of Indian scientists led by Praveen Anand also noted this genetic sequence in May of 2020, when they "reported that SARS-CoV-2 has evolved a unique S1/S2 cleavage site, absent in any previous coronavirus sequenced, resulting in the striking mimicry of an identical FURIN-cleavable peptide on the human epithelial sodium channel α-subunit (ENaC-α)."[39]

To discover if government-funded research on EnaC at Ralph Baric's University of North Carolina lab might have allowed Shi's experiments to utilize or force the same genetic sequence into a precursor of COVID-19 is a line of questioning congressional investigators *must* follow. I intend to pursue the truth relentlessly in the coming months.

Sachs and Harrison point out, "Special concerns surround the presence of an unusual furin cleavage site" because COVID-19 is, to date, "the only identified member of the subgenus *sarbecovirus* that contains an FCS [furin cleavage site], although these are present in other coronaviruses."[40]

The discovery of this unusual furin cleavage site in COVID-19 was exactly what had initially caused Fauci's yes-men such consternation. This conclusion did not alarm outliers or partisans only. Most of the scientific world was astonished by this furin cleavage site, particularly since the genetic coding for it turns out to be the coding often used in lab experiments but uncommonly found in coronaviruses.

As Sachs and Harrison put it, "From the first weeks after the genome sequence of SARS-CoV-2 became available, researchers have commented on the unexpected presence of the FCS within SARS-CoV-2—the implication being that SARS-CoV-2 might be a product of laboratory manipulation."[41]

While Sachs and Harrison would not say with absolute certainty that the FCS was inserted into a SARS-like virus as part of a laboratory experiment, they pointed out that the deliberate introduction of FCS sequences into such viruses was the defined objective of a 2018 research grant proposal called DEFUSE, which was submitted by a partnership of the EcoHealth Alliance, the Wuhan Institute of Virology, and the University of North Carolina. While the proposal, which was submitted to the U.S. Defense Advanced Research Projects Agency (DARPA), "was not funded," it is unknown whether some of the proposed research was done in 2018 or 2019 using an alternate form of funding.[42]

A Cover-Up from the Beginning

How did the public learn of this proposal to add a furin cleavage site to a coronavirus? Did Tony Fauci, Francis Collins, or anyone from the NIH reveal this voluntarily? Absolutely not. A whistleblower, U.S. Marine major Joseph Murphy, informed his military superiors, and this information was then leaked to Charles Rixey of DRASTIC (Decentralized Radical Autonomous Search Team Investigating COVID-19).[43]

The Courage of Whistleblower Major Joseph Murphy

Murphy is a true hero in uncovering the deception of the great COVID cover-up. Not only did Murphy brief his superiors on the DEFUSE experiments and their similarities to COVID-19, he also forwarded his analysis to the inspector general of the Department of Defense. Presumably, Major Murphy included the inspector general because he felt the DEFUSE documents were being hidden. By including the inspector general, Murphy also smartly put in place the necessary paperwork for him to be considered a whistleblower.

In Murphy's opinion, COVID-19 is "likely" a "precursor, deliberately virulent, humanized recombinant SARSr-Cov that was to be reverse engineered into a live attenuated SARSr-Cov bat vaccine."[44] Many other scientists also believe this scenario is possible.

Again, according to Murphy, the purpose of the EcoHealth proposal DEFUSE "was to inoculate bats in the Yunnan, China[,] caves where confirmed SARS-CoVs [SARS-like coronaviruses] were found. Ostensibly, doing this would prevent another SARS-CoV pandemic; the bats' immune systems would be reinforced to prevent a deadly SARS-CoV from emerging. The specific language used is 'inoculate bats with novel chimeric polyvalent spike proteins to enhance their adaptive immune memory against specific high-risk viruses.' Being defense-related, it makes sense that EcoHealth submitted the proposal first to the Department of Defense, before it settled with NIH/NIAID."[45]

Murphy's report concludes that "DARPA rejected the proposal because the work was too close to violating the gain-of-function (GoF) moratorium," despite arguments by Peter Daszak that the DEFUSE project was not gain-of-function.[46]

Murphy's report then reveals that these documents were placed in a top secret folder. But Murphy maintains the folder sat empty until July 2021. So, the documents were hidden somewhere from 2018 until 2021. As Murphy describes it, "This folder was empty for a year. The files, completely unmarked with classification or distribution data, were placed in this folder in July 2021, which conspicuously aligns with media reporting, my probing, and Senator Paul's inquiry into NIH/NIAID gain-of-function programs."[47]

If Murphy is correct, someone at DARPA became worried after watching my cross-examination of Fauci and surreptitiously slipped the DEFUSE documents back into the folder where they belonged.

Murphy concludes that "the unmarked nature combined with the timing signals that the documents were being hidden."[48] Murphy had found proof that someone in the deep state didn't want the public to know that the Wuhan Institute of Virology had been asking for money to create a virus that, for all intents and purposes, looks just like COVID-19.

Murphy hypothesized that when Dr. Shi created this bat vaccine, the vaccine or its precursor ultimately leaked and became COVID-19. The documents that Murphy discovered showed that researchers wanted "to prevent a pandemic by vaccinating bats, not by halting its infections amongst people, but by halting the infections amongst the bats."[49]

According to Major Murphy, when things went awry, when the proposed bat vaccine leaked and became COVID-19, a cover-up ensued— "information suppression" was "executed by the government."[50]

When Murphy witnessed the fiery exchanges between Dr. Fauci and myself, he concluded that "an actual cover-up would be more disciplined with its paperwork." Murphy concluded that "unclassified files would be concealed on a higher network," and when he looked, he found the DEFUSE documents that some scientists conclude are a smoking gun indicating that Dr. Shi was indeed inserting furin cleavage sites into recombinant coronaviruses, creating what ultimately would become COVID-19.[51]

Murphy's insight and courage in discovering and revealing Baric, Daszak, and Shi's DEFUSE grant proposal is nothing short of heroic. If we ever get Democrats to read and understand the importance of this smoking gun, maybe then—just maybe—we grapple with restraining this out-of-control, risky research.

So, the public became aware that EcoHealth Alliance, UNC, and Dr. Shi in Wuhan were asking for money to create a chimeric SARS-like coronavirus with a furin cleavage site (essentially the same genetic structure ultimately found in COVID-19) *only* because a patriot in government leaked it to DRASTIC's investigatory team.

Similarly, Americans only learned that their government was unconstitutionally spying on its citizens when Edward Snowden revealed that secret FISA orders were written to act as general warrants to gather the metadata of every customer of every cell phone company in the country.

While Snowden may be the greatest whistleblower of all time, Major Joseph Murphy and the DRASTIC team deserve great respect for making public the DEFUSE grant application showing Baric and Shi requesting money to create a coronavirus with a furin cleavage site.[52]

Without a doubt, Fauci must have known of the DEFUSE proposal. Certainly, it was the job of his subordinate Auchincloss to comb through any proposals of Baric or Shi. And yet Tony Fauci chose to protect science and himself from the public gaining access to these revealing documents.

The Defense-Related Work-Around

For many scientists, the discovery that Dr. Shi was seeking U.S. military research money to create a coronavirus with a furin cleavage site one year before the pandemic was the smoking gun that finally destroyed the so-called consensus that Tony Fauci had so diligently created.

Would it have been unusual for our defense dollars, via DARPA, to fund the creation of viruses? You would think so, but the very first synthetic virus—polio—was created with DARPA funds in 2002 by scientists at Stony Brook.[53]

With the bombshell revelation of DEFUSE project, the tide was turning, and acceptance of the plausibility of COVID-19 having originated in a Wuhan lab became, virtually overnight, no longer just a "conspiracy theory." It didn't take a deep dive to realize that the researchers asking to insert a furin cleavage site into a coronavirus also had the wherewithal to actually succeed—after all, they had for years been creating chimeric coronaviruses, and several labs in Wuhan had been known to manipulate and insert furin cleavage sites.

According to Sachs and Harrison, the Wuhan researchers would also have been familiar "with the FCS sequence and the FCS-dependent activation mechanism of human ENaC α, which was extensively characterized at UNC."[54]

To Sachs and Harrison, the pieces of the puzzle fit once you realize that Wuhan researchers wanted DARPA funds to insert furin cleavage sites: "For a research team assessing the pandemic potential of SARS-related coronaviruses, the FCS of human ENaC—an FCS known to be efficiently cleaved by host furin present in the target location (epithelial cells) of an important target organ (lung), of the target organism (human)—might be a rational, if not obvious, choice of FCS to introduce into a virus to alter its infectivity, in line with other work performed previously."[55]

My Pledge to Review This Information

I am determined to review EcoHealth Alliance research data and any and all relevant communications between their scientists and U.S. agencies that fund research, including DARPA, USAID, NIH, DTRA, and the Department of Homeland Security. We must have transparency if we are to understand the source of the pandemic, even if it reveals an uncomfortable truth about U.S.-funded research being responsible. I continue to be astonished at the lack of curiosity among Democrats and the mainstream media who for two years viewed COVID as such a great threat to humankind that it warranted the denial of civil liberties and education to millions of Americans. And now, they shrug their collective shoulders and ask us all to "move on." I, for one, will not.

I join Sachs and Harrison in calling for a bipartisan investigation. They point to a treasure trove of documents that would aid investigators: "[L]aboratory notebooks, virus databases, electronic media (emails, other communications), biological samples, viral sequences gathered and held as part of the PREDICT project and other funded programs, and interviews of the EHA-led research team by independent researchers, together with a full record of US agency involvement in funding the research on SARS-like viruses, especially with regard to projects in collaboration with Wuhan-based institutions."[56]

As of the delivery for publication of this book, not one Democrat committee chairman has cosigned the release request for COVID records from the Biden administration.

PART II

Fatal Conceit

CHAPTER 6

First Encounter with Fauci

On March 3, 2020, I had my first encounter with Anthony Fauci. I had no preconceptions and no previous interactions with him. World news was grim. It appeared that COVID-19 would spread everywhere.

I sincerely looked to the committee hearing as a time to learn where we stood with the pandemic, but also to explore what we might do to save lives.

The hearing was entitled "HELP Committee Hearing: An Emerging Disease Threat: How the U.S. Is Responding to COVID-19, the Novel Coronavirus."

On February 25, the week before the hearing, the news was filled with reports that Dr. Bruce Aylward of the World Health Organization had stated that remdesivir, originally intended to treat

Ebola, was showing promise in treating patients infected with the novel coronavirus.[1]

With these facts in mind, I asked my first question of Anthony Fauci.

The Wages of Arrogance and Error

"Dr. Fauci, you mentioned remdesivir, and I'm intrigued by the fact that they say it's effective against MERS and SARS in animal models," I said. "Do you take that as a very encouraging sign that it may work in humans too?"

Fauci responded, "Yes, I do, I do."[2]

(In the end, though, remdesivir likely was less effective than a very old, generic steroid—dexamethasone).

Early reports were that children in China were less severely affected by COVID-19 and that the most vulnerable to COVID-19 were the elderly. So, I asked Fauci, "With regard to the children, I think it's fascinating that there aren't many cases, and I would suspect that it would be improbable that they're not being infected, that somehow they have some blanket immunity. One important thing of maybe putting this into perspective, and maybe putting a better look on the overall outbreak, would be if we had numbers. I don't know if someone would suggest to China that they do some random testing of kids in a real hotbed where there's a huge number to see, because if we got ten thousand kids who weren't getting sick, or one hundred thousand kids, our percentage on fatality would go way down."

Dr. Fauci answered, "Right."

So far, Fauci seemed to be responding to questions in a reasonable fashion without politicizing his answers. Another panelist, Dr. Anne Schuchat responded as well: "Yes. There are some data about that, that attack rates may not be zero in children, but they may be asymptomatic. So there are data from a few places that are looking at that."

My questioning continued: "So it's more likely that they're asymptomatic, or less symptomatic."

Dr. Fauci responded, "I think we're going to get some data from the Chinese. They have actually been quite cooperative in sharing data. We had a group that was under the auspices of the WHO that went to China. There was an individual from the CDC and an individual from the NIH who have now returned, and we'll soon get a good look at the report of what they've had, and that was one of the questions we asked because, as you mentioned, Senator, that's a very important issue."[3]

This response may well have been Fauci's first lie to Congress. History will record that the Chinese were not very cooperative in sharing data. In fact, a truthful answer would note that the Chinese were secretive and manipulative in providing any data at all.

With regard to Fauci's reference to the WHO delegation sent to China, the lie is in what he left out. Sure, a group of investigators traveled to China, but China rejected the three scientists *we* chose and only accepted Peter Daszak, the scientist known to have a pecuniary interest in continuing U.S. funds to Wuhan.[4]

A senator's questions are timed, and my five minutes were coming to a close, but I wanted to address one more topic. Many people are aware of the "flesh-eating" Streptococcal infection that about 50 percent of the time leads to multiple amputations. I don't know if my life experience with this disease is extraordinary, but I know at least three people who survived a flesh-eating Strep infection. One man who lost all four limbs, but never let the disease defeat him, lives in my hometown and is a drywaller. He must have a great sense of humor—he has performed as a chain-saw victim in local haunted houses. (That's a whole "nother" story, as they say).

The daughter of one of my great supporters in Northern Kentucky also lost all four limbs but survived. And a good friend of mine from medical school, an orthopedic trauma surgeon at Vanderbilt, also contracted this horrible disease from an infected patient he was operating on. Miraculously, my friend survived and was able to return to continue his practice of orthopedic surgery. The difference in his outcome may have been early, high-dose IV steroids.

So, when I asked Fauci my next question, it came from both my medical background and personal experience: "With regard to treating the severe and potentially fatal cases in bacterial or viral infections, [the difficulty] is often in fighting off the cause of the infection as well as the body's immune response to [the infection]." I explained to Fauci that sometimes it isn't the disease that finally kills you but the patient's overwhelming immune response. The final common pathway of death is often ARDS (Adult Respiratory Distress Syndrome), where the lungs fill with fluid and even mechanical ventilation often fails. I noted that "in some bacterial infections, like with the flesh-eating strep," sometimes massive steroids are employed, in the setting of an infection, and some of these people survive.

But when I asked if they were finding that IV steroids were helpful in the severe COVID cases, Dr. Fauci responded with typical hubris: "They've done it [IV steroids] in an empiric, non-controlled way, and there doesn't seem to be any difference, that there's any effect positive or negative."[5]

Indeed, within two months, Fauci would be proven wrong yet again. In June, a British study called RECOVERY was published showing that a steroid, dexamethasone, was capable of reducing death by 36 percent.[6] In fact, some physicians believe that IV steroids are really the only therapeutic of value in cases of severe COVID.

The Consequence of Medical Deceit
But Fauci's proclamation that steroids didn't seem to make any difference would have real-world consequences.

Wyche Coleman, M.D., a family doctor in Shreveport, was on the front lines treating hundreds of patients suffering with COVID-19. In his clinical experience over decades, he had concluded that steroids were generally effective in treating viral pneumonia. When COVID-19 arose, Dr. Coleman began treating patients, as he had previously, with steroids. But he distinctly remembers in the spring of 2020 when Fauci was dismissive of steroids that the hospitals and their rigid algorithms followed suit, and it became more difficult to get patients treated with steroids.[7] (This scenario would repeat itself with monoclonal antibodies that were also controlled from the top down through rigid algorithms that forbade in-patient treatment with monoclonal antibodies. I literally had desperate family members of patients very sick with COVID and heading toward mechanical ventilation calling me asking how to get their family members access to the monoclonal antibodies, which were being denied.[8])

This is when I realized we had entered a frightening new era of medicine, where the training and expertise of one's physician are secondary to the rigid rules and edicts of government bureaucrats.

One husband called me distraught. His wife had just been admitted to the hospital with COVID-19 pneumonia. He'd heard me talk about the monoclonal antibody treatment, but her doctors said it was forbidden to give the treatment to in-patients. The husband wanted to know if he should discharge his wife and return to the emergency room in order to qualify for the monoclonal infusion. It was madness—and utterly immoral—to deny sick patients access to potentially lifesaving treatments with zero potential risk.

Discussions like this were heartbreaking. It's difficult as a physician to give advice that might mean life or death without actually seeing the patient. You hate to be rash and have someone's loved one die after leaving a hospital against medical advice. But the rigidity of the medical algorithms coming from Fauci's centralized fiefdom in Washington was appalling.

I urged the husband to ask the doctors again to allow his wife to receive the monoclonal antibodies. Ultimately, the doctors compromised and gave her a less specific monoclonal antibody. It was touch and go for weeks, but she survived. While it is likely her survival was as much attributable to not putting her on the ventilator as it was to IV steroids and the monoclonals, it is dangerous to make doctors little more than cogs in the medical delivery machine; we must allow physicians the freedom to use their knowledge and skill to serve each unique patient and situation.[9]

Indeed, doctors who dared utilize their own training and experience rather than simply blindly follow the approved government healthcare edicts found themselves attacked as outliers, quacks, or dangerous "deniers."

In another example, Dr. Richard Bartlett from Midland, Texas, was seeing success with early intervention using a common inhaled steroid used for COPD, asthma, and bronchitis. The medical industrial complex, of course, attacked him as well.[10]

Immediately local broadcaster NewsWest9 sought to dispel any notion that inhaled steroids worked. "A controversial treatment for COVID-19 used by an Odessa doctor, Richard Bartlett, who calls it the 'silver bullet' has been brought in front of the world," they reported.

They referenced anonymous "others in the medical profession" to imply to their viewers that the consensus believed that the use of inhaled steroids was "not...what it is cracked up to be."

The local hospital administrator at Midland Memorial was a critic as well: "People are out there saying it works, but there's no scientific proof, no carefully evaluated peer review studies that prove the efficacy of those treatments."

While immediately critical of Dr. Bartlett, the hospital administrators were wildly supportive of remdesivir, now acknowledged as ineffective. The vice president of medical affairs at his local hospital attacked

Dr. Bartlett with ridicule and sarcasm: "Do your homework, we're not making things up in this country…it's not a conspiracy theory."[11]

Do inhaled steroids lessen symptoms, speed up recovery, or decrease hospitalization and death? The studies are equivocal, just as the studies for other early treatments are equivocal.

When you have a disease like COVID-19 where 99.7 percent of the entire population survives and where 99.99 percent of the younger population survives,[12] most early treatments appear at first blush to work because almost everyone gets better with or without treatment.

Caution is justified when anyone proclaims they have a treatment for any disease. Controlled studies are necessary to rule out the placebo effect, where the psychology of taking a treatment, any treatment, sometimes improves outcomes. Controlled studies are very much needed, especially when a disease such as COVID-19 has such a low death rate.

If 99.7 percent of people recover from a disease, which is true averaging all age groups for COVID-19, then any study will have a 99.7 percent survival rate. In other words, if you give inhaled steroids, ivermectin, remdesivir, or any other therapeutic to prove efficacy toward lessening mortality, the drug would have to statistically improve on a 99.7 percent survival rate—hence the problem of "proving" therapeutics in a largely non-deadly disease.

One way around this is to take a subset of very sick patients who, left unattended, may have a 30 or 40 percent mortality rate. In those cases, it is easier to witness any life-saving efficacy.

For inhaled steroids used as early treatment, studies don't show a definite improvement in mortality, likely because it's hard to improve on 99.7 percent (or even higher if the cohort is younger and healthier). But mortality isn't everything. In people with confirmed COVID-19 and mild symptoms who are able to use inhaler devices, studies found moderate-certainty evidence that inhaled corticosteroids probably reduce the combined endpoint of admission to hospital or death and increase the resolution of all initial symptoms at day fourteen. In other words, they very well might have helped.[13]

Even the NIH's own COVID-19 treatment guidelines reveal that inhaled steroids may have value. Referencing "Inhaled Corticosteroids," NIH states that "inhaled budesonide reduced time to reported recovery but not COVID-19-related hospitalization or death."[14]

But it would make logical sense that inhaled steroids were a benefit early in the disease because we do know that IV steroids in the high mortality cases of COVID-19 reduced mortality by about a third. (Although the beneficial effect of IV steroids was less significant in patients that did not require mechanical ventilation.)

Use of remdesivir, on the other hand, became accepted practice largely at the behest of Tony Fauci, but has not been shown to reduce mortality. It had only been shown to shorten the time until recovery in hospitalized patients.[15]

So, the one treatment shown to reduce *mortality*, the chance of death, in severely ill COVID-19 patients was IV steroids. This was the very same treatment that Fauci confidently dismissed when I questioned him about it in March of 2020. It was a terrible mistake that likely cost lives. Equally as bad was Fauci's decision not to immediately conduct large randomized studies of early treatment. I remain, to this day, agnostic on whether inhaled steroids, ivermectin, or hydroxychloroquine reduce mortality, mainly because I recognize the statistical challenge of reducing a mortality that is already 0.3 percent.

Bad Policies Compound the Problem

One way to get around this problem would be to discover what genetic or metabolic anomaly puts certain people at risk. Studies show that age, obesity, and various other comorbidities are risk factors. One

French study of 5,795 patients showed that obesity doubled the mortality in patients hospitalized for severe COVID-19.

Early on in the pandemic, this was becoming obvious. Obesity and its common comorbidities, diabetes and heart disease, were common denominators in young people with severe COVID disease.[16] What was the government response? Take away all healthy ways to burn calories and boost mental health. Shut down hiking trails. Take nets off of outdoor basketball goals and tie chains around them. Shutter gyms. Put police tape around outdoor playgrounds in cities and arrest people who dared use them.

In Gavin Newsom's California, authorities not only closed outdoor trails, they filled some skate parks with sand.[17] Can't have any rogue kids skateboarding in fresh-air freedom. The Los Angeles County Sheriff's Department arrested a young man daring to paddleboard in the ocean.[18] For city dwellers especially, there was no way to exercise or get natural vitamin D from the sun. Children were forced in front of screens for two years in blue states.

Americans were fed a diet of nonstop media fearmongering, Netflix escapism, and loneliness. The result? Obesity, alcoholism, domestic violence, and addiction surged. Children have lost an estimated two years of learning, and standardized test scores dropped to levels not seen in thirty years.[19] The virus did not do this. This was done by government, by our "public health experts," and by teachers' unions.

Consider that many thought it perfectly safe for teens to work in fast food restaurants or deliver pizza…but unsafe to attend school. Of course the laptop class and their children were much less affected by the forced denial of outdoor play, sunlight, and learning. Gavin Newsom's kids attended their private schools in person.[20] Those with financial means could enjoy private country-club swimming pools, tennis courts, and golf courses. But millions of middle class and poor children in Democrat-run states, dependent on public facilities, faced a cruel lack of options for their physical and mental health.

The Democrats kept telling us we were "all in this together," as one by one they were revealed to be doing everything they publicly forbade:

- Celebrating with elderly relatives at Thanksgiving? Check! (COVID response team's Dr. Deborah Birx)[21]
- Sending your kids to private schools in person while demanding the public schools remained closed? Check! (Newsom and practically every other Democrat official)[22]
- Getting your hair done in a salon while demanding others stay shut down and actually imprisoning business owners who refused? Check! (Nor did eighty-two-year-old Nancy Pelosi look too worried as she swanned around mask-less getting her in-person beauty treatments)[23]
- Going boating and enjoying nature while closing garden centers and telling your constituents they cannot buy plants or seeds? Check! (Governor Gretchen Whitmer)[24]
- Sending law enforcement to take down the license plates of people going to church on Easter Sunday but leaving bars and liquor stores open? Check! (Governor Andy Beshear)[25]

In response to the utter hypocrisy of government and public health officials, Vinay Prasad, M.D., M.P.H. and professor of epidemiology and biostatistics at the University of California, San Francisco, tweeted, "Public health wasn't always a dystopian hellscape intent on using police and military power to maximize compliance with interventions are based on zero RCTs. But it is now!"

Dr. Prasad's tweet contained a link to a video of Deborah Birx lamenting, "I wish that when we went into lockdown, we looked like Italy...People weren't allowed out of their houses, and they couldn't come out but once every two weeks to buy groceries…they had to have a certificate that said they were allowed."[26] Birx's authoritarian desire for military-enforced home imprisonment of all Americans is especially shameless in light of the fact that she couldn't even follow her own lockdown rules when she celebrated Thanksgiving with three generations, including elderly parents. Never forget that people who issue edicts for the "public good" nearly always find a way to exempt themselves.

A Lack of Studies, but a Wealth of Political Posturing

Rather than try to perform studies with the large numbers necessary to discover an improvement with early treatment, Fauci did what he could to stymie the discussion. A phase-one NIH study of hydroxychloroquine was canceled because of "lack of enrollment."[27]

To my thinking, one of the most important areas of research regarding COVID-19 or any other infection that seems to selectively kill would be to sift through large amounts of genomic evidence to try to discover if there is a genetic marker within the DNA of some people, but not others, that would predict who will become severely ill. This selectivity of COVID-19 is not unique. The Streptococcus A infection commonly known as "the flesh-eating bacteria" has a high mortality and amputation rate but also can infect people without any significant symptoms of illness. It seems that it is an idiosyncratic and overly exuberant immune response that kills some and spares others.[28]

Researchers are exploring the connection between one's genetic makeup and susceptibility to COVID-19. Scientists at Hospices Civils de Lyon "hypothesize that pathogenic variants in genes coding for crucial factors involved in the HOST PATHOGEN interaction could explain the susceptibility of some patients to severe disease, even in the absence of comorbidities."[29]

Looking for a genetic predisposition to COVID-19 or Strep A "flesh-eating" bacterial infections is, indeed, looking for a needle in a haystack and would require a large study presumably of the size that a government organization like the NIH might undertake. We might narrow the haystack in which we are searching for a needle by looking at the genomes of patients who died from COVID with no comorbidities, say thin, thirty-to-forty-year-olds with no health issues. Scientists could run through their genomes looking for similarities.

One group of researchers at Russia's HSE University has in fact discovered a genetic predisposition to severe COVID-19. Their results were published in the journal *Frontiers in Immunology.*

The scientists found that people susceptible to a severe case of COVID-19 consistently showed specific genetic markers on certain T cells. T cells are part of the immune response to infections. In viral infections, T cells take the lead and are thought to be more important than the antibody response.

One T cell that recognizes and presents the virus for destruction is the human leukocyte antigen class I (HLA-1). HSE University professors found that patients that possessed certain genetically coded HLA-1 cells had minor infections and patients who had more severe infections had different genetically coded HLA-1 T cells.[30]

This information could potentially allow clinicians to know in advance which patients will become severely ill with COVID-19 and perhaps pre-treat them with an anti-inflammatory therapeutic.

Yet Tony Fauci remained so obsessed with universal vaccination that this strategy of discovering the vulnerable before they became too ill was never really brought to clinical practice.

Studying genetic predisposition to certain diseases could obviously help find new therapeutics, but it's not hard to imagine that an unscrupulous adversary could study genetic predisposition in order to develop a weapon that selectively attacks genetically "other populations," rather than their own.

I am still astonished that there is not more anger, especially from the young, over the years lost and memories stolen out of fear of a disease that for them, was 99.999 percent survivable and overwhelmingly presented with no illness or mild flu. Indeed, it is now acknowledged that the seasonal flu of past years had a higher mortality rate than COVID for children.[31] What was done to them in the name of "safety" is unconscionable. The anger and resentment are there, but for many of them, it is misplaced. Many are not angry at the government "leaders" who locked them down. They are angry at their fellow citizens who refused to comply, who did not obediently discard precious years of their lives out of fear. "I'm going to remember who partied during COVID," one young woman tweeted after spending nearly two years of her twenties on the sofa. She felt righteous that she was doing the right thing, but perhaps she has learned that there is much more to life than fearfully shielding oneself from other people in order to avoid sickness.

CHAPTER 7

COVID Up-Close and Personal

Sunday, March 22: My COVID Illness

I was one of the first public figures to contract COVID, and the hatred and vitriol directed at me were emblematic of our government's divisive and medieval tactics during the pandemic. The blaming and shaming of people for becoming sick, for contracting a virus that is impossible to contain, was utterly inhumane. When I announced that I had tested positive, Democrats and the media were practically salivating in their glee that I would suffer greatly for my sins of questioning, non-compliance, and free thought.

Current Democrat shill and former Bush staffer/waterboarding enthusiast Nicolle Wallace of MSNBC said on air that it was "more difficult" for her to hope that I would recover from COVID.[1] (Still not as bad as MSNBC's Kasie Hunt laughingly describing my 2017 assault and serious injuries as "one of [her] favorite stories" on air.[2])

My saga began on the afternoon of Thursday, March 12, when I had a mild stomachache. I had succumbed to the dessert (again!) at the Republican lunch and had two glasses of tea. I recall taking a Pepcid and lying down on my office sofa. I felt better in a couple of hours and flew home that night to Kentucky.

That weekend in Bowling Green was a typical one for Kelley and me. I felt great and worked in the yard, getting our landscape and deck ready for spring. I did have a few sniffles by Sunday night, but I suffer from seasonal allergies, and that is common for me when I'm outdoors that time of year.

On Sunday evening, Kelley and I were watching the news with growing alarm as we viewed the terrible images of Italian hospitals being overwhelmed with a mysterious new virus. Doctors were describing the swift cascade of symptoms as patients' lungs filled with fluid and drug-resistant pneumonia required artificial ventilators. At that time, there was little else we knew about who was most vulnerable to COVID, but we saw that the body's immune response could result in life-threatening pneumonias.

Kelley was worried about me, as she thought my damaged lung might make me more susceptible to the COVID pneumonia we were seeing on the news. I had suffered multiple bouts of pneumonia over the past three years, and Kelley had been my steadfast support and caregiver as I struggled to heal after being assaulted by a disturbed leftist in November of 2017.[3]

My injuries included six broken ribs, three of them displaced, and a damaged lung. Just six months earlier, in August of 2019, I had undergone surgery at Vanderbilt to remove a part of my lung that was damaged in the assault. After the surgery, I developed a life-threatening lung infection that resulted in a week's stay at Vanderbilt Hospital. There I was attached to a machine to drain fluid off of my damaged lung. I had already suffered two serious pneumonias in that lung and had coughed up blood for months prior to the surgery. Kelley had rushed me to the hospital in the early morning, after I awoke with acute pain and shortness of breath. She watched helplessly as an emergency chest tube was inserted with no anesthesia. She worried and prayed and suffered right along with me, and I never would have made it without her.

As we watched the news, Kelley suggested I take a COVID test when I got back to D.C. the next morning, given that I was alone there during the week and only flew home on the weekends. She asked me, "What if you catch it and get sick in D.C. and there is no one up there to help you?"

As she made the case for me to be tested, she reminded me that we had been in California at large events in the weeks just before things shut down, shaking hundreds of hands. We had also attended the Speed Museum event in Louisville, Kentucky, on March 7 where two people had tested positive, although we'd had no contact with either of them and public officials were not recommending testing for attendees. I promised her that even though I didn't meet the criteria for a test and felt fine, I would ask the next morning if testing was available through the Senate physician.

I flew to D.C. Monday morning, March 16, with Kelley's words on my mind. My chief of staff mentioned that the Senate physician's office was offering the newly arrived COVID testing, but you had to have symptoms to get the testing.

After thirty-three years of marriage, I have learned to listen to my wife's advice, so I decided to take the test. When the doctor asked me about what symptoms I had, he looked somewhat askance at me when a list of symptoms didn't roll off my tongue, so I added a report of my stomachache from the previous week and my sniffles from the night before as my symptoms. At that time, most test results were coming back in forty-eight hours; mine would not come back for six days. (Government medicine at its finest!)

The nature of COVID-19 put me—and us all—in a Catch-22 situation. I didn't meet the criteria for either testing or quarantine. The day of testing, I had zero symptoms of illness and no known exposure to the virus. I had, however, traveled extensively in the United States and was required to continue doing so to vote in the Senate. That, together with the fact that I had a compromised lung, led me to seek testing. Since nearly every member of the U.S. Senate travels by plane across the country multiple times per week and attends lots of large gatherings, my risk factor for exposure to the virus was similar to that of my colleagues, especially since multiple congressional staffers on the Hill had already tested positive weeks ago.

I took the test and moved on with my week, feeling fine. I worked out at the gym every day as usual. I didn't hear a word concerning my test results for the entire week. For those who want to criticize me for lack of quarantine, realize that if the guidelines on testing had been followed, I would never have been tested at all. It was purely my extra precaution, out of concern for my damaged lung, that led me to get tested to begin with.

The following Saturday was beautiful, and I played eighteen holes of golf with my oldest son, William, and two others. I remember we had a great round and that former president Obama utilized his executive privilege (which apparently doesn't end with the term in office) to cut in front of us on the fourteenth hole. If the media had known how close the sainted ex-president had come to encountering the "danger" of a golfer who might have had an asymptomatic infection the week before, they would have gone ballistic.

Little did I know that the very next morning, Sunday, March 22, the proverbial waste matter would hit the fan when the Senate physician called to inform me that the test I had taken nearly a week earlier had come back positive.

Shocked, I called Kelley immediately.

"Get home now," she said.

I jumped in the car and drove straight home from D.C. to Kentucky. Kelley left the garage doors open and had set up the basement bedroom for me to stay in during my quarantine. She immediately tested herself twice, since she had been with me constantly up to the moment I was tested. Her tests, and those of everyone on my staff, were negative. Our son and fellow golfers were also negative. Despite the hysteria of the D.C. media accusing me of trying to kill off the nation's elderly senators, nobody I encountered in the Senate that week became infected. It's disturbing to consider, but I sensed some disappointment in the worst of the media jackals about that.

D.C. is a place full of hype and hyperbole, but I really didn't anticipate the hysteria that ensued.

Allan Smith reported the news: "Rand Paul, R-Ky., on Sunday became the first senator known to have tested positive for COVID-19."

I tweeted out that I was "fine," "asymptomatic and was tested out of an abundance of caution due to...extensive travel and events."

I tweeted that I expected "to be back in the Senate after [the] quarantine period ends and will continue to work for the people of Kentucky at this difficult time."[4]

The left-wing media, never missing a chance to skewer a conservative, trolled me mercilessly. Why didn't he quarantine *after* he got tested? Well, I had no symptoms. Then why did I get tested? My chief of staff responded, "[He] decided to get tested after attending an event where two individuals subsequently tested positive for COVID-19, even though he wasn't aware of any direct contact with either one of them."[5]

Seung Min Kim, White House reporter for the Associated Press, tweeted out that "during the Senate GOP lunch today, Moran told colleagues that Rand was at the gym this morning...and that he was swimming in the pool."[6]

My staff responded to @seungminkim: "We want to be clear, Senator Paul left the Senate IMMEDIATELY upon learning of his diagnosis. He had zero contact with anyone & went into quarantine. Insinuations such as those below that he went to the gym after learning of his results are just completely false & irresponsible!"[7]

Even though I didn't receive my COVID test results till after I'd finished my morning workout, Kyrsten Sinema, the senator for Arizona, immediately threw me to the wolves via Twitter by saying my decision to be around people while my test was pending was "absolutely irresponsible."[8] (A year later, senators were walking around the Senate floor having just tested positive for COVID-19 wearing masks, as if the masks were really protecting us. Oh, how attitudes had changed.)

Lost on these armchair "Karens" was the fact that if you count a stomachache as a COVID symptom, it had been ten days since I'd had any iota of illness. Even by the CDC's current guidelines, I should have been beyond the window for quarantine. As time went on, the CDC would ultimately adopt a regimen that people could return to work *in a hospital* once they were symptom free for three days. The CDC ultimately even allowed physicians who were newly diagnosed as positive to return almost immediately with a mask. But heaven forbid a physician or nurse should decide not to get the vaccine. The government continued to fire healthcare workers who had already recovered from COVID but opted not to get vaccinated. But hey, in D.C., the facts are less important than the blood sport of condemning others.

At home, I settled into our basement, where I dutifully quarantined for two weeks even though I'd already been asymptomatic for ten days. By the end of my quarantine, I'd been asymptomatic for nearly twenty-four days. Kelley put food and drinks at the top of the stairs for me. We visited with her sitting on the top stair and me at the bottom. Every day she asked if I had started to feel sick in any way, and every day I reported that I felt fine.

I read, worked, and tried not to notice the barrage of death wishes coming at me from all sides. The weather turned nice, and one of my friends in the neighborhood set up a golf turf mat for me down by our boat dock. I used it to pitch golf balls so I wouldn't go stir-crazy stuck in the basement.

I was never sick—though President Trump did call to wish me well.

After two long weeks, our public health czars required that I show two negative PCR tests, the deep and uncomfortable nasal probe. Both were negative. I'll never forget bounding up the stairs that afternoon! Kelley and I celebrated on our deck by grilling steaks and toasting with some good Kentucky bourbon at sunset.

Our son Robert was home because his college had closed due to the virus. (He was a junior at Duke at the time. Our older two sons, William and Duncan, had graduated from the University of Kentucky, so we support both the Wildcats and Blue Devils). Robert had been on spring break when the campus closed and students were told not to return. One of his friends, Issac Wong, was from Hong Kong and stranded, so we invited him to stay with us for a few months until he could get home. Robert's degree is in mechanical engineering, and he and Issac built their own makeshift gym in the garage. We played a lot of Scrabble and cooked together. We really enjoyed getting to know Issac, and he still sends cards to Kelley that he signs, "from your adopted Chinese son."

Congress was meeting only sporadically in the next few weeks, so I volunteered at our local hospital.

I rounded on the COVID ward and helped the doctors and nurses reposition COVID patients that were on ventilators. I wanted to help because I knew what has been recognized for centuries—now that I had recovered, I had immunity.

I wasn't afraid to care for COVID patients and wanted to reduce the exposure of other healthcare workers to the illness.

Little did I know that even the universally accepted facts of basic immunology would be discarded by public health zealots concerned more with submission than science.

Kentucky's governor, Andy Beshear (I call him DWP, "drunk with power," Beshear) enforced mandate after mandate. He sent government agents to a church on Easter Sunday to take down license plate numbers of anyone defying his order to cancel church services.[9] Cars parked outside liquor stores were unmolested. He outlawed meetings and gyms, dictated restaurant hours, and commanded that anyone daring to travel across state lines self-quarantine.[10]

The federal courts struck down nearly every one of these mandates, and ultimately the state legislature came in and clipped his wings, legislating that his emergency edicts would expire in thirty days unless approved by the people's representatives, the legislature.[11]

We should never forget the hysteria and political venom in the air at this time. One particularly vicious episode occurred after I played golf at my local course once my quarantine had ended. Congress was meeting only irregularly, so I had time on my hands. Some partisan called the *New York Times* and claimed I was playing while still positive for COVID. The club demanded to see my medical records, ostensibly so that I would be allowed to play again, despite the fact that I had already been volunteering at the local hospital. I'm still angry about that invasion into my privacy, particularly since the next several hundred golfers who subsequently got COVID were not forced to divulge their test status.

This kind of snitching was happening all over the country. Our government's response to COVID unleashed the worst instincts in many people. Envy, suspicion, and fear caused people to report friends, neighbors, and businesses to the police for noncompliance. Our own government actively encouraged this behavior.

Kelley was furious when she called the Kentucky COVID hotline set up by Governor Andy Beshear in late 2020. She called to find out information about vaccine availability for her elderly parents—but the first line of the recording stated something along the lines of "If you know of a business that is not complying with Governor Beshear's COVID guidelines, please press one...." She got no information about vaccine availability—but there was a snitch line available for turning in her fellow Kentuckians! In other words, Beshear's tactics appealed to people's worst instincts, enabling them to turn in friends and neighbors out of envy and malice—oops, I meant to say out of their "upstanding concern for public health." Fortunately, Beshear's authoritarianism was reined in by the Kentucky State Legislature.

Never forget the dubious priorities of politicians with your tax dollars. The more they take, the more they seek to diminish your liberty.

A Government Spending Rampage

On March 27, 2020, while I was still in quarantine, Congress passed the Coronavirus Aid, Relief, and Economic Security Act (CARES). I voiced my opposition, but was little heard as I could not be present. The price tag? $2.2 trillion, nearly half of the entire budget from the previous year. A budget that returned a trillion-dollar annual deficit and now Congress was adding over $2 trillion more, all borrowed. The bill was 880 pages and was described as "the largest economic relief bill in history."[12]

It is doubtful if anyone actually read it, as many members weren't even in town.

Big government Republicans like Lamar Alexander explained their support: "The government has temporarily shut down the economy because of this disease, and the government must help those who are hurt by it."[13] During a July 28, 2020, Republican Senate lunch, Lamar further explained himself: "We will need to rise above principle to support whatever it takes to keep business afloat."[14]

Only a handful of us voiced the worry that the trillions being borrowed and spent would ultimately come back to bite us.

McConnell was described as "somber and exhausted as he announced the vote."[15]

The establishment of both parties never debated or considered the alternative of *not* locking down the entire economy and combatting the disease the way medicine and common sense has always historically responded, by isolating and taking care of the sick and at risk.

Meanwhile, Treasury secretary Steven Mnuchin was already admitting that the administration might soon be back asking for more money. When asked how long before more aid would be needed, he responded, "We've anticipated three months. Hopefully, we won't need this for three months."[16]

The bill gifted $1,200 to individuals and $2,400 to married couples. It didn't matter if you were retired or still employed with no loss of income, you still got a check. Of course, within months, we discovered that noncitizens and dead people received checks as well.[17]

When I tried to get the Senate to unanimously pass my bill to end government checks for dead people, a Democrat senator came running to the floor to object…but was minutes too late. We passed the bill. As with so many Pyrrhic victories in the Senate, that senator called a Democrat colleague in the House and soon blocked passage of my bill in that legislative body. Ultimately, all we got was a watered-down version that may or may not actually stop checks from being sent to dead people. This is your government at "work."

So-called small businesses were eligible to receive forgivable government loans, also known as grants. Subsequent review, of course, found Big Business quickly lapping up the dollars as well, including pro sports teams like the Los Angeles Lakers.[18]

About a month later, on April 24, Congress reconvened to pass the Paycheck Protection Program. After only one month, most of the small business so-called free money had run out. Three-quarters of the new appropriations went to replenish the PPP. The total tab was $484 billion.[19]

Later, as of January 2021, we would make the predictable discovery that $341 million was stolen from the PPP program: "Loot paid for with PPP loan money included two Lamborghini Huracan sports cars, a Rolex Presidential watch, a 5.73-carat diamond ring, a diamond bracelet, two Tesla cars, a 26-foot Pavati Wake Boat, a 33-foot Cruiser yacht, two Rolls-Royces, a Lamborghini Urus luxury SUV, a Kia Stinger, a Ford F-350 pickup truck, at least three Bentleys, and an assortment of other pricey vehicles and boats."[20]

In March 2020, the Senate passed an unparalleled $2.2 trillion economic rescue package steering aid to businesses, workers, and healthcare systems affected by the coronavirus pandemic.

As the pandemic fears mounted, Congress passed four enormous stimulus laws. The first was the Coronavirus Preparedness and Response Supplemental Appropriations Act on March 6 with a total cost of $8.3 billion.[21]

When Congress met to pass this legislation, the full impact of the pandemic was not yet apparent. Government's disastrous decision to lock down (and destroy the economy) for a mere "fifteen days to flatten the curve" had not yet occurred.

The appropriations were for vaccine development and public health. At this point, only eleven Americans had died from COVID-19,[22] and the hysteria was not yet palpable. Yet I was the only senator to oppose the bill.

I opposed the bill for the same reason I usually do: because it contravened Senate rules. The pay-go rules enacted a decade before demanded that new spending be offset by cuts in current spending. Congress routinely ignores this rule, but I typically force them to vote. In 2017, while I supported the tax cuts, I also insisted on voting to adhere to pay-go rules that would demand spending cuts if the deficit rose. Predictably, only three Senators joined me in a vote for fiscal responsibility.

This time I introduced an amendment to pay for the legislation by cutting foreign aid. Surely, in this time of pandemic, other Senators would vote to cut welfare to foreign countries to pay for vaccine development at home? Wrong and wrong again. The one concept that unites both parties, yours truly excepted, is spending taxpayer money without ever cutting or offsetting the new spending.

Even when I pointed out that some of our foreign aid funded ridiculous things like a school for circus arts in Argentina, I got little support. Your legislators do not care. They lack the spine to cut anything, no matter how absurd. In fact, Senate Minority Leader Chuck Schumer loudly complained that my amendment was "a colossal waste of time."[23] And so our $32 trillion debt increases, our dollar is devalued, and the threat to our security as a nation grows.

My press release at the time said, "I support our government's efforts to fight the coronavirus. We also owe it to the American people to do it in a way that avoids piling billions more in debt on their backs. My amendment responsibly uses taxpayer resources by reducing waste to pay for this new spending."[24]

Fiscal sanity lost yet again as the Senate voted 81–15 to table my amendment. On final passage, I was the only senator to oppose this new deficit spending.[25]

On March 18, Congress was back to spend more money. The Families First Coronavirus Response Act was passed as President Trump declared a national emergency. The total cost was $104 billion. The price tag for the government response to COVID-19 seemed to have no limit.

The bill mandated that private insurance and Medicare cover COVID-19 testing, though it was never clear that typical insurance rules wouldn't have sufficed. This bill essentially enacted a multibillion-dollar subsidy to Big Insurance as COVID costs would now be paid for by the taxpayer, not the incredibly profitable private health-insurance companies. What a gift to them! As in everything COVID, the rich got richer. Congress also decided to supplement the typically state-run unemployment insurance with a federal add-on of one billion dollars and mandated paid sick leave. The mounting waste was as spectacular and mind-boggling as the outlay had been.[26]

Once again, the new spending was not offset with spending cuts and would simply be borrowed. I voted with seven other Republicans against the bill. Republicans introduced an amendment to strike the sick leave mandates for fear that this mandate would actually encourage more job terminations. The amendment garnered forty-eight mostly Republican votes but failed.[27] That would be the last in-person vote cast in the Senate for a while. Fear gripped the nation, and where we needed calming and reasoned voices, alarming sirens of hysteria dominated the airwaves. A free people let down their guard and the impulse to authoritarianism sprouted and multiplied.

CHAPTER 8

Naturally Acquired Immunity and Political Witch Hunts

In 2004, Fauci was on C-SPAN when a woman called in and said she had had the flu for fourteen days, had been quite sick, but had avoided taking the flu vaccine because of her previous adverse reactions to the flu vaccine. The host then asked Dr. Fauci, "But she's had the flu for fourteen days—should she get a flu shot?"

In those days, before the pandemic politicization of all public health, Fauci was swift and certain in his response. "Well, no. If she got the flu for fourteen days, she's as protected as anybody can be, because the best vaccination is to get infected yourself.... If she really has the flu, she definitely doesn't need a flu vaccine," he stated. Surviving the infection itself created more immunity than the vaccine. In fact, the immunity gained from infection was better than any vaccine.[1]

A Contagion of Know-Nothingism

But by the spring of 2020, when I returned from my COVID sabbatical, all previous knowledge of immunity seemed to have been discarded. This contagion of "know-nothingism" could not be missed. On my return to the Capitol after recovering from COVID, I was met by a gaggle of young journalists, the ones who occupy a spot between the Capitol subway and the escalator to the Capitol. They barreled up to me with multiple masks on their twenty-something-year-old faces and demanded to know why I wasn't wearing a mask.

I calmly explained to them that the benefit of having survived COVID-19 was that I now had immunity. They challenged me, saying that I didn't know how long my immunity would last. I responded in kind, replying that they didn't know my immunity *wouldn't* last.

The week before I returned from quarantine, I had donated my blood to researchers at the University of Louisville for analysis. They found that I had a robust antibody response to three different sites on the COVID-19 surface.

The reporters, none of whom had a science degree (nor had any of them likely even passed an advanced science course), angrily and self-righteously excoriated me for my "ignorance" and my "dangerous noncompliance." What they did not do was challenge my position in any meaningful way by citing scientific studies based on randomized controlled trials showing any efficacy of masking for viral infection. No. The ignorance of today's "journalists" is staggering. They only know how to repeat the dogma fed to them.

Mask Hypocrisy and Ignorance

I tried to reassure the poor flat-earthers that "of all the people you'll meet today, I'm probably the safest person in Washington. You won't catch COVID-19 from me!" Their eyes visible above their "BLM" and

"Trust Science" masks only narrowed in angry and impotent disbelief. Our media repeatedly and stupidly conflated the use of masking in clinical and surgical settings involving body fluid spatter and bacterial infection with effectiveness against viruses ten times smaller than the smallest bacteria in public settings.

And Anthony Fauci played along. (Except, of course, in his private email, where he advised a personal friend not to bother masking since, of course, "The typical mask you buy in the drug store is not really effective in keeping out virus, which is small enough to pass through material."[2]) Of course, while he was writing this privately, he was sanctimoniously lecturing me in a Senate hearing wearing a ridiculous Washington Nationals cloth mask. When I rightly called him out for his public health theater, he angrily and huffily denied that it was theater.[3] I am still shocked at the childishly ignorant and emotional responses he gave, and by the media's fawning response to it.[4]

I told the press and anyone who might be interested via Twitter statements and press releases of the randomized controlled studies around the world, including the large and telling DANMASK study.[5] Even the *New York Times* admitted, "Researchers in Denmark reported on Wednesday that surgical masks did not protect the wearers against infection with the coronavirus in a large randomized clinical trial."[6]

As Anthony Lazzarino, M.D., commented in *British Medical Journal*, "The DANMASK-19 study proved that surgical facemasks have limited air filtering capacity with respect to SARS-CoV-2."[7]

I offered them a large, randomized-controlled mask study of influenza from Vietnam that showed the cloth mask–wearing group had more infections than the control group wearing no masks. As Dr. A. A. Chughtai and his coauthors concluded, "Rates of infection were consistently higher among those in the cloth mask group than in the medical mask and control groups."[8]

I would point out that the pores of a surgical mask were six hundred times larger than the virus. But, to these young nonscientists, I was portrayed as the person who did not "believe the science." Never mind that science is about objective provability, not belief. Yet in America, under the cult of personality around Fauci, science was bastardized into something akin to religion. And yet the media accused anyone who challenged the dogma of somehow "politicizing" the virus.

Indeed, to this day, there are zero randomized trials that justified the masking stupidity, and a major new international research study recently published in the peer-reviewed Cochrane Database of Systematic Reviews concluded that masks offer no protection against transmission of the virus. The study cited research from seventy-eight studies conducted in Canada, Australia, Italy, the United Kingdom, and Saudi Arabia. And yet our CDC still calls for masking in areas with medium-to-high rates of transmission.[9] Our "guidelines" are being defined by idiots.

Researchers also showed that mask mandates didn't slow down the spread of COVID-19. Damian Guerra and Daniel Guerra showed that "Mask mandates and use [were] not associated with slower state-level COVID-19 spread during COVID-19 growth surges."[10]

Many others, including noted epidemiologist Paul Alexander, Ph.D., found over 170 comparative studies and articles on the ineffectiveness of masks, and not one mainstream journalist bothered to read or attempt to refute the findings.[11] Instead, the chosen strategy was to attack people not wearing masks as lacking "empathy."

Even CNN's Leana Wen, one of the worst offenders in spreading misinformation about COVID and the importance of masks, eventually admitted on air that they are "little more than facial decorations," and that masking contributed to the developmental speech delays in her young son.[12]

However, before the about-face of CNN's Wen, I was kicked off YouTube for the Stalinist sin of spreading "disinformation" for saying exactly the same thing in 2020. No apologies forthcoming from CNN's Leana Wen for her disinformation—nor from CNN's Brianna Keilar for her childish tantrums, calling me an "ass" and a "bloviator of misinformation" for the crime of citing objective, provable facts that didn't conform to the script she had been given to recite.[13] So much for dispassionate and unbiased reporting.

As one by one we skeptics were censored by Big Tech and vilified in the media during what can only be referred to as the COVID witch trials, voices of scientific reason and bravery emerged. One of them was the brilliant Vinay Prasad, M.D., M.P.H., a professor at UCSF. Dr. Prasad spoke out often on the lack of randomized trials to justify our worst and most damaging public health responses: forced masking, lockdowns, and mandatory vaccinations, especially of young and healthy individuals given the risk of myocarditis and pericarditis from the vaccine. Dr. Prasad tweeted, "Medicine is only better than witchcraft if we subject our interventions to randomized trials. If we don't, we are just as stupid as our primitive ancestors. And this [masking] is the case of that. Some people think masking protects the immunocompromised. Sorry, untrue. Zero RCTS [randomized controlled studies] support that claim. Also we never did for years pre-covid. Things were comparable then."[14]

And yet there are no corrections, let alone apologies from the *Washington Post* for their massive misinformation campaign during the course of the pandemic. This included headlines such as "Rand Paul's False Claim That Masks Don't Work,"[15] (which was embarrassingly published in December of 2021, after randomized controlled studies had proven exactly that). None of this was new information. If the *Washington Post* had cared to do the slightest fact-checking, they would have quickly come across a 2019 WHO review that had already concluded, "Ten RCTS [randomized controlled trials] were included in the meta-analysis, and there was no evidence that face masks are effective in reducing transmission of laboratory-confirmed influenza."[16]

This conclusion was not surprising to me or anyone in medicine not utterly cowed by the Fauci machine. Indeed, the WHO conclusion was the consensus opinion pre-COVID. All U.S. pandemic preparedness information, prior to the COVID pandemic, discounted mask-wearing by the healthy. It had long been accepted by the medical community that masks are ineffective in the public square. The WHO meta-analysis had been written prior to the epidemic,[17] and it would not have been thought controversial—that is, not until Fauci's famous flip-flops on masks from calling them not advised and not effective to his ridiculous ultimate position of wearing two or three masks at the same time.[18]

Indeed, the media steadfastly ignored results from the May 2020 University College London study, which included meta-analysis of eleven randomized controlled studies (RCTs) and ten observational studies and concluded, "Available evidence from RCTs is equivocal as to whether or not wearing face masks in community settings results in reduction in clinically- or laboratory-confirmed viral respiratory infections."[19] No, the *Washington Post* and the *New York Times* preferred to ignore actual, inconvenient scientific studies and continue to worship at the Altar of Fauci. That cult needed a villain.

By refusing to comply with something I knew was a lie, I became that villain.

The Media's Frenzied Collusion in Cover-Up Shifts to Full Gear

In the Twitter files, revealed by Elon Musk, we know now that the government was pressuring Big Tech to censor any speech that questioned the official dogma concerning COVID.[20] Scientists, politicians, and anyone else who wanted to debate the lab-leak possibility, the superiority of natural immunity, and masking and masking mandates were all swiftly silenced and banned for "misinformation."

When I posted a video citing the very same scientific studies mentioned above, YouTube swiftly suspended me for violating its "COVID-19 medical misinformation policy." Their policy literally banned any questioning of mask efficacy. Never mind that my comment in the video—"The masks you get over the counter don't work. They don't prevent infection"—was literally stated by Fauci before his flip-flop. It was now verboten at YouTube to make "claims that masks are ineffective in preventing the contraction or transmission of COVID-19."[21]

We were living in a dystopian novel.

I called my suspension a "badge of honor" and linked my video to Rumble, which I have used exclusively since. In my statement at the time, I called YouTube's decision a "continuation of their commitment to act in lock step with the government," and said, "I think this kind of censorship is very dangerous, incredibly anti-free speech and truly anti-progress of science, which involves skepticism and argumentation to arrive at the truth."[22]

Of course, every major news outlet jumped on my suspension as proof of my villainy and uniformly blasted headlines like "Rand Paul Suspended from YouTube Video Full of Covid Lies" (*The Independent*—U.K.) and "YouTube Suspends Rand Paul after Misleading Video on Masks" (Associated Press).[23]

The *New York Times* wrote an article criticizing me, of course. Ironically their article was full of demonstrably false statements such as, "In fact, masks do work, according to the near-unanimous recommendations of public health experts." Leaving no room for the plethora of inconvenient studies and dissenting scientists, the *New York Times* wanted you to know it's all "near-unanimous."[24] No need to think, to question, or to ever hear the blasphemous words of those not in lockstep agreement. Take your Soma, America. Go to sleep.

I wonder if any of the media talking heads who accused me of "misinformation" or "not trusting science" ever had a moment of curiosity that another great COVID heretic, also routinely censored on YouTube and Twitter, was my friend and fellow Kentuckian congressman Thomas Massie. I have an M.D. from Duke, completed an internship in general surgery, and completed my residency in ophthalmology at Duke. I practiced eye surgery for twenty years. Thomas holds both a B.A. and a master's in engineering from MIT. He is a brilliant scientist with twenty-nine patents to his credit. His prizes and inventions are too numerous to mention, but he won the Lemelson-MIT student prize for inventors. Massie was a seventh grader in Vanceburg, Kentucky, when he watched that contest on television and vowed to go to MIT and win it. Was there ever a dark night of the soul for a single reporter who was directed to condemn Massie and me as idiots?

The Witch Hunt Spreads

The pitchforks were out for anyone who challenged the Fauci-controlled "consensus." This wasn't only limited to the media. For refusing to comply with the lie that masks were effective, I was scolded on the Senate floor by my fellow senator Sherrod Brown (D-OH). My refusal to wear the costume, to participate in the theater, called for dramatics, and Senator Brown relished his role on the stage. His angry righteousness was so strong that he believed it within his rights to demand my compliance. But he didn't stop there. Senator Brown, whose scientific literacy is limited to his B.A. in Russian Studies, told reporters that I was "kind of a lunatic."[25] Coming from a scientific illiterate like him, I took this as a compliment.

Here's a full report on Brown from a fawning *Cincinnati Enquirer* interview: "Brown, asked about senators who don't wear face coverings, acknowledged that most of them are before mentioning Paul, a Republican from Bowling Green. 'One of them that's an M.D., isn't, but he's kind of a lunatic,' Brown, a Cleveland Democrat, said during a Tuesday visit to a Columbus mass vaccination site. He added: 'He thinks he wants to be different but it doesn't serve the public interest.'" The *Enquirer* made sure to piously check all the approved boxes when they intoned that "Brown, who is fully vaccinated, wore a mask during the entirety of his 45-minute event. Brown said he does so to 'make sure everyone is safe and to set that tone.'"[26]

I refused to stoop to the level of Senator Russian Studies and reply in kind to his ignorant insults, but I did put out a statement that said that "Vaccine-deniers [that is, immunity-deniers] who dispute immunity after natural infection and after vaccination, should refrain from name-calling and perhaps try to get informed."[27]

I couldn't help but recall the quote from Steve Jobs, who famously stated in 2011 (back when dissent was allowed on tech platforms), "Here's to the crazy ones, the misfits, the rebels, the troublemakers, the round pegs in the square holes…the ones who see things differently— they're not fond of rules, and they have no respect for the status quo. You can quote them, disagree with them, glorify or vilify them. About the only thing you can't do is ignore them. Because they change things."[28]

I wonder what Jobs would have to say about the obeisance of our tech overlords to the government and their willingness to abandon the First Amendment and censor the "ones who see things differently."

We were silenced. We were vilified. But in the stirring words often attributed to Saint Augustine, "The truth is like a lion; you don't have to defend it. Let it loose; it will defend itself."[29] While the government and their cronies in the media and Big Tech tried to shackle it, and sadly succeeded long enough to cause great damage to our nation, the truth is finally being let loose.

The Real Scientific Consensus

In this upside-down world, in some ways mimicking the Middle Ages, scientific knowledge, once commonplace, appeared to be lost. Reporters had forgotten how routine it was to acknowledge immunity. Take this quote from the *Washington Post* in 1978: The Russian flu does not seem to be affecting "those persons in the 23- to 33-year-old age group [because they] have some resistance against the virus because they were probably infected by a very similar H1N1 virus in the late 1940s and the 1950s. Therefore they have antibodies against that type of infection." No need for doubt or argument that "antibodies might fade over time." No, it was simply recognized as a basic fact that previous infection explained why anyone older than twenty-three likely had immunity.[30]

For the next few months, I would try to get Trump's White House health team to grasp the value of immunity. I told them ad nauseam to comprise Trump's Secret Service detail with agents who had recovered from COVID. I never got any indication that they listened. Until a vaccine was available, the best safety precaution known for a public figure would be to surround him or her with people already immune to COVID-19. The same logic could have been applied to nursing homes. Forty percent of all COVID deaths came from nursing homes.[31] In the year before the COVID vaccine, assigning caregivers recovered from COVID could have saved thousands of lives. But it never happened, primarily because Fauci downplayed and disparaged naturally acquired immunity.

HuffPost, not known for dispassionate analysis or scientific acumen, joined the melee to mask me up. They chose as an authority an ER physician from *Brown*. Hmmm? A doctor with no immunology expertise from a university whose student body is so leftist they once voted to be given suicide pills to take in case of nuclear war?[32] Seems on brand!

This Dr. Megan L. Ranney stated that it was unknown when people become "non-infectious to others." Ranney also opined that the current requirement was that "health care workers are required to test negative for the virus twice before being allowed to return to work."[33] Well, yes, without any scientific evidence as support, two weeks had been made the initial mandate from our government agencies. But as the absurdity and costs mounted, that mandate would be altered again and again. It ultimately dwindled down to allowing doctors and nurses to practice even with a positive COVID test.

But at the time, even with zero science supporting a two-week quarantine for a patient already ten days past his symptoms, such that they were, I did as I was told, quarantined, and then took two PCR tests before I volunteered to work in the COVID ward at my local hospital.

Over the next few weeks, I helped reposition COVID patients who were on the ventilator. Internists had discovered the hard way that heavily sedated patients on a ventilator did better if rotated onto their stomachs periodically. Belatedly, clinicians also learned that mechanical ventilation might have actually brought down the survival rate. Doctors began describing "happy hypoxics"—that is, COVID patients with O_2 saturation in the dangerously low 80 percent or even in the 70 percent area, clearly short of oxygenation but not laboring such that they had to be ventilated.

The two big discoveries that came out of the COVID-19 ICUs were to try to delay mechanical ventilation as long as possible and to use high-dose IV steroids. Ultimately, these two insights would save thousands of lives.

The Madness of Vaccine Mandates

For the first ten months of the pandemic, before the vaccine was available, doctors and nurses risked their lives daily to take care of COVID patients. How did Fauci and public health treat these heroes?

Well, they summarily fired many healthcare workers who had already survived COVID and rationally understood they had immunity and therefore elected not to vaccinate.

The rigidity of the COVID overlords resulted in the fining of thousands of doctors and nurses and the firing of many more. Ultimately, after hospitals had spent months firing unvaccinated nurses and doctors, the Omicron COVID surge arrived and the policy miraculously changed to allow a worker's return once asymptomatic for ten days.[34] There were even reports of hospitals allowing doctors and nurses to work while having tested positive for COVID. The CDC even provided for COVID positive doctors to see patients: "If shortages continue despite other mitigation strategies, as a last resort consider allowing HCP to work even if they have suspected or confirmed SARS-CoV-2 infection, if they are well enough and willing to work, even if they have not met all the contingency return to work criteria described above."[35]

Justice delayed is still injustice, but a New York court eventually ruled that these medical workers who were fired for not choosing the COVID vaccination should get their jobs back with pay.[36]

Congress, with my loud advocacy, passed a law in late 2022 to strike down the military mandate for the COVID-19 vaccine.[37] Republicans supported reinstating all soldiers discharged for lack of vaccination with back pay. Unfortunately, most doctors and nurses that were let go never got their jobs back.[38]

This is particularly galling when you realize these doctors and nurses risked their lives for nearly a year caring for COVID patients when no vaccine existed. Many of them survived COVID and had natural immunity. They were summarily fired anyway with not one iota of discussion about the need for vaccination after previous infection.

Not only that. Young males are at increased risk for vaccine-induced myocarditis, a serious inflammation of the heart, and yet hospitals and universities rigidly adhered to one-size-fits-all mandates despite potential harms. Reporting in The Defender, Suzanne Burdick, Ph.D., quotes Vinay Prasad, M.D. Ph.D.: "With emerging data from the UK it was clear that for some products and some doses, myocarditis post vax exceeded myocarditis post illness."

"Prasad said he believes COVID-19 vaccine mandates were 'always unjustified' and that he strongly supports the repeal of any such law—especially college vaccine mandates that were created by 'some mid-level bureaucrat' who had no scientific expertise. College students who were required for attendance to get the COVID-19 vaccine and now have myocarditis or pericarditis should be able to sue that college, he said."[39]

Though the CDC was mute about the benefits of naturally acquired immunity and the risks of myocarditis, they did acknowledge that it was not desirable to be vaccinated within three months of a previous COVID Infection.[40]

Presumably this was because it was not smart to provoke a new vaccine-induced immune response when you were still in the midst of a natural immune response. What else could be the reasoning? Indubitably, though, thousands of people who should not have showed up at their local chain pharmacy and got the jab within that three-month period.

One young man on my staff got a bad flu-like syndrome with COVID. His doctor, perhaps forgetting the part about a physician being sympathetic, berated him for not being vaccinated and asked accusingly, "Well, I guess now you'll get vaccinated?"

My staff member came back at him quickly: "I think I just got inoculated by the disease itself! Didn't I?"

The doctor glared back without apologizing.[41]

The Mask as a Ritual Talisman

The medical establishment's recommendations for what to do after testing positive for COVID evolved. When I got COVID in March 2020, I was told to quarantine for two weeks and have two negative COVID tests before returning to normal interaction. By 2022, people were only told to avoid people if they were symptomatic and to wear a mask. Did the "science" change? No. The politics did.

Instead of hiding away in sheer terror at the thought of encountering people, it now became commonplace to see senators on the floor with masks who were actually positive for COVID. This was a far cry from the hysterical cries from my colleagues and their liberal allies in the media when I tested positive.

In the fall of 2022, Senator Tom Carper came up to me on the floor of the Senate with a mask on. He is invariably friendly and loquacious, but his speech—at least to this hearing-impaired senator—is sometimes hard to make out. So, as he greeted me and spoke to me, I indicated that I could not understand him through the mask. He obligingly pulled it down to apologize and leaned in close to me and said, "Sorry, I've got COVID and the doctor told me to wear this mask."[42] Wonder if any of these senators remembered how they'd accused me of literally trying to kill them by not quarantining when I was asymptomatic without a positive test?

HuffPost evidently felt they hadn't scolded me sufficiently with their pseudoscience, so they tried chastising me for my lack of manners: As their Brown University ER doc, Megan L. Ranney, said, "Paul should be setting a better example for his constituents by wearing a mask either way."[43] So this ER physician (with no special expertise in the matter) felt it was her duty to scold me—not about the science of mask-wearing but *because I was displaying bad public manners.*

Their non-expert expert continued: "Regardless of whether he has been infected or not, he is a political leader, and his constituents look to him for guidance. He owes it to all of us to model best public health practice—in other words, to wear a mask in public."[44]

What it came down to was this doctor/"Karen" wanted me to wear a mask as a mere talisman of good manners.

Lest you think I am jumping to conclusions, consider that during this period of time, a letter to the *New England Journal of Medicine* addressed the idea of mask-wearing as a talisman and concluded that masks were ineffective outside of the hospital setting:

> It is also clear that masks serve symbolic roles. Masks are not only tools, they are also talismans that may help increase health care workers' perceived sense of safety, well-being, and trust in their hospitals. Although such reactions may not be strictly logical, we are all subject to fear and anxiety, especially during times of crisis. One might argue that fear and anxiety are better countered with data and education than with a marginally beneficial mask, particularly in light of the worldwide mask shortage, but it is difficult to get clinicians to hear this message in the heat of the current crisis.[45]

One might, indeed.

The *NEJM* letter went on to conclude the following:

> We know that wearing a mask outside health care facilities offers little, if any, protection from infection. Public health authorities define a significant exposure to Covid-19 as

face-to-face contact within 6 feet with a patient with symptomatic Covid-19 that is sustained for at least a few minutes (and some say more than 10 minutes or even 30 minutes). The chance of catching Covid-19 from a passing interaction in a public space is therefore minimal. In many cases, the desire for widespread masking is a reflexive reaction to anxiety over the pandemic.[46]

The conclusion that masks are merely a talisman and don't work outside the hospital setting seems straightforward.[47] But as the *NEJM* letter lit up Twitter, someone got to the authors and they made an about-face. The authors amended their letter to say the opposite of what they had originally written. They now wrote, "The intent of our article was to push for more masking, not less." They altered their original letter to now say, "[W]e intended this statement to apply to passing encounters in public spaces, not sustained interactions within closed environments."[48] Makes you wonder who got the authors to make such a public reversal.

Anyone who looks for truth from fact-checkers is looking in the wrong place. Most journalists work for far-left publications and are anything but unbiased. In fact, fact-checkers are not really fact-checkers at all. For the most part, they are simply opinion writers masquerading as experts.

HuffPo's fact-check writer spilled much ink attacking my immunity claims but didn't mention what her scientific qualifications were to make such a judgment.[49]

In fact, a COVID fact-checker at PolitiFact was ultimately exposed for having no scientific credentials or background. @TexasLindsey let the Twitterverse know that this fact-checker was not a scientist, did not have a Ph.D., was not a doctor, and had no medical background whatsoever, yet PolitiFact put him forward to debunk and dispute anything and everything that contradicted the company line of universal, unquestioned mandatory vaccination.[50]

HuffPo's fact-checker complained that I couldn't know that I was no longer infectious without two negative PCR tests.[51] As we all soon found out, the testing requirement standards changed with each month. Initially, they demanded two deep sinus swabs for a PCR test. Until one day when they didn't require two tests.[52] As the hysteria waned, COVID-19 patients were told they could return when they'd been without symptoms for three days. For all the grief these so-called journalists heaped on me, it was never made clear by any authority how many days you should stay away from people if you were COVID positive but asymptomatic.

The media and our public health mouthpieces never clearly informed people that the PCR test detected remnants of RNA, not active virus. The hysterics blathered on about positive PCR tests on hand railings and surfaces only to have scientists finally disabuse them of the notion that the virus lived for long periods on such surfaces.

Billions of dollars were spent sanitizing surfaces, and people were told to disinfect their groceries. It was all part of the fearmongering to justify closing schools and shutting down the economy.

The HuffPo fact-checker also alleged "that [my] claim of immunity has not yet been proved."[53] But really, wouldn't it be equally valid to say that my claim of immunity was consistent with the historical scientific record? The degree of immunity or length of time of COVID immunity might be open to debate, yet it was frankly a lie to deny a century of evidence for naturally acquired immunity and the accumulating record for COVID-19.

2020: The Year Long-Term Flu Immunity Became Controversial

We have over a hundred years of knowledge of communicable disease and the body's ability to produce an immune response upon survival. Why was this insight ignored? To these flat-earthers, I offered the case of a 102-year-old woman who lived through the Spanish flu in 1918 who also survived COVID in 2020. Angelina Sciales was born in 1918 on a ship coming from Italy to New York. Her mother died in transit from the Spanish flu. Angelina contracted the Spanish flu as a newborn but survived. Incredibly, scientists have discovered that patients like Angelina still have active antibodies *ninety to one hundred years later.*[54]

In 2008, two studies showed that elderly patients in their nineties and hundreds still had antibodies to the Spanish flu and that those antibodies could still effectively neutralize a similar virus in mice.[55]

This is not proof that all immunity lasts, but shouldn't it be incumbent on critics to prove that survivors *don't* have immunity rather than that survivors do?

Microbiologist and coauthor of one of these studies Christopher Basler commented, "What this shows is that these [immune] responses can last pretty much the entire human lifetime."[56]

Another survivor of the influenza with long-term immunity was Michael Mosley, born in Calcutta, India, in 1957. As a newborn, he became incredibly ill from the H1N1 flu, a variant of the 1918 flu. Fifty-five years later, his serum still shows antibodies to the 1957 flu.[57] But in 2020, this knowledge was forgotten or purposefully ignored in order to accomplish what Fauci and his ilk would call the greater good.

Knowledge of long-term immunity to influenza viruses was dangerous to the goal of universal submission to vaccination and therefore needed to be suppressed. Hence the hundreds of requests by government to the media, experts, Big Tech, and the population at large to censor discussion of naturally acquired immunity.

When Fauci was finally deposed by Attorneys General Jeff Landry and Eric Schmitt, he played the role of the mentally debilitated mafia don and responded dozens of times that he could "not recall." Under oath, they asked him repeatedly about his meetings with social media companies to enlist them as "surrogate-censors" to take down any posts espousing naturally acquired immunity and any voices opposed to universal, mandatory vaccines. "I don't recall," he repeated, again and again.[58]

He showed no awareness of the mountains of scientific evidence of naturally acquired immunity. He seemed oblivious to studies showing that patients who recovered from the first coronavirus epidemic, SARS1, retained T cell immunity seventeen years later.[59] Duke-NUS Medical School in Singapore evaluated twenty-three SARS1 patients and found that all of them still had T cells specific for SARS1.

Researchers noted that finding long-term immunity in SARS1 patients supported "the notion that Covid-19 patients will develop long-term T cell immunity."[60]

It is certainly true that not all infections provide life-long immunity or protection. While some infections such as smallpox, chickenpox, and measles provide lifelong protection from reinfection, infections from other viruses such as the common cold do not prevent subsequent infection, but previous infection does create memory immunity that likely lessens symptoms in subsequent infections. But it is, without question, the accepted norm in immunology that previous infection provides some form of immunity.

In 1721, Dr. Zabdiel Boylston of Boston brought the discovery of the smallpox vaccine—or *variolation* as they called it at the time—to America. Boylston first heard of the idea from the Puritan preacher Cotton Mather, who had gained the knowledge from his enslaved servant, an African man named Onesimus.

In many parts of Africa and the Middle East, people had observed that survivors were immune to further infection, and would take the scabs of smallpox survivors, grind them up and rub the skin of never-infected people with small needle punctures, usually on the back of the hand. They had discovered that those who were "variolated" usually experienced a much milder form of smallpox, with only a few pustules at the inoculation site, and would more easily survive. More importantly, they were "forever free from fear of contagion."[61]

Dr. Boylston was immediately met with great hostility from the establishment medical community, many of whom feared the smallpox variolations would only spread the disease. It took great courage to inoculate his own son first with the live vaccine, using the disease itself as the inoculum. Zabdiel also inoculated between 180 and 250 other Bostonians.

Opposing physicians created an outrage mob that threatened Boylston's family. He was arrested soon after inoculating his son, and only freed after promising to "only inoculate with government permission."[62]

During the great smallpox epidemic of 1721, people were placed under guard in an attempt to keep the disease from spreading—to no avail. As Steve Templeton wrote in an article for the Brownstone Institute,

> By mid-June of 1721, the city was overwhelmed with cases, and as historians Otho Beall and Richard Shryock wrote in 1954, "…the disease was free to take its natural course." They concluded, "One has here a nice illustration of the ineffectiveness of isolation procedures as then practiced, once a serious infection had spread beyond a few original foci." In modern pandemic parlance, there is a point when high disease prevalence makes "flattening the curve" impossible. To stop the smallpox outbreak and/or to prevent it from returning, the best option was to increase immunity in the population. Yet proponents of variolation encountered fierce resistance.[63]

Indeed, Boylston faced intense "backlash" for promoting the inoculation. As Templeton wrote, "Some physicians had circulated horror stories about variolation in Europe, further terrifying and cowing the public (one can easily imagine them with Twitter accounts, over 100K followers, and recommended as 'experts'). By November, popular passions were such that a bomb was thrown into Mather's home. When the disease continued to spread throughout Boston, Boylston's inoculations were blamed. Boylston himself calculated that inoculated individuals developed smallpox with one-sixth the frequency of uninoculated individuals. But his opponents, driven by emotion, could not be convinced."[64] Realize also that Boylston introduced this "vaccine" against the consensus of medical opinion. In fact, a great many scientific discoveries came about because a brave scientist stood up and opposed consensus, conformity, and groupthink. Today's overlords of misinformation might want to consider the history of science before decreeing what the latest scientific consensus must be and silencing the speech of critics.

It is indeed ironic that centuries later, during the COVID-19 hysteria, the public health establishment would ignore the very science the smallpox vaccine (and every other vaccine since) is based upon: the body's natural immune response to infection with disease.[65]

Within two generations, though, the vaccines, even with the risk of contracting smallpox from the vaccine, became accepted by most knowledgeable people. George Washington insisted that Martha be inoculated before she came to visit him in the Revolutionary War camps.

George Washington, himself, however, did not choose to be vaccinated. Why? Because he had already had smallpox as a teenager in Barbados. I'm guessing no mouth-breathing journalist from Philadelphia had the temerity to question why Washington considered himself immune despite a lack of "randomized controlled studies."

Two hundred fifty years later, fact-checkers found legions of public health wonks willing to disparage naturally acquired immunity and opine that we just don't know. Sad that what was once common sense in the days of George Washington had succumbed to a bureaucratic desire to "universally mandate vaccines," common sense be damned.

Nevertheless, scientists continued to produce evidence that immunity after COVID infection was real and long lasting. One intriguing hypothesis that might explain why children recover so easily from COVID is that previous infection with common cold coronaviruses may provide the protection that allows many patients to have few or no symptoms when infected with COVID-19.

"Scientific studies have shown people who have had a common cold in the past two years have T cells that display 'cross-reactive protection' against Covid-19."[66] Children get more colds than adults, which might explain why children seem to be less symptomatic with COVID-19.

Another study from Guangzhou, China, found that patients infected with SARS1 in 2003–2004 still had IgG antibodies to SARS1 twelve years later.[67] So, instead of no evidence of my having immunity to COVID-19 after my infection, the opposite was true. All the evidence known suggested that I and others infected with COVID would have some form of immunity. And yet in 2020, this was kept from the public.

Even as early as March 20, 2020, while I was still in quarantine, studies came out showing that macaques infected with COVID-19 could not be reinfected, at least in the short-term.[68]

As the months rolled on, study after study continued to show that infection with COVID would lead to long-lasting immunity.

NIH scientist Margaret Smelkinson, Ph.D., pointed out in her May 2023 testimony to the House Oversight Committee that already "in September 2020, a study from Qatar estimated a 0.01% reinfection rate within a few months from the first infection with none of those reinfected having a severe illness."[69]

Instead of no evidence of naturally acquired immunity, as the media claimed, the evidence was abundant and pointed toward lasting immunity. A study in *Journal of the American Medical Association* showed a 0.3 percent rate of reinfection compared to a 3 percent infection rate for individuals not previously infected.[70]

By the spring of 2021, large studies, such as the SIREN study from England, were showing that prior infection reduced the risk of reinfection by 84 percent.[71]

A May 2021 *Nature* paper showed that recovered COVID patients still had anti-S protein antibodies at eleven months. Indeed, as the pandemic stretched month after month, scientists consistently were able to detect antibodies to COVID.[72]

Nevertheless, the scientific illiterates virtuously posing with three masks (also known as the Capitol press corps) demanded that I must prove I had immunity or else submit to useless masking.

In June of 2021, Marty Makary, M.D., of Johns Hopkins wrote in the *Wall Street Journal*, "After treating Covid for 16 months, we haven't seen significan[t] incidence of re-infection. In Italy no re-infection clusters have been observed. In a large study from Denmark, less than 0.7% of people who tested positive for Covid, including those who were asymptomatic, ever tested positive again—a 'breakthrough infection' rate similar to that of vaccines."[73]

Yet, Dr. Fauci, the CDC, and the government public health complex continued to downplay naturally acquired immunity, arguing that there were too many unknowns and that everyone should just submit to vaccination and repeat vaccination and boosters and repeat boosters.

But wouldn't it be reasonable to want to understand how protective natural immunity was? Did previous COVID infection provide protection? Did previous COVID infection count as the equivalent of a booster vaccine?

Finally, in January of 2022, the CDC admitted what most objective observers had suspected—natural immunity was actually more protective than vaccination. The incidence of COVID-19 infection among those vaccinated alone (without prior COVID-19) was 6.2-fold lower in California and 4.5-fold lower in New York. The rates among those with natural immunity were 29.0-fold lower in California and 14.7-fold lower in New York. So, while during the Delta wave of COVID infections the vaccine decreased your chance of getting COVID, previous infection actually decreased the incidence of COVID three to four times better than the vaccine.[74]

The CDC's own data from over one million people showed that previous infection was protection against severe illness as well. In the study, people who were vaccinated were 19.8 times less likely to be hospitalized than people who were unvaccinated. But people who had recovered from COVID were 55.3 times less likely to be hospitalized than people who were unvaccinated.[75]

Clearly, naturally acquired immunity was not only equal to vaccination but in this study exceeded the value of vaccination. The vaccine disciples on the Left, even with this information, abruptly changed tactics to state that COVID infection is not worth the immunity you obtain. Well, exactly no one was arguing that it was. The point I was making was that once you've recovered from COVID, you had protective immunity. It was never an argument not to be vaccinated or to choose infection.

However, it was valuable information to consider, particularly if you were young and healthy, about whether to be vaccinated if you'd already recovered from COVID. It would also be useful information if you'd been vaccinated and had also had COVID. Did a twenty-year-old who'd had two vaccines and natural COVID need a booster? Certainly not, yet colleges were mandating it despite significant risks of vaccine-induced myocarditis. The CDC presumably has that data but refuses to release it because it might lead to less mass submission to endless booster vaccines.

The Media Trolls On

HuffPo's "resident expert," also known as the Brown ER doctor—not an expert in immunology—claimed that serum "antibody tests were 'unreliable, and the value of antibodies is still under debate.'"[76]

As the Left piled on with their criticisms of my refusal to wear a mask, I tweeted back at them, "The fake news can't stand that some people might not need to submit to the new authoritarianism of the left because they are immune to coronavirus. Modern science disagrees."[77]

For good measure, I mocked them with Lord Fauci's own words:

Dr. Fauci: "We know with infections like this, that at least for a reasonable period, you're gonna have antibodies that are protective… if we get infected in February/March and recover, next September, October, that person who's infected—I believe—is going to be protected. To be clear, most experts do think an initial infection from the coronavirus, called SARS-CoV-2, will grant people immunity to the virus for some amount of time. That is the case with acute infections from other viruses, including other coronaviruses."[78]

HuffPost complained that it was a partial quote and pointed to another flip-flopping Fauci quote in which he said that it "has not been proven" that infected coronavirus patients have immunity."[79]

Is that a true "fact-check"? It does not indicate in any way that Fauci disagrees with me. It is obvious that he, like his left-wing cronies at HuffPost, fears people might put two and two together and decide for themselves that they may not need to further feed Big Pharma's bottom line once they have recovered from COVID. But it's about much more than that. In medicine, there is always a trade-off when you put something in your body that it may not need. There is a risk/benefit analysis.

People depend on their doctors to help them decide if they actually need a drug. During the COVID hysteria, the public health overlords shamed young people, recovered people, and other individuals for assessing their own low risk and choosing not to expose themselves to an mRNA vaccine for which we have no long-term studies. Doctors were threatened with the loss of their medical licenses and board certifications for noncompliance with the official edicts. Doctors were ordered to give the same treatment to an eighteen-year-old healthy boy as an eighty-year-old man with heart disease and diabetes. Just take two vaccines! Take two boosters! Do not question. Do not use your medical judgment about the patient's risk. Ignore the centuries of scientific knowledge we have about natural immunity. This was just one of the many injustices brought against the American people.

Never one to back down from a fight, particularly one with the scientifically naïve and uneducated Washington media, I tweeted, "Modern medicine shows us that immunity is based on having antibodies. Why do they think medicine is trying so hard to get a coronavirus vaccine? Immunity. I have taken an antibody test and am positive for long term Covid-19 antibodies."[80]

I could have added that immunity actually comes in many forms, not just antibodies. In addition to humoral immunity (antibodies), the body also responds with cellular immunity (T cells). And these two wings of the immune response have both an immediate response and a delayed response that typically involves immune system memory cells being kept ready for reinfection.

While not all immunity prevents reinfection, it typically provides some protection against serious infection the second time around. Ironically, this is exactly the argument that government vaccine proponents would make when they were forced to defend a vaccine that doesn't prevent infection or transmission. These vaccine advocates shifted their argument from prevention to "protection against serious disease."

So, the argument that previous infection would either stop reinfection or at least attenuate a subsequent infection was rejected by the vaccine promoters but then promoted by them (in support of continued vaccination) when it turned out their vaccine didn't protect against infection or transmission.

The level of misinformation assailing the American people in 2020 was staggering. For months, I fought these flat-earthers and their relentless attacks. A typical headline from November 2020 was

FactCheck.org's harangue: "Paul Misleads on Natural Infection and COVID-19 Vaccines."[81]

The great thing about Twitter is knowing the scientifically illiterate Left will freak out if you point to studies that challenged the universal vaccine mandate.

So, on November 17, 2020, I tweeted,

> Great news!
> - Pfizer vaccine 90% effective
> - Moderna vaccine 94.5% effective
> - Naturally acquired COVID-19 99.9982% percent effective*
> * (estimating 200 reinfections out of 11 million Americans, which is likely an overestimation of actual reinfections)[82]

I followed up with this tweet: "Why does the left accept immune theory when it comes to vaccines, but not when discussing naturally acquired immunity?"[83]

Like so many media outlets, FactCheck.org relied upon straw-man arguments like this one from quoted virologist Angela Rasmussen: "We don't really know how many reinfections there have been." Jessica McDonald, the author of the article, noted Rasmussen's contention "that many reinfections have not been confirmed and that efficacy of naturally acquired immunity 'isn't a thing.'"

"It's true that reinfections so far appear to be rare," McDonald went on to say, "which bodes well both for a vaccine and for people who may have immunity as a result of infection. But no one knows yet how the immunity from each will compare."

She goes on to admit that "most vaccines do not offer quite as good protection from a pathogen as a natural infection will—but of course, a person has to survive or suffer through the infection to get that future protection, sidestepping the entire function of a vaccine. It's therefore largely irrelevant whether or not vaccine immunity is superior to that from natural infection."[84]

Never mind that exactly no one was arguing about a choice of taking a vaccine versus waiting for natural immunity to occur. My point had always been about the proper medical advice to give patients who had *already recovered* from COVID.

McDonald somehow believes that discussion is "irrelevant"? If your child has had COVID-19, would it be irrelevant to ask whether that infection now protects him or her from reinfection—particularly since the mRNA treatment had no long-term safety studies and was only approved under an emergency authorization?

Realize that the current CDC policy is that if your child has had COVID he should be vaccinated. If he is vaccinated and is hospitalized for myocarditis caused by the vaccine, the parents are to wait until he recovers and then vaccinate him again. Insanity.

And these idiots wonder why Americans have "vaccine hesitancy"? To any CDC "experts" reading this text, know this: no informed parent will subject his or her kid who has already survived COVID and now survived myocarditis from the vaccine to *yet another vaccine*!

I included a link to an article in the *New York Times* that reported:

"But these cases [reinfection] make the news precisely because they are rare, experts said: More than 38 million people worldwide have been infected with the coronavirus, and as of Monday, fewer than five of those cases have been confirmed by scientists to be reinfections."[85]

If you extrapolate five reinfections out of thirty-eight million and apply the ratio to eleven million Americans, you get about one and a half reinfections per eleven million. To be generous, I showed what the reinfection rate would be if you rounded up to about two hundred per eleven million. The idea was to demonstrate that, yes, natural immunity is a reality, and, if compared to vaccination, shows similar efficacy.

Now over time, reinfection rates would become less important when the Omicron variant arrived on the scene. Reinfection became quite common among the vaccinated and among those previously infected.

But even after Omicron, a meta-analysis of nineteen studies published in the *Chinese Medical Journal* showed that the pooled reinfection rate after surviving COVID-19 infection was 0.65 percent or less than 1 percent. The analysis also showed significant protection against symptomatic reinfection. The authors concluded, "The rate of reinfection with SARS-CoV-2 is relatively low. The protection against SARS-CoV-2 after natural infection is comparable to that estimated for vaccine efficacy."[86]

Of course, FactCheck.org misinformed its audience by reporting that I "misleadingly suggested that immunity from '[n]aturally acquired' COVID-19 was better than that from a vaccine."[87] I said no such thing. I simply pointed out that the data, at the time, showed only very rare reinfection.

FackCheck.org went on to scold, "The entire point of a vaccine is to offer immunity without the risk of getting sick."[88] No kidding! Once again, I was never arguing that it was better to get COVID. What I was maintaining, and still do, is that if you've had COVID-19 and survived—as approximately 99.7 percent of those infected did—you have immunity.

I couldn't help giving the Twitterverse another nudge: "More great news on immunity for people who've survived COVID! To the haters—I'm not arguing against vaccines. Simply pointing out the good news that COVID+ patients, some of whom suffered almost to dying, can celebrate immunity if lucky enough to survive."[89]

I also tweeted a link to an article that opened with this: "How long might immunity to the coronavirus last? Years, maybe even decades, according to a new study...."

The article referenced the research of Shane Crotty of La Jolla Institute of Immunology, who had found that "eight months after infection, most people who have recovered still have enough immune cells to fend off the virus and prevent illness, the new data show."[90]

The article quoted Crotty: "That amount of memory would likely prevent the vast majority of people from getting hospitalized disease, severe disease, for many years."[91]

In a transparent attempt to debunk challenges to their "must vaccinate all" narrative, FactCheck.org published this quote from Crotty "quoting his manuscript": "That led us to speculate...that 'it may be expected that at least a fraction of the SARS-CoV-2-infected population with particularly low immune memory would be susceptible to re-infection relatively quickly.'"[92]

Quite hilarious when the fact-checker actually provides a fact that actually doesn't support her case. The quote instead clearly implies that everyone else not included in that small fraction *does* obtain significant immunity from having had the infection.

This type of selective quoting in order to present a "science is settled" narrative has been the rule throughout COVID. Crotty was quite explicit that immunity from prior COVID infection "particularly protects against hospitalizations and severe illness."[93]

Crotty warned that natural immunity may not provide as much protection against variants of COVID.[94] Which also turned out to be true for the vaccines. But for the initial, most deadly variant and its successor, the deadly Delta variant, the CDC finally admitted in a study of over a million patients, during the Delta wave, that, yes, prior infection was not only protective against hospitalization but actually more than twice as effective as the vaccine.[95]

According to PolitiFact, Crotty argued that "those who receive a vaccine shot have a much more consistent number of immune cells, since everyone receives the same dose amount."[96]

While that is likely true, it is an argument for vaccinating the vulnerable, a policy I agree with. Time would ultimately show that healthy individuals who were previously infected and not vaccinated would have virtually zero hospitalizations or deaths.

I responded to this liberal onslaught with an op-ed in the Louisville *Courier-Journal*:

It's long past time for us to say no more to the science deniers.

It's time for us to stand up to Washington bureaucrats who think you're not smart enough to make your own decisions. It's time for us to stand up to people who write columns ignoring 100 years of immunity science just to score cheap—and incorrect—political points.

These petty tyrants in government and their enablers in the media always think they know best. They deal in the currency of fear, hoping to scare the American people into submission.

For months, I've heard your pleas for a return to normalcy, and for months I've raised the alarm—loudly, publicly, and armed with studies that Dr. Anthony Fauci and the media have mostly chosen to ignore—studies showing that we can in fact safely send our kids back to school and reopen the economy.

Now they're finally coming along, slowly.

But once again—from masks to vaccines, from variants to natural immunity—they have the scientific method upside down. Scientists aren't supposed to ban or demand behavior based on a lack of knowledge. An objective scientist would defer from making pronouncements one way or the other until there is ample evidence.

To dictate that a person recovered from COVID-19 with natural immunity also submit to a vaccine—without scientific evidence—is nothing more than hubris. If you have no proof that people who acquired natural immunity are getting or transmitting the disease in real numbers, then perhaps you should just be quiet.

People are not getting re-infected in large numbers. And that's not me saying so, that's the Centers for Disease Control and Prevention, quietly admitting that on its website.

One thing they also admitted, while at first trying to hide it, was that there are no studies showing that getting the vaccine if you already have natural immunity is of *any* benefit at all. They can't show that, because it has not yet been studied. It took my friend Congressman Thomas Massie to make them admit this, by the way. They originally denied their own studies on this.

So, when I go out to the media and say that I, as a recovered COVID patient, will not get a vaccine that is not proven to help me nor proven that I even need—the science deniers, bureaucrats and media typically go nuts.

But facts are facts. I'm no more likely to get or transmit COVID than someone who is vaccinated.

We *know* this. Doctors know this. Scientists who design vaccines know this. Vaccines are created to attempt to replicate the immunity we get from having been infected with a disease.

I want all the science deniers to read that again. Vaccines are a *replacement* for natural immunity. They aren't necessarily better. In fact, natural immunity from measles confers lifelong immunity and the vaccine immunity wanes over a few decades.

I choose to follow the science with COVID, rather than submit to fear-mongering.

We are simply not seeing any numbers that tell me otherwise.

In a recent British study, David Wyllie and others found no symptomatic re-infections from COVID-19 after following 2800 patients for several months. In fact, there have been no reports of significant numbers of re-infections after acquiring COVID-19 naturally.

Shane Crotty, a virologist at the La Jolla Institute for Immunology, concludes from his experiments that, "The amount of (immune) memory (gained from natural infection) would likely prevent the vast majority of people from getting hospitalized disease, severe disease, for many years."

In this study which was published in *Science*, Crotty showed that antibody levels stayed relatively constant with only "modest declines . . . at 6 to 8 months."

Crotty reports that, "Notably, memory B cells specific for the Spike protein or RBD were detected in almost all COVID-19 cases, with no apparent half-life at 5 to 8 months after infection." In other words, Crotty found significant evidence of long-term immunity after COVID infection.

Furthermore, Crotty notes, "B cell memory to some other infections has been observed to be long-lived, including 60+ years after smallpox vaccination, or 90+ years after infection with influenza."[97]

We have begun to study this, though we already know the answer—natural immunity against COVID-19 appears to be at least as good as vaccine immunity.

In one extensive recent study in *The Lancet*, Dr. Florian Kramer of the Icahn School of Medicine notes, "The findings of the authors suggest that infection and the development of antibody response provides protection similar to or even better than current used SARS COV-2 vaccines."[98]

Rather than doubting that people gain immunity after they've had COVID, studies argue for significant optimism. Because what we *do* know is that there have been no scientific studies arguing or proving that infection with COVID does *not* create immunity.

Before the emergence of the Omicron variant, virtually no studies showed significant numbers of reinfection. Of the thirty million Americans who have had COVID, only a handful of reinfections have been discovered.

Additionally, a recent study published in the *Journal of the American Medical Association* shows that vaccines and naturally acquired immunity do effectively neutralize COVID variants. Participants who had previously been either vaccinated or infected were exposed to four variants of the coronavirus, and researchers found "neutralizing activity of infection- and vaccine-elicited antibodies against 4 SARS-CoV-2 variants, including B.1, B.1.1.7, and N501Y. Because neutralization studies measure the ability of antibodies to block infection, these results suggest that infection and vaccine-induced immunity may be retained against the B.1.1.7 variant."[99]

Before Omicron came to prominence, CDC Director Rochelle Walensky publicly stated that "our data from the CDC today suggests that vaccinated people do not carry the virus, don't get sick, and that it's not just in the clinical trials, but it's also in real-world data."[100]

The CDC website quietly offered similar information for those who have natural immunity, but it was never promoted in any meaningful way by the public health experts.

The bureaucrats wanted to "simplify the message" in order to achieve maximum compliance. I believe their persistent use of the "noble lie" not only undermines faith in public health, but informed consent itself.

The American public should have been better informed on these real scientific studies on natural immunity, the uselessness of masks, and lockdowns, as well. It's almost as if some in power saw the benefit of not doing so. As Marty Makary tweeted,

> Rochelle Walensky has been known for her kindness & collegiality in academia. When she started as @CDCDirector she spoke freely—saying schools can be open[ed] safely. The next day, the White House (Jen Psaki) condemned her comments saying, "she was speaking as a private citizen." Since then, Dr. Walensky has obediently supported all Biden Covid policies, often with flawed research and non-disclosure of critical data on things like the breakdown of child deaths for healthy kids vs. those with special medical conditions, deaths from Covid vs. deaths with an incidental Covid+ test, & hospitalization rates among boosted people <50 vs. those with the primary vaccine series alone.
>
> Her agency also worked to censor others as the CDC put out misinformation on myocarditis, long-Covid, masking toddlers (except when they nap for up to 2hrs, or eat food), boosters in young people, and school closures.
>
> I wish her well in her next endeavor and pray that future CDC directors will speak their minds and stand up for science rather than use it as political propaganda.[101]

This was in response to Jay Bhattacharya's pointed comment that "Rochelle Walensky's legacy will be the shattered dreams of a generation of American kids, especially poor and minority kids, whose futures she marred by working to keep schools closed in 2021."[102]

Revealing the COVID cover-up misinformation and challenging the bureaucrats' spin was not without danger. The same day my *Courier-Journal* op-ed ran, white powder was delivered to our house.

The Threats Get More Personal, Menacing—and Threaten My Family

On a beautiful spring day, Kelley walked out to retrieve the mail, not realizing what awaited her in the mailbox. As she retraced her steps to the house, she remembers the exact moment: "I was walking up to my front steps and I started shuffling through the mail. I looked down and saw an envelope with a horrible doctored image of a wounded Rand with a broken neck and a gun against his head."

"It had writing that said, 'I'm going to finish what the other guy started, you MF-er.' I just was terrified and froze."

The letter was referring to the 2017 felony assault and threatened to finish the attack that left me with six broken ribs and a permanently damaged lung.

Kelley remembers, "I went to sort of throw the letter down—I didn't open it—but as I did, I could feel something that sounded like sand, like a weighty substance. I could feel it moving in the letter."

"I dropped it and ran inside. I washed my hands. Of course, I was terrified. You know, you think of anthrax, you think of the poisonings that happened years ago when people sent poisons in the mail, ricin or anthrax. I immediately called Rand, the FBI, the sheriffs."

"Everyone told me, 'take off all your clothes,' because I had been holding the mail up against my chest and to 'get in the shower.' I spent several anxious hours before I found out that it was non-toxic, convinced that I might have been poisoned. It was a very thin paper envelope so I kept thinking, 'Have I absorbed something through my hands?'"

"I was frightened and shaken up. It's pure terrorism. People are trying to terrorize us into silence for being a public servant."[103]

The FBI ultimately determined several hours later that the powder was not anthrax.

Stephen Colbert apparently thought the whole episode was good fun.[104]

Maria Bartiromo interviewed me and asked about Colbert's taste-less sense of humor: "We have people on the Left who think it's just hilarious. Comedian Stephen Colbert thinks it's great to make fun of the injuries I had. I had six broken ribs, a damaged lung, part of my lung removed."[105]

When Colbert, Bette Midler, Cher, and countless other leftists with "empathy" and "love all" in their bios ridiculed my assault and injuries, they truly embodied the hatred they claim to revile.[106] They loudly condemned Trump for incivility while engaging in something a thousand-fold worse: literal vicious delight in another person's human pain and suffering.

Even worse, these celebrities with huge platforms encourage their fans to become desensitized to violence. They and their fans feel justified with an almost religious zeal in fomenting and committing violence against people they disagree with because, of course, those people are "on the wrong side." This sentiment is the root of genocide throughout history.

Nancy Pelosi's daughter, Christine (who also conveniently works as her political strategist) literally tweeted that the man who assaulted me "was right."[107] There is no way to interpret Christine Pelosi's words other than an endorsement of my attack and ensuing injuries. Not a soul in the Democratic Party criticized her.

I once had respect for Stephen Colbert. I had appeared on his show a few times, and he treated me fairly. But like so many on the Left, he was so angry at Trump's election that he could no longer simply make jokes about my political views, but resorted to gleefully ridiculing my injuries. And he did so with absolutely zero criticism from the media.

And so when Colbert and all these other people who think they're so funny and enjoy getting everybody on the internet ginned up—guess what? They encourage crazy people across the country.

Of course, his lawyers made sure that Colbert make the generic disclaimer that there's "never any excuse for violence or threats of any kind at any time against anyone for any reason," meanwhile doubling over laughing that I had the temerity to call out left-wing internet trolls who were encouraging someone to finish the assault that almost killed me.[108]

Richard Marx is one of those trolls. He tweeted, "I'll say it again: If I ever meet Rand Paul's neighbor I'm going to hug him and buy him as many drinks as he can consume."[109]

To Colbert, support for my assailant was just hilarious.[110] I don't recall him laughing when Paul Pelosi was nearly killed by a crazy intruder with a hammer. He apparently feels zero compassion when conservatives are attacked and injured.

Twitter in the pre–Elon Musk era did nothing to stop Marx's or Pelosi's advocacy for violence against me. The service only removed the tweet later when we reported them, with no further action against their accounts.[111]

Speaking with Bartiromo, I didn't pull any punches: "We got the white powder the day after some has-been songwriter...encouraged people to come over and finish the job and says he's going to buy drinks for anybody that'll come and assault me again."[112]

Amidst this craziness and anthrax scare, I tried to continue a rational debate about naturally acquired immunity. Fauci and his merry band continued to argue that they didn't have to prove that the vaccine prevented infection. All they had to do was prove that the COVID vaccine stimulated patients to make antibodies.

That a vaccine causes a patient to consistently make antibodies indicates an immune response, but it does not necessarily indicate that the vaccine is necessary. To prove efficacy, a vaccine or a booster must show real-world results such as a reduction in either infections, hospitalizations, or death. That a vaccine causes a patient to create antibodies is a supportive finding but final proof of nothing.

For example, this lame argument was used to approve booster COVID vaccines for kids. Inject them with a booster and voilà! The kids make antibodies. While true, this fact ignores whether the booster lessens infections, hospitalizations, or death. Likewise, the original studies showed reduced hospitalizations when comparing patients inoculated with the COVID vaccine versus no vaccine.[113] You can't claim efficacy by simply reporting that a booster vaccine causes antibodies to be generated. Researchers must prove that kids risk reinfection and hospitalization or death after two vaccines, and that a booster reduces that risk.

When the CDC began pushing boosters for children, they simply ignored any need to release efficacy data and argued that kids have been shown to make antibodies when boosted.[114] Without tangible evidence of efficacy, this means exactly nothing.

In the case of boosters for children, there is no scientific evidence of a reduction in infections, hospitalizations, or death. When Fauci was challenged on this question, he mumbled something like "There you go again."[115] This is an insult to millions of American parents who deserve real data before injecting their children with an experimental drug.

In fact, when the CDC promoted this false interpretation of the data, two long-time members of its vaccine committees resigned—Marion Gruber and Philip Krause.[116]

Paul Offit, a professor of pediatric medicine and a member of the FDA advisory committee on vaccines, joined Gruber and Krouse in a *Washington Post* editorial criticizing the lack of evidence for universal COVID boosters:

We don't think boosters for all are necessary, even with the emergence of the omicron variant. Two of us—Krause and Gruber—were co-authors of a recent article in the Lancet, a medical journal, that summarized all available studies and concluded that the data did not support widespread boosting; the other—Offit—is a member of the FDA vaccine advisory committee that did not support widespread boosting at either of its most recent meetings on this topic, in September and October. While boosting can further increase already very high levels of protection against even mild illness, the only people who really need an additional dose of vaccine are those who are at high risk of serious disease (including the elderly) or who might expose vulnerable household or workplace contacts if they got infected.[117]

Offit famously told the media he would not recommend the COVID booster to his twenty-year-old son. Another infectious disease expert, Dr. Monica Gandhi of the University of California, also advised her teenage son not to get the COVID booster, because "vaccinated teenage boys have a low risk of hospitalization, but the likelihood of myocarditis, an inflammation of the heart, is higher." Both scientists maintained that "the benefits of a booster for teen males are outweighed by the possible side effects."[118]

Despite these warnings from scientists, colleges and our military were forcing the vaccine and boosters on all our young people, placing them at real risk for life-threatening myocarditis.

On a Fox News appearance around this time, I decided to bring some good news to the seemingly endless trail of pessimism. I told the audience that people who've recovered from COVID can "celebrate" immunity.[119] And sure to irk the Left, I went on to say, "We should tell them to throw away their masks, go to restaurants, live again, because these people are now immune."[120] You could virtually hear their chins hitting the floor when the clip finally got replayed on a left-wing outlet.[121]

When the large Cleveland Clinic study came out, I couldn't resist throwing more chum into the Twitterverse. I tweeted, "Great news! Cleveland clinic study of 52,238 employees shows unvaccinated people who have had COVID 19 have no difference in re-infection rate than people who had COVID 19 and who took the vaccine."[122]

In a normal world, that news should have been greeted with cheers. It assured that the millions of people around the world who had survived COVID either before the vaccine was available or by choice could now rest easy.

Also, knowing that prior COVID infection was protective would free up millions of doses of vaccine for those at risk in places with vaccine shortages like India.

I followed up by again tweeting a quote from the study: "The immune response to natural infection is highly likely to provide protective immunity even against the SARS-CoV-2 variant.... Thus, recovered COVID-19 patients are likely to better defend against the variants than persons who have not been infected but have been immunized with spike-containing vaccines only."[123]

The Cleveland Clinic study found no reinfections among patients who were unvaccinated but had previously been infected with COVID. Likewise, infections were similarly low among those who were vaccinated. In the unvaccinated patients with no previous COVID infection, the study found significant evidence of new COVID infections.[124]

PolitiFact requested a comment from the study's lead researcher, Dr. Nabin Shrestha, a Cleveland Clinic infectious diseases physician, as to whether he believed my tweet had interpreted his study results factually.

Shrestha responded that "it was an accurate interpretation of the study's findings."[125]

But fact-checkers are virtually never content to judge a Republican tweet as truthful.

The fact-checker moved to the next study that I quote-tweeted. Hard to fathom how a tweet that *quotes directly from a source* can be rated false—but this was the Twitterverse before Elon Musk.

The fact-checker acknowledged that "Paul quotes directly from the study's 'discussion' section: 'The immune response to natural infection is highly likely to provide protective immunity even against the SARS-CoV-2 variants.... Thus, recovered COVID-19 patients are likely to better defend against the variants than persons who have not been infected but have been immunized with spike-containing vaccines only.'"[126]

It requires a certain chutzpah to take a quote-tweet back to a study's author in order to elicit a rebuttal of her own quote.

According to the fact-checker, "Kristen Cohen, a senior staff scientist in the Vaccine and Infectious Disease Division at the Fred Hutchinson Cancer Research Center in Seattle, acknowledged that Paul's tweet was a direct quote from the study. Still, she said, in her view the quote was taken out of context and presented to suit Paul's objective—but does not accurately reflect the overall take-home message from the study's findings."

Cohen went on: "We wrote that recovering COVID patients are 'likely' to better defend against variants than those who have just been immunized, but it's not saying they do.... It's not saying they have been known to. It's making a hypothesis or basically saying this could be the case."[127]

Exactly.

I had quoted her verbatim.

I used her word "likely," but her reaction revealed an animus deep enough for her to attempt to retract her own words.

Cohen goes on to complain, "We did not intend to argue that infected people do not need to get vaccinated or that their immune responses are superior." Well, I didn't make that point either. I simply quote-tweeted from her study.

Cohen was so shaken by being quote-tweeted by a Republican that she pledged to the fact-checker that since "the sentence was confusing when taken out of context [that] she will eliminate it from the paper when it gets submitted for publication."[128]

Gotta love it. I had posted a quote-tweet, not *my* words, but *the author of the study's* words. And yet the disease of wokeness is so strong that the author ended up disputing and editing her *own* quoted conclusions.

Cohen, like others, argued that the vaccine elicits antibody production even in patients who have already been infected. Which, of course, is true, but not necessarily meaningful. Several studies show that people who have been previously infected will make still more antibodies if they are vaccinated. This may well mean nothing. Making antibodies isn't, in and of itself, evidence of a benefit. Evidence of a benefit would be that a vaccination, after previous infection, leads to less infection, hospitalization, and death in patients who are previously infected but not vaccinated.

Cohen's lack of insight is astounding but not unique. To state the truth once again, when Fauci and others began to push booster vaccines for kids, the government based the advice on the fact that kids given booster vaccines make antibodies. The scientific response to this should have been "So what!" Evidence that a booster vaccine is needed can only be proven with clinical data in a controlled study.

Yet, Fauci and the CDC knew that the booster vaccines could not be proven to lessen infection or the severity of the illness, so they relied on actual, scientifically acceptable data—that is, evidence of efficacy. Showing that boosted kids make more antibodies is a red herring at best.

CHAPTER 9

Congress Embraces Lockdowns and Borrows Trillions

On April 21, 2020, when I returned to Washington, I was the only passenger on the plane: just me, the flight attendants, and the pilots. The airport was an eerie ghost town. All of the airport restaurants were shuttered. A dystopian sense of doom pervaded the lonely, long walk down empty airport corridors.

Late in the afternoon of April 21, 2020, Congress convened to heap even more money on the lockdown economy. Almost no senators were in the Capitol that day. On the House side, Representative Thomas Massie bravely requested a roll call vote that forced representatives to actually do their jobs and show up to vote. His colleagues responded with outrage.

The Surreal April 21 Senate Floor Debate
That Spent Billions

I went to the Senate floor to speak against the Paycheck Protection Act. Only three members were present on the floor: Myself, Senator Lee, and Senator McConnell. Mike Lee's desk is next to mine. Though he too warned of the consequences of the massive COVID spending, when it came time to vote, I was the lone voice in opposition. But it takes only one senator to object to a voice vote. A voice vote requires unanimous consent of all senators. As one of only three present, I could have objected, and on principle I normally would on a bill such as this one that entailed such tremendous expense to the people. But this time I didn't. I allowed them to vote by voice because I knew that in the current climate of COVID hysteria the media would blame me if any elderly senator returned to vote and contracted COVID. But I was present that afternoon, and just before 5:00 p.m. gave this speech:

No amount of money—not all the money in China—will save us from ourselves.

Our only hope of rescuing this great country is to reopen the economy. If you print up billions of dollars and give it to people, they're unlikely to spend it until you end the quarantine.

The good news though is that the scientific community has facts instead of conjecture. The models that used 3.4 percent mortality were fortunately very wrong. Random samples now show that thousands of people now have antibodies to COVID and therefore immunity to coronavirus.... The number of people who have already developed antibodies to the coronavirus is twenty-five to fifty times higher than the number that is being reported as infected.

This is great news. Since the death rate is deaths divided by the number of infected, this study shows that the number of people infected has been grossly underestimated such that the mortality rate may well be twenty-five to fifty times less deadly than previously thought.

The virus is still dangerous, and we shouldn't ignore the risks, but we should put those risks in perspective. These randomized tests indicate that instead of a 3.4 percent mortality, the rate could be as much as only a tenth of a percent or two-tenths of 1 percent. [As of the fall of 2022, the death rate turned out to be about 0.3 percent.[1]]

We now have scientific evidence from randomized studies that we can treat this disease without a draconian lockdown of the country....

So today I rise in opposition to spending $500 billion more. The virus bailouts have already cost over $2 trillion. Our annual deficit this year will approach $4 trillion. We can't continue on this course. No amount of bailout dollars will stimulate an economy that is being strangled by quarantine.

It is not a lack of money that plagues us but a lack of commerce. This economic calamity only resolves when we begin to open the economy. Opening the economy will require Americans to rise above partisanship, to understand that deaths from infectious disease will continue but that we cannot indefinitely quarantine.

Make no mistake about it, this has been a difficult month for our country. For many of us, we have not seen a greater challenge. I'm encouraged to see how our communities have responded.

In Kentucky, we have seen tremendous collaboration. People from all walks of life have come together to help each other. We have worked to identify and supply additional protective gear, masks, and gloves to protect our doctors and nurses who risk their lives on a daily basis.

UPS has set up an airlift operation out of Louisville that includes a healthcare facility for FEMA. It allows FEMA to make deliveries from anywhere in the country. Over three million masks and other equipment have been shipped to the Louisville airport by UPS. We have worked with facilities to produce hand sanitizer....

When protective equipment was in short supply, we discovered a way to use industrial masks and supported legislation that allowed them to bring some thirty thousand masks into the community. When the FDA wouldn't approve COVID tests...we introduced legislation that circumvented the FDA and red tape to get testing done quicker.

Over the years, the U.S. has accumulated more than $23 trillion in debt, though, spending money that we do not have, borrowing from our kids and our grandkids' future. The gargantuan federal bailout that just passed, over $2 trillion, brings us closer and closer to a point of no return, a point at which the world loses confidence in the dollar, a point at which our debt becomes an existential threat to our security.

The United States was already having to borrow simply to pay our promises to senior citizens. The U.S. is borrowing about $1 trillion a year just to pay for everyday obligations. This was before the pandemic bailout. The U.S. was already borrowing nearly $2 million every minute. With the recent

$2 trillion bailout, we are borrowing faster than we have ever borrowed before.

Had we practiced sound budgeting in the past, we would have been significantly better positioned to weather this storm. Congress's failures of the past coupled with the pandemic crisis of the present could seriously jeopardize our economic future.

In this moment we need to think carefully about what we do next. To stop the threat of the virus, commerce has been disrupted, businesses have closed, and millions have lost their jobs. Right now that number is over twenty million unemployed. The job losses will continue no matter how much money you throw at it until you reopen the economy. Our government has intervened with unprecedented scale to prop up our economy. We've injected $2 trillion.

I don't believe it makes sense for the government to provide support to all businesses and families. I do believe it makes sense for the government to provide support to businesses and families that can't make it through this.

I've supported expanding unemployment benefits to workers displaced by government quarantine, including self-employed individuals that have lost their businesses.

But make no mistake, the massive economic calamity we're experiencing right now is caused by government.

Passing out $1200 checks indiscriminately to people who haven't lost their jobs will do nothing to rescue the country. If we were going to make discreet payments, direct payments, the criteria should have been sending checks to people who needed it, people who lost their jobs, people furloughed, people who had wage cuts. Instead of directing help to the unemployed, though, some of these bailout checks will go to couples who earn nearly $200,000 a year.

You could give everybody in the country $12,000 and it wouldn't end this recession. A recovery only comes when the quarantine has ended. Experts will disagree on the exact date that we should reopen the economy, but sane, rational counsel should continue to push for the quickest end possible.

Opining about never shaking hands again is a recipe for keeping the economy closed until no one dies from infectious disease. The infectious disease experts should be queried and so too should economists. We should seek counsel about balancing the harm-to-health caused by disease with the harm-to-health caused by imposing dysfunction on the economy. Not easy decisions.

Most importantly, leaders in each state should weigh in on the problem.... We need to get past a one-size-fits-all approach to infectious disease.

Realize that most of this money that's being loaned to small business is not really a loan. Most of this money will not be repaid. It will ultimately be considered grants that will be added to our national debt. Let's be honest about this. Applications for the program opened to overwhelming initial demand. The current data indicates that the money is gone.

So now here we are again with leadership from both parties saying let's do another $300 billion. What's another couple hundred billion?

But realize the money desired is not money that we have saved for a rainy day. This money doesn't exist anywhere. It will be created or borrowed.

Even more alarming than the money is the idea that one senator can stand on the floor and pass legislation spending a half a trillion dollars and have no recorded vote and no debate.

I understand the hardships of senators returning from around the country, so I have not invoked the Senate rules to demand a recorded vote.

I did return today, though, so that history will record that not everyone gave in to the massive debt Congress is creating.

My hope is that across the country there will remain a vibrant voice for limited government for our constitutional Republic. I don't want to see this massive accumulation of debt destroy this great country.

So my advice to the Senate and to the American people is let's be aware of what we're doing by creating all this new debt, and let's think before we jump to a terrible, terrible conclusion.[2]

Senate Majority Leader Mitch McConnell took to the floor to gloat: "This is even more money than we had first requested a while back." Nowhere in his remarks was there any alarm at the unintended consequences of borrowing so much money in such a short period of time.[3]

Senator Mike Lee was the only other senator on the Senate floor that day. Mike began his speech by expressing concern that these enormous sums of money were being spent while Congress was technically in recess and few if any senators were present in Washington.

"…And yet, Congress is in recess. This, Mr. President, is simply unacceptable. If COVID-19 requires Congress to act, then it requires Congress to convene…."

But in this crisis, we doubled down on that decades-long bad habit.

In many cases...we've empowered party leaders to nego-
tiate in secret, asking us to rubber-stamp...these take-it-
or-leave-it proposals without individual members being
able to read them, let alone have meaningful input in their
negotiation, and reducing the role of each individual elected
lawmaker in the law-making process to a series of tweets
and press conferences. This isn't legislating....

Well, most of us were not part of that process. Most of us
saw this legislative package, this bill, only within the last few
hours. That, Mr. President, isn't a true negotiation. It's not
a true legislative process. I understand that we're in unusual
circumstances, but we can't let it happen this way again. This
is not acceptable. We should not be passing major legislation,
especially legislation providing nearly a half trillion dollars
in new spending, without Congress actually being in session,
without members actually being here to debate, discuss,
amend, and consider legislation and vote on it individually
rather than on an absentee basis, rather than by delegating
that power to someone else.

This crisis is too big to leave up to a small handful of
people. Different parts of the country will face different
kinds of threats and therefore have different kinds of needs.
Different industries will need different kinds of help in order
to recover the health of the economy.

And as long as Congress remains in recess, Democrats
are free to politicize and stifle legislation with impunity, as
they did just a couple of weeks ago. Only returning to work,
and, indeed, actually working, will give the American people
the government they deserve.

The American people need to know who is helping them
and who is simply playing politics. We can't allow them to

know that if we're not in session. We can't just spend another half trillion dollars every week or two or three and hope and pretend that it's going to turn out okay.[4]

I returned to the floor at 5:06 p.m. to respond to Mike Lee's point that Congress should not pass such enormous spending bills without debate and without senators actually being present:

No virus, not even a plague, should cause us to forget that our freedom is a result of resisting the concentration of power in the hands of the few.

Recently, there has been dangerous talk of the president adjourning Congress. I'm reminded of the long English battle to forbid the king from dissolving Parliament. In fact, Charles I lost his head partly because he insisted on dissolving Parliament.

In those days, Parliament did not take Charles's royal power grab lying down. When Charles I dissolved parliament in 1629, members took matters into their own hands. They descended on the speaker John Finch and *sat on him.* Since he could not rise, the Parliament could not close. While he squirmed and was held down, Parliament passed several motions condemning the king's power grab. Ultimately, the English Parliament would change their charter to forbid the king from dissolving Parliament.

Now, I'm not suggesting we hold the president of the Senate down and commandeer the Senate...But the idea has crossed my mind....

Whatever path of resistance we take, talk of the administration adjourning or temporarily dissolving Congress should loudly be resisted as if the Republic depended on it.

Perhaps more alarming than allowing a president threatening to dissolve Congress is that Congress currently has allowed itself to become more of an oligarchy than an assembly. A few members of the leadership are set to pass legislation, spending nearly a half a trillion dollars without any recorded vote or debate.

Shouldn't someone shout "Stop!"? Shouldn't someone point out the terrible precedent of having a few members speak for all the members?

I for one believe that there exists too much danger *not* to have Congress in session. And if there exists too much danger to have Congress meet in person, we should allow emergency voting remotely.

In that vein, I offer the following resolution. I ask unanimous consent that the Senate proceed to consideration of my resolution at the desk—to allow senators to vote from their home states.[5]

McConnell stood up and objected to my resolution to allow remote voting until senators could safely return to Washington.

Seconds later, McConnell rammed through the half-a-billion-dollar bill with only a handful of senators even present in Washington. Rule by the elite few had become a reality.

"The Senate vote was by voice vote, a procedure typically used for relatively noncontroversial legislation, in which no record of individual senators' votes is recorded."[6] But I returned to make sure there was a record of at least one senator's opposition to the bankrupting of America. I stood on the floor of the Senate and loudly proclaimed my solitary opposition to the largest government program ever created.

Meanwhile, the COVID Cover-Up Continued

Just days before this debate on the Senate floor, Peter Daszak sent Anthony Fauci this email: "I just wanted to say a personal thank you on behalf of our staff and collaborators, for publicly standing up and stating that the scientific evidence supports a natural origin for COVID-19 from a bat-to-human spillover, not a lab release from the Wuhan Institute of Virology."[7]

What was unspoken in the email was "Thanks for saving the business of science!" Ensuring that the world did not realize that COVID might have come from a lab funded by Fauci and the NIH would preserve the millions of dollars that the organization continues to funnel to EcoHealth Alliance.

CHAPTER 10

Fauci Balks at Sending Kids Back to School

On May 12, 2020, I had my second encounter with Anthony Fauci. The hearing was entitled "COVID-19: Safely Getting Back to Work and Back to School."

I began by reminding Dr. Fauci that evidence was already accumulating that COVID infections would provide immunity:

> Scientists have shown that rhesus monkeys that are infected with COVID-19 cannot be re-infected.
>
> Several studies have also shown that plasma from recently infected coronavirus patients neutralizes the virus in lab experiments. In addition, infusion of convalescent plasma is based on the idea that recovering coronavirus patients are developing immunity and that it can be beneficial as donated.

Studies show that the recovering COVID-19 patients from the asymptomatic to the very sick are showing significant antibody response.

Studies show that SARS and MERS, also coronaviruses, induce immunity for at least two to three years, and yet the media continues to report that we have no evidence that patients who survive coronavirus have immunity. I think actually the truth is the opposite. We have no evidence that survivors of coronavirus don't have immunity, and a great deal of evidence to suggest that they do.

The question of immunity is linked to health and economic policy. Workers who have gained immunity can be a strong part of our economic recovery. The silver lining to so many infections in the meat processing industry is that a large portion of these workers now have immunity. Those workers should be reassured that they likely won't get it again instead of being alarmed by media reports that there is no evidence of immunity.[1]

There was a reason I confronted Fauci with the statistics on meat processing workers and COVID. He could have chosen to calm fears with a rational assessment of the risks to in-person essential workers who had recovered from COVID. Instead, Fauci fanned the flames and encouraged the emotionalism across the networks.

It was certainly a tragedy that many meat-processing workers died from COVID. But the social panic brought on by faulty information regarding immunity played a role in endangering our nation's food supply.

In July 2020, CDC reported that data from twenty-three states showed 16,233 cases of COVID-19 outbreaks in "meat and poultry processing facilities" and 86 COVID-19–related deaths, resulting in a death rate of about 0.5 percent.[2] All of these early studies underestimated the denominator of number of cases by failing to record legions of asymptomatic cases.

Likely, the final death rate would be less than the population rate of 0.3 percent, because their ages skewed younger and their comorbidities less than average. But the deaths of these workers was well known because they continued to work throughout the pandemic. They had to, or the food supply would have been in peril.

By the fall of 2021, the House Select Subcommittee on the Coronavirus Crisis estimated that over fifty-nine thousand meat processing workers had contracted COVID-19 with 269 deaths, or a 0.46 percent fatality rate. However, seroprevalence studies—that is, studies of bodily serum tests—to detect antibodies to COVID from patients who never tested positive or never became ill indicate that the fifty-nine thousand number of the reported infected workers could easily have been seven times that in actual cases, thus making the mortality number seven times less than 0.46 percent, or about 0.06 percent fatality.[3]

Knowing they have acquired natural immunity also has a profound and positive psychological effect on people. This was denied them.

Without doubt, meat-processing workers deserve our respect and did risk their lives to put food on the table for America, but by discounting their naturally acquired immunity, Fauci and his friends robbed the over 99 percent who survived of the great comfort of knowing that they were now protected.

The great disservice to these workers was not that they continued working but that Fauci and his yes-men did not have the decency to assure these workers that once they had recovered—as 99.5 percent or more would—they were now safe from the danger of COVID. Instead, the talking public health heads on CNN continued to feed the hysteria and say, *We just don't know about naturally acquired immunity.* They did, but it conflicted with the desire to enforce public health mandates of lockdowns and total vaccine enforcement. And, of course, there was the ever-hoped-for ratings boost. The truth didn't fit their narrative.

The data accumulated quickly. Reinfection was rare and rarely led to serious illness when it did occur.

As Jeffrey Klausner, M.D., of the University of Southern California Keck School of Medicine, noted, a study in Austria showed "that the frequency of re-infection from COVID-19 caused hospitalization in only five out of 14,840 (0.03%) people and death in one out of 14,840 (0.01%)."[4]

Wouldn't it have been great if these brave workers on the front lines of healthcare and food processing had been told this?

Instead, Americans were being treated to a daily dish of hysteria by CNN and MSNBC. Our citizens and workers deserved better. There was no context, only a daily death-toll meter to frighten people into compliance. The effect was to politicize COVID to the point that mere factual discussion of its high survival rate and low risk to children angered the Left.

Fauci Hems, Haws, and Hedges

I tried to get Dr. Fauci to give Americans hope. I continued my questioning: "You have stated publicly that you would bet it all that survivors of coronavirus have some form of immunity. Can you help set the record straight that the scientific record as it is being accumulated is supportive that infection with coronavirus likely leads to some form of immunity? Dr. Fauci?"

> **Dr. Fauci:** Yep. Thank you for the question, Senator Paul. Yes, you are correct that I have said that, given what we know about the recovery from viruses, such as coronaviruses in general, or even any infectious disease with very

few exceptions, that when you have antibody present, it very likely indicates a degree of protection.

I think it is in the semantics of how this is expressed. When you say, "Has it been formally proven by long-term, natural history studies?" which is the only way that you can prove, one, is it protective—which I said and would repeat is likely that it is—but also, what is the degree or titer of antibody that gives you that critical level of protection, and what is the durability?

As I have often said, and I again repeat, you can make a reasonable assumption that it would be protective, but natural history studies over a period of months to years would then tell you definitively if that is the case.

Senator Paul: A better way of describing the immune response to COVID would be that the vast majority of these people will *have* immunity, instead of saying there is no evidence. The WHO fed into this misinformation by saying "no evidence of immunity" after COVID infection—and the media ran with it as fact. In reality, there is ample evidence of immunity accumulating. In fact, a lot of the different studies have shown that re-infection is very unlikely in the short term.[5]

One thing that was left out of that discussion is mortality [especially in regard to going back to school]. Shouldn't we at least be discussing what the mortality of children is? This [question] is for Dr. Fauci, as well.

The mortality between ages zero and eighteen in the New York data approaches zero. It is not going to be absolutely zero, but it does approach zero.

Between eighteen and forty-five, the mortality in New York was ten [deaths] out of a hundred thousand....

We need to observe with an open mind what went on in Sweden where the kids kept going to school. The mortality per capita in Sweden is actually less than France, less than Italy, less than Spain, less than Belgium, less than the Netherlands, about the same as Switzerland.

I don't think there is anybody arguing that what happened in Sweden is an unacceptable result. I think people are intrigued by it, and we should be. I don't think any of us are certain when we [project outcomes by modeling.] There have been more people wrong [using] modeling than right. As we begin to open the U.S. economy, I hope that people who are predicting doom and gloom and saying, oh, we can't do this, there is going to be a surge, will admit that they were wrong if there is not a surge. Because I think that is what is going to happen....[6]

I went on to make the argument that the one-size-fits-all lockdown strategy that keeps the schools closed is ridiculous, that we really should be individualizing our approach, examining each school district one by one to allow the schools to re-open. The power over the decisions to open schools needs to be decentralized, the power needs to be dispersed amongst many people. Because of human fallibility, because experts often make wrong predictions, we should not centralize all the decision-making. One needn't look very far afield to see the profound errors of prediction during this pandemic. A prime example, I noted, is the statistician Neil Ferguson from England.[7]

Before locking down the economy, someone might have reviewed his previous predictions.

Likely no mathematician is treated more deferentially than Britain's Neil Ferguson, despite his having a prediction record worse than throwing random darts at numbers. His horrendous record would simply be laughable if government nannies in the United Kingdom and the United States hadn't given them credence and concluded that lockdowns were the only answer.[8]

Preposterous Predictions

I didn't have time to recount Ferguson's record during the questioning, but it is abysmal. Here is a small sampling: In 2002, Ferguson said that there could be up to 50,000 deaths from mad cow disease. The actual deaths were 177. In 2005, Ferguson predicted that up to 200 million people might die from the bird flu. Yet the actual number of people who died from the bird flu across the globe over a six-year period was 282. In 2009, Ferguson forecast that the "worst-case scenario" for swine flu deaths would be 65,000 deaths. The actual number of deaths in the United Kingdom turned out to be 457.[9]

Renowned Stanford epidemiologist John Ioannidis described Ferguson's Imperial College as "a highly competent team of modellers. However, some of the major assumptions and estimates that are built in the calculations seem to be substantially inflated."[10]

Inflated? These overestimates are absolutely ridiculous. They should be disqualifying.

Like many other lockdowners, Ferguson would ultimately get his comeuppance. After being the biggest cheerleader for lockdowns, he was caught visiting his mistress, breaking the very isolation rules he was championing.[11] Hypocrisy is the one sin the public doesn't soon forget. Just ask Gavin Newsom about his extravagant dinner at the French Laundry, an excursion he took while forcing us commoners to "shelter in place."[12] Or who will soon forget the ultimate "Karen"—Governor Gretchen Whitmer—ordering Michiganders to stay at home and banning citizens from buying fertilizer and garden tools? Meanwhile her husband took a trip to their vacation home to do a little boating.[13]

Ferguson's hypocrisy ultimately brought down his reputation,[14] but it should have been his terrible track record of predictions and his current COVID prediction mistakes instead of personal hypocrisy that did it.

Alistair Haimes of *The Spectator* explains that Ferguson's boast that lockdowns dramatically reduced the infection rate for COVID is utterly false. Haimes shows very clearly that the rate of infection had peaked before the lockdowns and that the rate of infection fell in countries such as Sweden that did not follow the lockdowns of the United Kingdom or the United States.

According to Haimes, "All three countries [United Kingdom, Germany, and Sweden] were at R of 2.5–3.0 early on in the epidemic, peaked before lockdown, declined fast, dropped below 1.0 (signifying the peak of the epidemic) around the third week of March and are currently around 0.8 to 0.9 and have bumbled around just under 1.0 for the past couple of months."[15]

In May of 2020, John Fund noted in *National Review* that "Ferguson's Imperial College model has been proven wildly inaccurate. To cite just one example, it saw Sweden paying a huge price for no lockdown, with 40,000 COVID deaths by May 1, and 100,000 by June. Sweden now has 2,854 deaths and peaked two weeks ago. As Fraser Nelson, editor of Britain's *The Spectator*, notes: 'Imperial College's model is wrong by an order of magnitude.'"[16] Even after a year and a half of COVID, Sweden's deaths were only 15,000, about one-fifth of what Ferguson had predicted.[17]

Ferguson predicted that by the fall of 2020, "more than 500,000 people in Great Britain and two million people in the U.S. would die as a result of COVID-19" without any action by government.[18]

Government decisions to impose lockdowns in both the United Kingdom and the United States were based in large part on Ferguson's predictions.

Ferguson's model estimated about a million deaths if the United States used strategies such as "enhanced social distancing" and "shielding the elderly."[19] In the end, the United States did have about a million deaths, so Ferguson can claim at least one successful prognostication. However, proving that mitigation strategies actually cut the deaths from two million to one million doesn't follow.

In fact, the original argument by lockdowners was that they would "flatten the curve"—but the area under the curve would be the same. That area represented the number of deaths. The evidence that mitigation, masks, social distancing, and so forth flattened the curve is weak. Inevitably, though, most people did get infected despite masking up and standing on socially distanced stickers in public.

While some will argue that masks and social distancing slowed the spread and allowed the virus to mutate to a form of lesser virulence, allowing time for the vaccine to be introduced, no one can or will ever know if mitigation markedly changed the ultimate death count.[20]

Getting caught breaking his own lockdowns didn't stop Ferguson. In the summer of 2021, he was admonishing English government officials not to lessen the lockdown. He predicted that the daily cases would skyrocket.[21] The reality was much different, leading the British radio host Julia Hartley-Brewer to remark, ". . . the Government should stop listening to advisors like Neil Ferguson on SAGE who predicted that it was almost inevitable we'd have up to 100,000 cases a day and possibly even 200,000—Yesterday, the case rate was 21,952...."[22]

Why spill so much ink over this one statistical modeler? Because many analysts say Neil Ferguson and his doomsday models were the primary factor in convincing President Donald Trump and British prime minister Boris Johnson to embrace the lockdowns.[23]

The Disastrous Effects of Lockdowns on Children

I didn't have enough time to get any response from Fauci on why he heeded Ferguson's folly of predictions. But I did have time to address his support for closing down our schools.

I continued my committee questioning of Fauci:

> So, I think we ought to have a little bit of humility in our belief that we know what is best for the economy. And, as much as I respect you, Dr. Fauci, I don't think you are the end-all. I don't think you are the one person that gets to make this decision. We can listen to your advice, but there are people on the other side saying there is not going to be a surge and that we can safely open the economy.
>
> And the facts will bear this out, that if we keep kids out of school for another year, what is going to happen is the poor and underprivileged kids who don't have a parent that is able to teach them at home are not going to learn for a full year.
>
> And I think we ought to look at the Swedish model, and we ought to look at letting our kids get back to school. I think it is a huge mistake if we don't open the schools in the fall....[24]
>
> **Dr. Fauci:** Well, first of all, Senator Paul, thank you for your comments. I have never made myself out to be the end-all and only voice in this. I am a scientist, a physician, and public health official. I give advice according to the best scientific evidence. There are a number of other people who come into

that and give advice that are more related to the things that you spoke about, about the need to get the country back open again and economically. I don't give advice about economic things. I don't give advice about anything other than public health. So, I wanted to respond to that.

The second thing is that you used the word "we should be humble" about what we don't know. I think that falls under the fact that we don't know everything about this virus and we really better be very careful, particularly when it comes to children. Because the more and more we learn, we are seeing things about what this virus can do that we didn't see from the studies in China or in Europe. For example, right now, children presenting with COVID-16—with COVID-19—who actually have a very strange inflammatory syndrome, very similar to Kawasaki Syndrome. I think we better be careful if we are not cavalier in thinking that children are completely immune of the deleterious effects.

So, again, you are right in the numbers that children, in general, do much, much better than adults and the elderly and particularly those with underlying conditions. But I am very careful, and hopefully humble, in knowing that I don't know everything about this disease, and that is why I am very reserved in making broad predictions.[25]

Fauci may have described himself as "reserved" in making broad predictions, but any routine viewer of the evening news would find that Fauci was never bashful about making pronouncements.[26]

When I asked him about trying to get kids back in school and showed him the data from several countries that had opened schools safely, he answered by tossing a grenade into the discussion. He brought up Kawasaki disease in an attempt to deflect my questions and instill fear in the public. He likely knew he was providing a juicy soundbite for the day.

Was the fear justified? Well, the media ran with it and breathless broadcasters wanted to know if, since I was obviously heartless enough to risk children dying from COVID (the evidence showed this risk was virtually non-existent), did I not care that Kawasaki disease might kill children? It sounded exotic. (It is. In twenty years of medical practice, I diagnosed exactly one case).

But was it a real concern—enough of a concern to keep the schools closed? If Fauci truly didn't consider himself to be the "end-all," he would have waited for the data before frightening people about a rare disease and falsely conflating it with COVID.

In June of 2022 the *JAMA Network Open: Pediatrics* reported that Kawasaki disease incidence "fell by 28 percent in 2020 and remained low during the peak pandemic period."[27]

In 2020, though, Fauci and the mainstream media were stoking the flames and scaring parents across the land based solely on one small, two-month French study. But many other studies did not show an increase in Kawasaki's disease. A 2021 study from Japan showed "Kawasaki disease remained stable during Japan's state of emergency from April to May 2020." "A 2021 study from the United States reported an overall decrease in instances of Kawasaki disease over the course of 2020, although cases peaked in May." Also in 2021, a study from Iran "found that hospitalizations for Kawasaki disease remained stable during the COVID-19 pandemic."[28]

Americans would have been better served if Fauci had actually shown some humility. The data on European schools showed that they could be opened safely. Instead, Anthony Fauci beat the drums for Kawasaki disease, a frightening scenario he falsely conflated with COVID. As a consequence, our kids lost up to two precious years of their education and life experiences such as sports, socialization, and normal life.

CHAPTER 11

Fauci, Hayek, and Fatal Conceit

B y June 2020, Anthony Fauci's true colors were apparent. He loved the limelight and had never met a mandate he wouldn't embrace or defend. The Senate HELP Committee requested his and others' comments on "Progress toward Safely Getting Back to Work and Back to School." When he appeared in committee, he came prepared to support maintaining the mandates and to resist opening the schools.

I came prepared to give him a piece of my mind.

Loaded for Bear with Hayek and Common Sense

I began by referring to Friedrich Hayek's discussion of "fatal conceit":

Fatal conceit is the concept that central planning with decision-making concentrated in a few hands can never fully take into account the millions of complex, individual interactions occurring simultaneously in the marketplace.

It is a fatal conceit to believe any one person or small group of people has the knowledge necessary to direct an economy or dictate public health behavior. I think government health experts during this pandemic need to show caution in their prognostications.

It is important to realize that if society meekly submits to an expert and that expert is wrong, a great deal of harm may occur when we allow one man's policy or that of one group of small men and women to be foisted on an entire nation. Take, for example, government experts who continue to call for schools and daycare to stay closed, or who recommend restrictions that make it impossible for a school to function. For a time, there may not have been enough information about coronavirus in children, but now there is. There are examples from across the United States and the world that show that young children rarely spread the virus.

Let's start in Europe. Twenty-two countries have reopened their schools and have seen no discernible increases in cases.

Behind me, my staff quickly arrayed a series of charts on easel boards showing schools across Europe opening up without any increase in COVID infections.

These graphs behind me show no surge when schools opened. The red line is where the schools opened. There is data from

Austria, Belgium, Denmark, France, Germany, Netherlands. No spike when schools are opened.

Contact-tracing studies in China, Iceland, Britain, and the Netherlands failed to find a single case of child-to-adult infection.[1]

In fact, data would ultimately show that no schoolchildren died in Sweden despite the schools being open nearly the whole time and without mask mandates. In addition, studies indicated that teachers did not become infected at a greater rate than any other occupation in Sweden.[2]

Here at home, childcare for essential workers continued to be available in some states throughout the pandemic. Brown University researchers collected data on daycares that remained open during the pandemic. Over twenty-five thousand kids in their study, [which] found that only 0.16 percent got COVID. And when you look at the confirmed cases for staff, there was about 1 percent of more than nine thousand staff.

The YMCA also has put forward statistics. Of forty thousand kids at eleven hundred sites, there were no reports of coronavirus outbreaks or clusters.

Dr. Joshua Sharfstein of Johns Hopkins writes, "There is converging evidence that the coronavirus doesn't transmit among children like the flu," that it is a lower risk.[3]

Just yesterday, the American Academy of Pediatrics says we have to get kids back in school. We want them physically present in school. They even cite mounting evidence that children are less likely to contract the virus.

Ultimately, this all comes down to the fatal conceit that central planners have enough knowledge somehow to tell a nation of 330 million people what they can and cannot do.

Perhaps our planners might think twice before they weigh in on every subject.

Perhaps our government experts might hold their tongue before expressing the opinion whether we can play NFL football or Major League Baseball [in the fall].

Perhaps our experts might think twice before telling the whole world that a COVID vaccine likely won't provide herd immunity.

We don't know. Why weigh in with these opinions that we have no knowledge of? These are forecasts that may well be wrong.

Perhaps our experts might consider the undue fear they are instilling in teachers who are now afraid to go back to work.

No one knows the answers to these questions. We should not presume that a group of experts somehow knows what is best for everyone.

Hayek had it right. Only decentralized power and decision-making based on millions of individualized situations can arrive at what risks and behaviors each individual should choose. That is what America was founded on, not a herd with a couple of people in Washington all telling us what to do and we, like sheep, blindly follow.[4]

President Eisenhower, in his farewell address, warned of the "danger that public policy could itself become captive of a scientific-technological elite."[5]

Asking the Questions No One Else Would

Lecturing Fauci on Hayek was likely a lost cause, but Americans deserved to hear a critique of a public health bureaucrat besotted by his own supposed expertise.

I turned my attention to questioning Fauci on opening the schools:

> When are we going to tell the people the truth, that it is okay to take their kids back to school? Dr. Fauci, every day, virtually every day, we seem to hear from you things we cannot do, but when you are asked, "Can we go back to school?" I don't hear much certitude at all. I hear, "Well, maybe, it depends."

I tried to show Fauci that the evidence from schools around the world demonstrated that there was no surge. Indeed, all of the evidence shows that it is rare for children to succumb to COVID-19. But COVID had become so politicized that it was politically incorrect to even question the dangers of continued school closures. I pointed out that there was a WHO scientist who had the temerity to admit that mortality is rare among children. What happened to this scientist who challenged the so-called "consensus"? She was blackballed and her report was memory-holed, disappeared. When you went to that scientist's speech and tried to click on the link, the WHO had screened it because it reported something that is not politically correct. Her heresy? Honestly reporting that it is rare for kids to transmit COVID-19. "But I hear none of that from you," I told Fauci.

> All I hear, Dr. Fauci, is we can't do this, we can't do that, we can't play baseball. Well, even that is not based on the science. I mean, flu season peaks in February. We don't know

that COVID is going to be like the flu season. It might be, but we don't know that. But we wouldn't ban school in October. You might close some schools when they get the flu. We need to not be so presumptuous that we know everything.

But my question to you is, can't you give us a little bit more on schools, that we can get back to school? That there is a great deal of evidence and that it is actually good—good evidence that kids are not transmitting this? It is rare, kids are staying healthy, and yes, we can open our schools?

Dr. Fauci: Mr. Chairman, do I have a little bit of time to—

The Chairman: I will give you a little. That was well over five minutes, but we will—

Dr. Fauci: Thank you, Senator Paul.

The Chairman: Go ahead and answer the—please answer the question.

Dr. Fauci: Yeah. So, very quickly, Senator Paul. I agree with a lot of what you say about, you know, this idea about people having to put their opinions out without data. And sometimes, you have to make extrapolations because you are in a position where you need to at least give some sort of recommendation.

But if you were listening, and I think you were, to my opening statement and my response to one of the questions, I feel very strongly we need to do whatever we can to get the children back to school. So, I think we are in lock agreement with that.[6]

Fauci, as usual, was agreeing with his own assumptions, not answering my question at all. In fact, he was dissembling. Journalist Jordan Schachtel reviewed Fauci's flip-flops on opening the schools.

According to Schachtel, in April 2020, Fauci criticized Florida governor Ron DeSantis, who was advocating to open schools. Fauci warned, "If you have a situation where you don't have a real good control over an outbreak and you allow children together, they will likely get infected."[7]

Which begs the question, yes, but will any of these children actually become sick? Are the students really a danger to teachers or parents at home? And, ultimately, the most important question, will these children all eventually get COVID-19 whether they are in school or not?

A month later, Fauci was still inflaming and exaggerating claims that COVID-19 is risky for children, and hyping media hysteria over "Kawasaki syndrome"[8]—which turned out to be quite rare.

And even though he now claimed to support my position that schools could open, he qualified his advocacy for reopening by saying that school's reopening depended on the "dynamics of the outbreak,"[9] which of course offered no quantitative criteria and meant whatever he took it to mean.

In July 2020, Fauci was still of two minds, communicating that he was in favor of "looking at schools on a case by case basis."

Schachtel reminds us that in July 2020, Fauci continued to "advance his vague ideas about school reopenings, but again makes clear that he opposes having schools open in areas where the coronavirus is spreading."[10]

Then in August 2020, Fauci went back to calling for the closure of schools "in areas with high transmission."[11]

According to Schachtel, Fauci was still playing both sides, showing concern that "schools could be vectors for transmission of COVID-19" and saying the United States may need "'many months' of virtual learning, in supporting keeping schools physically closed."[12]

In September 2020, Fauci returned to his line that schools could only open back up once the virus was "under control."[13]

But when November came, Fauci seemed to have recently discovered the data showing little transmission of COVID-19 in schools. This was the exact same data I had presented to him back in June. He told ABC, "But as I said in the past...the default position should be to try as best as possible within reason to keep the children in school or to get them back to school."[14]

No matter what tale he was spinning, Fauci defied the worldwide evidence that COVID-19 was very rarely deadly in children and instead fed the atmosphere of fear among parents and teachers in the United States.

As to Fauci's bizarre desire to opine not only on schools but professional sports, he responded in committee,

> The other thing that I would like to clarify very briefly is that I—when things get into press of what I supposedly said, I didn't say. I never said we can't play a certain sport. What happens is that people in the sport industry...ask me opinions regarding certain facts about the spread of the virus, what the dynamics are. I give it, and then it gets interpreted that I am saying you can't play this sport or you can't play that sport.
>
> I agree with you. I am completely unqualified to tell you whether you can play a sport or not.[15]

Yet if you look at *what he actually said* about Major League Baseball, you find Fauci rushing to provide his opinion despite absolutely no science to support it.

Fauci was quite specific: "...I would try to keep [baseball] in the core summer months and end it not with the way we play the World Series, until the end of October when it's cold."[16]

Not that anyone should arrogantly dictate the American baseball schedule, but if you were to estimate the worst season for COVID, you might look to the typical influenza seasonality which peaks in February, not October. But once the klieg lights click on, Fauci's concerns over nuance give way to his penchant for glorious edicts.

I concluded my questioning with one last appeal: "What we need, Dr. Fauci, is we just need more optimism. There is good news out there. We are not getting it from you."[17]

Indeed, Anthony Fauci was turning out to be more of a disaster for the country than COVID itself.

PART III

Confronting Deception

CHAPTER 12

Sweden, New York, and Lockdowns

On September 23, 2020, Anthony Fauci returned to the Senate for more drama, appearing before a committee upon which I serve, the Health, Education, Labor and Pensions (HELP) Committee, at a hearing entitled "COVID-19: An Update on the Federal Response."

I began my questioning by asking why the temporary lockdowns were still in effect:

> Initially, government officials were honest enough to admit that the goal of mitigation efforts, a.k.a. lockdown, was to flatten the curve. But the area under the curve, the total deaths from the virus, would likely be the same. In other words, the lockdown was to mitigate the spike in viral deaths so our hospitals would not be overwhelmed. But the same

amount of people would likely die with or without the lock-down. The media, and, frankly, government officials, seem to have forgotten this important caveat.

Flattening the curve morphed into a belief that we could change the course of the pandemic with an economic lock-down. This is unfortunate and has led to the protracted lock-down recession we are currently mired in. It is important that we examine the data, learn from the data, and try to avoid the man-made aspect of this calamity in the future. To those who argue that the lockdown flattened the curve in New York and New Jersey, the evidence argues otherwise. New York and New Jersey wound up with the sharpest spike or highest death rate in the world, at over seventeen hundred deaths per million [in population].[1]

In contrast, Sweden had a relatively softer touch, few mandates, and mostly voluntary guidelines. Sweden's death rate ended up about a third less than that of New York and New Jersey. Some might argue that Sweden and New York and New Jersey are different populations. Perhaps, but even the average death rate for the U.S. is now greater than Sweden. In fact, the U.S. death rate is quite comparable to less developed parts of the world where social distancing is virtually impossible, such as Brazil.... Which brings us to an important question: Is man really capable of altering the course of an infectious disease by crowd control?

The statistics argue a resounding no. The evidence [indicates] that mitigation efforts have failed to flatten the curve, that most countries, regardless of public health policy, suffered a significant spike in deaths and then a gradual decline. Now some will argue, what about Hong Kong, Taiwan, South Korea, Japan, each of which has had extraordinarily low death rates? Hong Kong, Taiwan, and South Korea certainly enforced strict quarantine and contact tracing rules . . . but Japan's rules were largely voluntary since their prime minister lacks the legal powers to enforce a lockdown.

One explanation for the low death rate in much of Asia is that the population may have a higher degree of exposure to coronavirus colds and therefore have more preexisting, cross-reactive immunity. If scientists were interested, there is a fascinating field of inquiry looking at susceptibility to COVID-19, an assessment of whether people may have preexisting immunity to similar coronaviruses. In fact, preexisting cross-reactive immunity to coronavirus may explain why we have so many people who have very [few or few severe] symptoms or are asymptomatic.

While there are still many things we need to learn about this pandemic, it is important that we the people not simply acquiesce to authoritarian mandates on our behavior without first making the nanny state prove its hypothesis. As for now, what we do know is that New York, New Jersey, Connecticut, and Rhode Island still experienced among the highest death rates in the world.[2] We also know that Sweden, which enforced few mandates, ended up with a death rate less than one-third of that of New York and New Jersey.[3]

We also know that the overall death rate for the U.S. now is essentially equivalent to that of South America, where social distancing and mitigation efforts are virtually impossible.

Dr. Fauci, today you said you are not for economic lockdowns, yet your mitigation recommendations—from dating to baseball to restaurants to movie theaters—have led to this economic lockdown.

Do you have any second thoughts about your mitigation recommendations considering the evidence that despite all the things we have done in the U.S., our death rate is worse than Sweden's, equivalent to death rates in the less developed world, an area unable to put in place any of the action that you have promoted? Do you have any second thoughts? Are you willing to look at the data that [show that] countries that did very little actually have a lower death rate than the United States?

Dr. Fauci: You know, Senator, I would be happy at a different time to sit down and go over detail. You have said a lot of different things. You have compared us to Sweden. And there are a lot of differences. And you said, well, you know, there are a lot of differences between Sweden, but compare Sweden's death rate to other comparable Scandinavian countries. It is worse. So I do not think it is appropriate to compare Sweden with us. Yes, we have—I think in the beginning, we have done things based on the knowledge we had at the time.

And hopefully, and I am, and my colleagues are, humble enough and modest enough to realize that as new data comes, you make different recommendations, but I do not regret saying that the only way we could have really stopped the explosion of infection was by essentially, I would not say shutting down—I mean essentially having the physical separation and the kinds of recommendations that we have made.

I interjected: You have been a big fan of Cuomo and the shutdown in New York. You have lauded New York for their policy. New York had the highest death rate in the world. How can we possibly be jumping up and down and saying, "Oh, Governor Cuomo did a great job"? He had the worst death rate in the world.

Dr. Fauci: No, you misconstrued that, Senator. And you have done that repetitively in the past. They got hit very badly. They have made some mistakes. Right now, if you look at what is going on right now, the things that are going on in New York to get their test positivity 1 percent or less is because they are looking at the guidelines that we have put together from the task force of the four or five things of masks, social distancing, outdoors more than indoors, avoiding crowds, and washing hands.

Senator Paul: Or they have developed enough community immunity that they are no longer having the pandemic because they have enough immunity in New York City to actually stop it. [Or because the vulnerable in New York City had already died and therefore, the rate of death will inevitably decline].

Dr. Fauci: I challenge that, Senator. Please, sir, I would like to be able to do this because this happens with Senator Rand all the time. You were not listening to what the director of the CDC said, that in New York it is about 22 percent. If you believe 22 percent is herd immunity, I believe you are alone in that.

Senator Paul: There is also the preexisting immunity of those who have cross-reactivity, which is about a third of the public in many estimates and studies—which would actually get you to about two-thirds.

Dr. Fauci: I would like to talk to you about that also because there was a study that recently came out that preexisting immunity to coronaviruses or that of a common cold do not cross-react with the COVID-19.[4]

Confronting Faulty Lockdown Logic

Contrary to Fauci's opinion, many studies do show evidence that a previous infection with a coronavirus cold may provide immunity that cross-reacts with COVID. Robert Sealy and Julia Hurwitz write in the journal *Microorganisms*, "One factor that may influence virus control is pre-existing immunity conferred by an individual's past exposures to common cold human coronaviruses (HCoVs)."[5]

Khalid Shrwani and his coauthors reported in the *Journal of Infectious Diseases* that a "significant proportion of children (up to 40%) had detectable cross-reactive antibodies" to COVID-19.[6]

Clearly other scientists were open to the idea that previous infections with coronavirus colds might explain why some people had little or no symptoms with COVID-19 infection. But as usual, Fauci was convinced that anything that gave hope to people, anything that might lessen the arguments for lockdowns, mask mandates, and universal vaccines must be dismissed out of hand.

CHAPTER 13

A Plague of Pandemic Thievery

By the fall of 2020, COVID deaths in the United States had reached about 280,000.[1] True to my predictions, the massive government welfare programs set up in the spring were attracting the usual liars and thieves. On November 9, I tweeted: "Your government sent 1.1 million dead people stimulus checks. Wonder how many of these folks also voted absentee?"[2]

I made the mistake of assuming the Twitter czars recognized snark and sarcasm. Apparently they didn't, and they flagged my tweet as misinformation.[3] So, I doubled down, of course, and tweeted, "Twitter is flagging my question: Your government sent 1.1 million dead people stimulus checks. Wonder how many of these folks also voted absentee? So, now it is unacceptable to pose questions?"[4]

Did a million dead people actually receive pandemic welfare checks? According to the U.S. Government Accountability Office, they did—to the tune of $1.4 billion.[5] Did a million dead people actually vote absentee? Well, of course not, one cannot expect a 100 percent turnout from the dead! Certainly the actual number of dead people voting would likely be well short of a million. (For any unemployed Twitter fact-checkers reading this, that's sarcasm).

It wasn't just dead people who were attracted to free money. Devron Brown of Philadelphia applied for and received almost a million dollars from the Paycheck Protection Program (PPP) for a company that didn't exist and for employees who didn't exist. What did he spend the money on? Well, diamonds, a motorcycle, an "all-terrain vehicle," a luxury car, and a new house in Florida. How did they finally catch him? He came back nearly a year later and applied for *another* million bucks.[6] The unknown is how many thieves evaded detection since the primary oversight was left to each individual applicant.

Not to be outdone, Rudolph Brooks was charged with stealing $3,560,855 from the PPP program to buy a new house, a Tesla, restaurant tabs, groceries, retail items, cash, and real estate in Baltimore and in Upper Marlboro, Maryland.[7]

The Justice Department revealed that "authorities have charged 57 people with stealing $175 million from an aid program meant to help small businesses weather pandemic lockdowns." And prosecutors apparently "have identified 500 individuals who may have defrauded the $660 billion Paycheck Protection Program (PPP)...."[8]

The list of thieves goes on and on. News reports from Texas and Illinois showed seven people stole $16 million in PPP funds dollars.

In Florida, a man illegally received "$3.9 million in PPP loans," which he used to purchase a $318,000 Lamborghini. Another Florida man stole nearly $2 million, using some of his ill-gotten gains to buy "a new Mercedes and a pickup truck."[9]

Clearly, the lockdowns were not bringing out the best in people.

Christmas 2020: Lockdowns and a Congressional Spending Spree

On December 22, 2020, I went to the Senate floor, annoyed that both Democrats and Republicans were still throwing good money after bad during the government-created lockdown. Particularly annoying was that President Trump approved this spending. He also encouraged two GOP U.S. Senate candidates mired in a run-off election to support the spending by issuing $2,000 per person in government checks.[10] The irony of GOP candidates campaigning for $2,000 checks for all while simultaneously warning voters that their Democrat opponents were "radical, extreme socialists" was not lost on independents and libertarians. They likely didn't perceive a dime's worth of difference between the Big Government spending sprees proposed by both parties.

Joseph Curl in a Daily Wire headline called my pre-Christmas remarks a "Viral Speech on Senate Floor Railing against Covid Bill." Curl's story led with a key quote from the speech: "When you vote to pass out free money, you lose your soul…."

Curl continued, "Sen. Rand Paul (R-KY) let loose on the Senate floor on Monday blasting the 5,593-page, $2.3 trillion COVID-19 relief and catchall spending bills in a speech that has gone viral."[11]

I didn't spare harsh words for members of my own party who were everywhere criticizing the socialism of Democrats: "If you vote for this spending monstrosity, you are no better," I said.[12]

My speech condemned the $900 billion coronavirus relief package attached to a $1.4 trillion spending bill. This COVID welfare bill was once again sending checks to everyone regardless of whether the individual had lost his job or not.

I expected this kind of profligate spending from Democrats. What particularly annoyed me was seeing it from Republicans. At our weekly Republican lunch, Senate leaders unveiled and lobbied for another COVID bailout bill. As I emerged from lunch, I couldn't help commenting to the media that I felt like I must have been at the Democrat caucus lunch because it sounded like a bunch of "Bernie bros" in there.

I told the *Washington Times*, "This is insane, they are ruining the country" with these fiscally irresponsible bailouts. I tweeted out: "Just came from Progressive Democrat—whoops—I'm mean Republican caucus: They're going to spend $105 billion more on education, more than we spend every year on the Dept. of Education. Anyone remember when Reagan conservatives were for eliminating the Federal Dept. of Education?"

I laid it on the line: "The majority of Republicans are now no different than socialist Democrats when it comes to debt. They simply don't care about debt and are preparing to add at least another trillion dollars in debt this month, combined with the trillions from earlier this summer."[13]

In my floor speech, I was similarly unsparing.

"If free money were the answer, if money really did grow on trees, why not give more free money? Why not give it out all the time? Why stop at $600 a person? Why not $1,000? Why not $2,000? ... Maybe these new free money Republicans should join the 'everybody gets a guaranteed income' caucus? Why not $20,000 a year for everybody, why not $30,000? If we can print out money with impunity, why not do it?"[14]

I let loose on the leaders of both parties. "We can't keep pretending that more debt is a sustainable policy course. Leadership is not passing on the problem until you reach someone who can't protest. Leadership is making the hard choices *now*. This is what we have to do. I will oppose this new debt, and I will continue to sound the alarm until we change our course here in Congress."[15] I knew that our country could be saved, that we could survive the pandemic if we pulled together—but adding more debt was a mistake, not the solution.

As Curl reported, "Paul said the government is not in the business of providing free money, adding, 'the only thing that can save us is opening the economy.'"[16]

Instead of bankrupting the country, I thought the Senate should debate the arbitrary and capricious nature of the lockdown edicts.

What the lockdowners did to restaurants was simply crazy. First the restaurants were shut down, then they were told they could serve outside, then they were told they could open with reduced seating. Never once was data shown to prove that any of these edicts worked. In fact, one of the most tragic-comic episodes of the lockdowns was New York governor Cuomo in his millionth press conference releasing a study showing where COVID was spread the most.

Not in restaurants. Wait for it—at home.[17]

I pointed out the insanity of telling bars that they can only serve alcohol if people are sitting, not standing, and only if the bars have heavy foods on their menus.

I railed at the stupidity of other lockdown regulations:

Restaurants are told they have to close at an arbitrary time determined by government officials—as though the virus only comes out late at night. A business in one zip code can open, but one in an adjoining zip code across the street has to close, as if the virus can't cross an imaginary line. Airlines are allowed to fly, but hotels have to limit their occupancy, so you may not have anywhere to stay when you get there. Mom and pop stores and specialty stores are forced to close, but big box store competitors are allowed to stay open.

How is any business expected to survive with this kind of arbitrary regulation that changes from day to day?[18]

When the time came to vote, five Republican senators voted with me against yet another COVID bailout: Rick Scott of Florida, Mike Lee of Utah, Marsha Blackburn of Tennessee, Ted Cruz of Texas, and Ron Johnson of Wisconsin.[19]

In addition to allocating $105 billion to support education and child-care, Senate Majority Leader Mitch McConnell said the Republican stimulus proposal included another wave of direct impact payments to individuals and funding to accelerate COVID-19 vaccine development.

I was livid with my fellow Republicans. I told them they "should apologize now to President Barack Obama for complaining that he was spending and borrowing too much."[20] Though President Donald Trump often did right by conservatives, on spending his backbone went missing. He happily signed one COVID bailout bill after another.

I pointed out that our exploding debt was not the result of lack of compromise. "Republicans and Democrats compromise every day of the year to spend money we don't have." In a Fox News interview, I described our debt situation: "We were already running a trillion dollars short just with our normal budgetary expenses for the year. We added $3 trillion, now they're talking about another $1 to $2 trillion. We're going to borrow [another] $5 trillion in five months." I warned that all this spending might turn off true conservatives and libertarians to the point that we "might just lose this election because Republicans are acting like Democrats now." Republicans went eight years criticizing Obama for deficit spending, I noted. "They should apologize now to President Obama for complaining he was spending and borrowing too much. He was a piker compared to their borrowing that they're doing now."[21]

Pompeo Reveals Wuhan Lab Illnesses *before* Public Cases

In the dying days of the Trump administration, Secretary of State Mike Pompeo decided that information the State Department had discovered needed to see the light of day. One of the bureaucratic tricks used in Washington is marking practically *everything* classified. This is done not to protect any truly sensitive secrets but to keep those secrets from Congress and the American people.

Secretary of State Pompeo decided to declassify as much as he could on the origins of COVID and let the American people decide what to think. Just a few days before Biden's inauguration, the State Department released its "Fact Sheet: Activity at the Wuhan Institute of Virology." The statement announced that "the U.S. government has reason to believe that several researchers inside the WIV became sick in autumn 2019, before the first identified case of the outbreak, with symptoms consistent with both COVID-19 and common seasonal illness. This raises questions about the credibility of WIV senior researcher Shi Zengli's public claim that there was 'zero infection' among the WIV's staff and students...."[22]

Pompeo recounts that he had to fight Anthony Fauci and the NIH at every turn to get the truth out. When Fauci asserted on MSNBC that "Americans shouldn't 'be accusatory' or be 'pointing fingers' at the Chinese Communist Party," Pompeo responded: "He implies good faith for the Chinese Communist Party. We are on the 32nd anniversary of the Tiananmen Square [incident]. For Dr. Fauci to go out and think the CCP cared that there were people in Wuhan who were dying...is just naive beyond all possible imagination."[23]

Jamie Metzl, a member of the WHO's advisory board, put it this way: "The Chinese have engaged in a massive cover-up that is going on until this day, involving destroying samples, hiding records, placing a universal gag order on Chinese scientists and imprisoning Chinese citizen journalists asking the most basic questions."[24]

And yet Fauci still felt compelled to do everything possible to defend China's reputation. The day cannot come soon enough when we will expose how the so-called "business of science" is powered not only with U.S. Treasury funds but also with funds from the Chinese government.[25]

CNN, ever the bellwether for disinformation, continued to broadcast in the spring of 2021 that the lab-leak hypothesis was "a controversial theory without evidence."[26]

Nevertheless, one of the first steps toward exposing the COVID cover-up had just been made via Pompeo and the Trump administration's declassification. It would take another year, until the GOP capture of the House, to begin to get more declassified information that would ultimately unravel the cover-up and reveal the facts surrounding the origins of COVID-19.

CHAPTER 14

Fauci and Natural Acquired Immunity

B y the spring of 2021, nearly six hundred thousand Americans had died either from COVID or with COVID.[1] On March 18, 2021, the HELP Committee met for an "Update from Federal Officials" on COVID-19.

I continued to see no evidence that Fauci or his yes-men had publicly acknowledged naturally acquired immunity, so I tried once again to elicit something useful—anything—from Fauci.

The Fauci Smokescreen Continues

Senator Paul: Dr. Fauci, in a recent British study, David Wiley and others found no symptomatic reinfections from COVID-19 after following 2,800 patients for several months. In fact, there have been no reports of significant numbers of reinfections after acquiring COVID-19 naturally. Shane Crotty, a virologist at La Jolla Institute for Immunology, concludes from his experiments that the amount of immune memory gained from natural infection would likely prevent the vast majority of people from getting hospitalized disease, severe disease, for many years. In this study, which was published in *Science*, Dr. Crotty showed that antibody levels stayed relatively constant with only modest declines over six to eight months.

Dr. Crotty reported that, notably, memory B cells specific for the spiked protein, or RBD, were detected in almost all COVID-19 cases with no apparent half-life at five to eight months after infection. In other words, Dr. Crotty found significant evidence of long-term immunity after COVID infection. Furthermore, Dr. Crotty noted that B-cell memory to some other infections has been observed for as long as sixty-plus years after smallpox vaccination or even ninety years after a natural infection with influenza. There was a woman who got the Spanish flu who still showed immunity ninety years later. So rather than being pessimistic towards people gaining immunity after they have had COVID or had a vaccine, studies argue for significant optimism.

And in fact, there have been *no* scientific studies arguing or proving that infection with COVID does not create immunity. There have been no studies showing significant numbers of reinfections. Of the thirty million Americans who have had COVID, only a handful of reinfections have been discovered. In fact, the *New York Times* reported last fall more than thirty-eight million people at the time worldwide had been infected with the coronavirus. And as of that date, fewer than five of these cases had been confirmed by scientists to be reinfections.

Scientists interviewed for the article concluded, that in most cases, a second bout with the virus produced milder symptoms or none at all. Given that no scientific studies have shown significant numbers of infections of patients previously infected or previously vaccinated, what specific studies do you cite to argue that the public should be wearing masks well into 2022?

Dr. Fauci: I am not sure I understand the connection of what you are saying about masks and reinfection. We are talking about people who have never been infected before—

Senator Paul: You are telling everybody to wear a mask, whether they have had an infection or a vaccine. What I am saying is they have immunity, and everybody agrees they have immunity. What studies do you have that people that have had the vaccine or have had the infection are spreading the infection? If we are not spreading the infection, isn't it just theater?

Dr. Fauci: No, it is not—

Senator Paul: If you have had a vaccine and you are wearing two masks, isn't that theater?

Dr. Fauci: No, it is not. Here we go again with the theater. Let's get down to the facts, okay? The studies that you quote from Crotty and Sette look at in-vitro examination of memory immunity, which in their paper, they specifically say this does not necessarily pertain to the actual protection. It is in vitro.

Senator Paul: And what can you point to that shows reinfection? There are no studies that show—

Dr. Fauci: Let me finish the response to your question, if you please. The other thing is that when you talk about the

infection and you don't keep in the concept of variance, that
is an entirely different ballgame. That is a good reason for a
mask. In the South African study conducted by J & J, they
found that people who were infected with wild type and were
exposed to the variant in South Africa, the 351, it was as if
they had never been infected before. They had no protection.
So when you talk about reinfection, you have got to make
sure you are talking about wild type. I agree with you that
you very likely would have protection from wild type for at
least six months if you are infected. But we in our country
now have variants that are circulating—

Senator Paul: What study shows significant reinfection,
hospitalization, and death after either a natural infection or
the vaccine? It doesn't exist. There is no evidence that there
are significant reinfections after the vaccine. In fact, I don't
think we have a hospitalization in the United States after the
two-week period after the second vaccination. I don't think
we have had a death in the United States [after COVID infection or vaccination].

Dr. Fauci: You are not hearing what I am saying about variants.
We are talking about wild type versus variants. Now we—

Senator Paul: And what proof is there that there are significant infections with hospitalizations and deaths from the
variants? None in our country, zero.

Dr. Fauci: Well, because we don't have a prevalence of a
variant yet. We are having one—can I finish? We are having
a 117 [new variant] that is becoming more dominant.

Senator Paul: But you are talking about conjecture. You are
making policy based on conjecture. You have the conjecture
that we are going to get variants—

Dr. Fauci: No, it isn't based on conjecture.

Senator Paul: So you want people to wear masks for another couple of years. You have been vaccinated and you parade around in two masks for show.

Dr. Fauci: No.

Senator Paul: …There is almost—there is virtually 0 percent chance you are going to get reinfected. And yet you are telling people that have had the vaccine, who have immunity—you are defying everything we know about immunity by telling people to wear masks who have been vaccinated. You won't get rid of vaccine hesitancy by telling people to wear a mask after they get the vaccine—you want people to get the vaccine, give them a reward instead of telling them the nanny state is going to be there for three more years and you've got to wear a mask forever. People don't want to hear it. There is no science behind it.[2]

Dr. Fauci: Well, let me just state for the record that masks are not theater. Masks are protective. And we—

Senator Paul: As immunity, they are theater. If you already have immunity, you are wearing a mask to give comfort to others. You are not wearing a mask because of any science.

Dr. Fauci: I totally disagree with you.

The Chairman: Dr. Fauci, if you could respond so that we could understand the difference between the virus itself and the variants and the reason for a mask.

Dr. Fauci: I am sorry, ma'am, I can't—

The Chairman: If you could respond to the question so that we could all understand the difference between the vaccine in controlling the wild type versus the variants that are out there and the reason for wearing a mask. I would appreciate it.

Dr. Fauci: Yes, I mean, yes. First of all, when you have a variant, you have an immunity that you get with convalescent sera and the same sort of thing. If I vaccinate you or me against a wild type, you get a certain level of antibody that's specific for a particular viral strain. If there is a circulating variant, you don't necessarily have it. You have some spill-over immunity, to be sure, but you diminish by anywhere from two- to eight-fold the protection.

So the point I am saying is that there are variants now circulating. The point that Senator Paul was making was that if you look at wild type only, there is some clear-cut credence to what he is saying. But we are living right now in a situation where we are having a dominance of 177 [a new variant], which was the original UK. We have a very trouble-some variant in New York City.... We have got two variants in California.... And we have a number of others. So we are not dealing with a static situation of the same virus. That was the only point I am making.[3]

And yet we did discover that prior infection with COVID no matter which variant *did* protect against severe disease, hospitalization, and death. So, once again Fauci's pessimistic outlook that naturally acquired immunity would ultimately fail, turned out to be false.

Masks Are, Indeed, Theater

My exchange with Fauci stirred up a hornet's nest, and his allies came buzzing in. My contention was that if vaccines effectively induce an immune response, just as an infection with COVID induces an immune response, there really isn't any need to wear a mask. Seemed pretty obvious to me.

My question to Fauci was that if the vaccinated and the previously infected aren't spreading the infection, isn't wearing a mask "just theater?"[4]

A few days later, H. Holden Thorp, the pompous editor in chief of *Science*, chimed in with an op-ed in his journal. Once upon a time, scientific journals stayed out of politics but not under H. Holden Thorp, who had publicly congratulated *Nature* for using its pages to endorse Joe Biden in the presidential race.

Thorp, in his smugness, had previously waded into politics when he announced, as the *Washington Examiner* summarizes, that scientists must "agree with me on climate change or don't get published."[5]

Responding to critics who admonish that scientists should stick to science and stay out of politics, Thorp tweeted, "'Stick to science' infantilizes scientists and tells us to sit at the kids table and let the adults decide. We must fight back."[6]

Thorp basically argues that science should be politicized to prevent wrongthink.

Thorp's tweet argues that if scientists sit on the sidelines, "this gives people the permission to say things like 'climate change may be real, but I don't think we should have government regulation to deal with it,' which is unacceptable. We can't concede that by letting people pick and choose."[7] Big words from a man who obviously thinks he can make better decisions than the common man. When the *Washington Examiner*'s Matt Lamb and others called him out on Twitter for this hubris, Thorp removed the tweet.

Vinay Prasad, M.D., Ph.D., and professor at UC San Francisco, chastised Thorp for his arrogance: "Holden [Thorp] has made it abundantly clear that as EIC of *Science*, *Science* is a journal for US democrats only. He writes many one-sided commentaries, and bizarre attacks.... Ok for me b/c I'm a progressive, just bad for the institution of science and society, which I still care about."[8]

Thorp doesn't seem to be gaining any humility over time, which is surprising considering that he was UNC chancellor during the worst scandal in their history—a scandal that ultimately led to his resignation.[9]

So when Thorp sat down to scold me, no one should have been surprised. Thorp titled his polemic "No, Senator, It's Not Theater."[10]

Well, if you're immune, wearing a mask *is* actually theater.

Thorp whines that we just don't know "whether vaccinated individuals can transmit the virus or whether the vaccines now in use will cover all of the viral variants currently circulating in the United States and around the world."[11]

What Thorp fails to discuss or to attempt to prove is whether masks work to prevent the spread of COVID. What we would find out over time is that the vaccines worked less well against each subsequent variant but that prior infection had a near perfect record of preventing hospitalization or death from a subsequent COVID infection. What we also knew, even before the pandemic, was that mask-wearing in the public sphere is ineffective in controlling the spread of aerosolized viruses.

Thorp was so proud of his op-ed slamming me that he previewed it before publication by email with Tony Fauci and Francis Collins—no doubt hoping to ingratiate himself. Thorp writes, "Letter in Science tomorrow...I just wanted you to be aware of the letter in case the misinformation forces try to use it to create more confusion, which I worry they will. Reporters have had the letter since Sunday night and we are working with them to provide context."[12]

(I suppose these are hand-selected reporters expected to parrot the party line.)

Thorp gushes in concluding, "Thanks again to you both for al[l] you are doing."

Collins responded to Thorp: "Holden, Agree 100% with Tony.... [Anyone] suggesting that we supported gain of function research on coronaviruses (we did not), is another example of a dark and dangerous misinformation campaign that seems to know no bounds of decency."[13]

Fauci likewise responds, "What I am not in favor of is the egregious misinformation and innuendoes related to the appropriate and necessary NIH funding of top USA [coronavirus] scientists who collaborate with respectable Chinese scientists to understand the evolution of emerging pathogens."[14]

No one should seem shocked. Francis Collins had, as the pandemic began, instructed Fauci to "take down" three prominent epidemiologists.[15] Condemn their ideas as misinformation. Don't bother with the facts. After seeing what they did to three world-famous scientists, it wasn't much of a leap to learn that Fauci and Collins were equally ecstatic about taking down a U.S. Senator.

The Shi Lab-Leak Revelations

In May of 2021, Nicholas Wade's article on Medium.com came out. It caught my attention and shaped my questions for my next committee encounter with Anthony Fauci. In Wade's origins article, he reviewed the experiments that Dr. Shi performed to determine whether her research at the Wuhan Institute of Virology was gain of function.

Wade explained that Dr. Shi created "novel coronaviruses with the highest possible infectivity for human cells." Shi created chimeric viruses that combined spike genes from one coronavirus variant with the backbone of another coronavirus to test for enhanced transmissibility.

According to Wade, "These chimeric viruses would then be tested for their ability to attack human cell cultures ('in vitro') and humanized mice ('in vivo'). And this information would help predict the likelihood of 'spillover,' the jump of a coronavirus from bats to people."[16]

These laboratory-created viruses were not found in nature but were intended to serve as templates for vaccines against future viral pandemics.

How did the mainstream media respond to Nicholas Wade's detailed examination of the lab-leak theory? *New York Times* science writer Apoorva Mandavilli tweeted that "Someday we will stop talking about the lab leak theory and maybe even admit its racist roots. But alas, that day is not yet here."[17]

Contrast the agenda-driven reporting of Mandavilli with a *New York Times* editorial from 2012 commenting on Fouchier's experiments that mutated avian flu to make it aerosolized and possibly infectious to humans. At the time, the *New York Times* perspective was, to put it gently, a bit more open-minded. The editorial staff wrote, "We respect the researchers' desire to protect public health. But the consequences, should the virus escape, are too devastating to risk."[18]

What happened to honesty and deliberative reasoning at the *New York Times*? Have wokeness, race-obsession, and partisan politics completely replaced common sense?

On May 11, 2021, a week after I had read Wade's prescient article, I got a chance to ask some very pointed questions to Anthony Fauci. At the time, over six hundred thousand people had died from COVID or with COVID in the United States.

CHAPTER 15

Fauci Funds Gain of Function in Wuhan

I opened the May 11, 2021, U.S. Senate HELP Committee hearing by restating what everyone knew but that Anthony Fauci still denied: that the U.S. Government had funded dangerous gain-of-function research in Wuhan.

> **Senator Paul:** Dr. Fauci, we do not know whether the pandemic started in a lab in Wuhan or evolved naturally, but we should want to know. Worldwide, three million people have died from this pandemic, and that should cause us to explore all possibilities.
>
> Instead, government authorities, self-interested in continuing gain-of-function research, say there is nothing to

see here. Gain-of-function research, as you know, is juicing up naturally occurring animal viruses to infect humans.

To arrive at the truth, the U.S. government should admit that the Wuhan Virology Institute was experimenting to enhance the coronavirus's ability to infect humans. Juicing up super-viruses is not new. Scientists in the U.S. have long known how to mutate animal viruses to infect humans.

For years, Dr. Ralph Baric, a virologist in the U.S., has been collaborating with Dr. Shi Zhengli of the Wuhan Virology Institute, sharing his discoveries about how to create super-viruses. This gain-of-function research has been funded by the NIH. The collaboration between the U.S. and the Wuhan Virology Institute continues. Doctors Baric and Shi worked together to insert bat virus spike protein into the backbone of the deadly SARS virus and then used this man-made super virus to infect human airway cells.

Think about that for a moment. The SARS virus had a 15 percent mortality. We are fighting a pandemic that has about a 1 percent mortality. Can you imagine if a SARS virus that has been juiced up and had viral proteins added to it, to the spike protein, if that were released accidentally?

Dr. Fauci, do you still support funding of the—NIH funding of the lab in Wuhan?

Dr. Fauci: Senator Paul, with all due respect, you are entirely and completely incorrect. The NIH has not ever and does not now fund gain-of-function research in the Wuhan Institute of Virology.

Senator Paul: Do they fund Dr. Baric?

Dr. Fauci: We do not fund gain—

Senator Paul: Do you fund Dr. Baric's gain-of-function research?

Dr. Fauci: Dr. Baric is not doing gain-of-function research. And, if it is, it is according to the guidelines, and it is being conducted in North Carolina, not—

Senator Paul: You do not think—

Dr. Fauci: —in China.

Senator Paul: —inserting a bat virus spike protein that he got from the Wuhan Institute into the SARS virus is gain of function?

Dr. Fauci: That is not—

Senator Paul: You would be in the minority because at least two hundred scientists have signed a statement from the Cambridge Working Group—

Dr. Fauci: Yeah.

Senator Paul: —saying that it is gain of function.

Dr. Fauci: Well, it is not. And, if you look at the grant and you look at the progress reports, it is not gain of function, despite the fact that people tweet that and—

Senator Paul: So, do you still—

Dr. Fauci: —write about it.

Senator Paul: —support sending money to the Wuhan Virology Institute?

Dr. Fauci: We do not send money now to the Wuhan—

This was of course a lie. The NIH and NIAID money was sent to Wuhan using the intermediary of EcoHealth Alliance and various U.S. universities. Even worse, in the fall of 2022, a House Republican intel committee report revealed that NIH and NIAID money was funding a military research institute in China.[1]

Senator Paul: Do you support—

Dr. Fauci: —Virology Institute.

Senator Paul: —sending money? We did, under your tutelage. We were sending it through EcoHealth. It was a sub-agency and a sub-grant. Do you support the money from NIH that was going to the Wuhan Institute?

Dr. Fauci: Let me explain to you why that was done. The SARS-CoV-1 originated in bats in China. It would have been irresponsible of us if we did not investigate the bat viruses and the serology to see who might have been—

Senator Paul: Or perhaps it—

Dr. Fauci: —infected in China.

Senator Paul: —would be irresponsible to send it to the Chinese government that we may not be able to trust with this knowledge and with these incredibly dangerous viruses. Government scientists, like yourself, who favor gain-of-function research—

Dr. Fauci: I do not favor—

Senator Paul: —maintain—

Dr. Fauci: —gain-of-function research in China.

Senator Paul: —that the disease arose naturally.

Dr. Fauci: You are saying things that are not correct.

Senator Paul: Government defenders of gain-of-function, such as yourself, say that COVID-19 mutations were random and not designed by man. But, interestingly, the technique that Dr. Baric developed forces mutations by serial passage through cell culture that the mutations appear to be natural. In fact, Dr. Baric named the technique the "no-see-um" technique because the mutations appear naturally.

Nicholson Baker of *New York* magazine said nobody would know if the virus had been fabricated in a laboratory or grown in nature. Government authorities in the U.S., including yourself, unequivocally deny that COVID-19 could have escaped a lab. But even Dr. Shi in Wuhan was not so sure.

According to Nicholson Baker, Dr. Shi wondered, could this new virus have come from her own laboratory? She checked her records frantically and found no matches.

"That really took a load off my mind," she said. "I had not slept for days."[2]

The director of the gain-of-function research in Wuhan could not sleep because she was terrified that it might be in her lab.

Dr. Baric, an advocate of gain-of-function research, admits the main problem that the Institute of Virology has is the outbreak occurred in close proximity. What are the odds?

Baric continued, "Could you rule out a laboratory escape? The answer in this case is probably not."[3]

Will you, in front of this group, categorically say that the COVID-19 could not have occurred through serial passage in a laboratory?

Dr. Fauci: I do not have any accounting of what the Chinese may have done, and I am fully in favor of any further investigation of what went on in China.

However, I will repeat again, the NIH and NIAID categorically has not funded gain-of-function research to be conducted in the Wuhan Institute of Virology.

Senator Paul: You do support it in the U.S. We have eleven labs doing it, and you have allowed it here. We have a committee to oversee it, but the committee [was bypassed and this research in Wuhan was never reviewed]. You are fooling with Mother Nature here. You are allowing super-viruses to be created with a 15 percent mortality. It is very dangerous, and it was a huge mistake to share this with China, and it is a huge mistake to allow this to continue in the United States. And we should be very careful to investigate where this virus came from.

Dr. Fauci: I fully agree that you should investigate where the virus came from. But, again, we have not funded gain-of-function research on this virus in the Wuhan Institute of Virology. No matter—

Senator Paul: You are parsing words.

Dr. Fauci: —how many times you say it, it did not happen.

Senator Paul: There was research done with Dr. Shi and Dr. Baric. They have collaborated on gain-of-function research where they enhanced the SARS virus to infect human airway cells, and they did it by merging a new spike protein on it. That is gain of function. That was joint research between the Wuhan Institute and Dr. Baric. You cannot deny it.

The Chairman: Senator Paul, your time is expired. Dr. Fauci, I will let you respond to that. We need to move on.

Dr. Fauci: Excuse me?

The Chairman: I will allow you to respond to that, and then we will move on.

Dr. Fauci: Yeah. I mean, I just wanted to say, we—I do not know how many times I can say it, Madam Chair. We did not fund gain-of-function research to be conducted in the Wuhan Institute of Virology.[4]

So, Fauci stated: "I will repeat again, the NIH and NIAID categorically has not funded gain-of-function research to be conducted in the Wuhan Institute of Virology."[5]

Democrat Denial

This moment should have been the end of any reputation that Fauci still had. The easel behind me displayed the actual NIAID number of the grant Fauci approved for Wuhan. And yet he lied to my face.

Unfortunately, Democrats turned away from the truth. They refused to read the 2012 direct quotes of Dr. Fauci supporting gain-of-function research, even if an accident performing such research should create a pandemic.[6] They refused to acknowledge that Fauci had exempted the research in China from the gain-of-function regulations.[7] And yet, the exchange exposed, without question, a chink in Fauci's armor.

I vowed that one day the whole world would know what all the evidence points to: that Anthony Fauci made the catastrophic decision to fund dangerous research in Wuhan that may have led to a lab accident that killed millions of people.

Despite later claiming that he'd never supported gain-of-function research, in 2012 Fauci wrote in the *Journal of the American Society for Microbiology*, "In an unlikely but conceivable turn of events, what if a scientist becomes infected with the virus, which leads to an outbreak and ultimately triggers a pandemic…. Should the initial experiments have been performed?… [T]he benefits of such experiments and resulting knowledge outweigh the risks."[8] So , it was a provable lie for Fauci to claim he'd never favored gain-of-function research. He had already contradicted his own statement in a major medical journal.[9]

And the mainstream media, with few exceptions, let him get away with it. Apparently, cover-ups are easier to accomplish when most of the broadcast media looks the other way.

The scales really tipped against Fauci when DRASTIC, the informal, extremely dogged internet sleuthing group, revealed the 2018 proposal by Daszak, Baric, Shi, and Linfa Wang for U.S. dollars to insert "appropriate human-specific cleavage sites" into SARS-CoV S gene sequences.[10] In other words, to create the genetic material that was ultimately found in COVID-19 and had never before been found in nature in the *sarbecovirus* family of SARS-like viruses. The Defense Advanced Research Projects Agency (DARPA) rejected Daszak's application, but we know that this group was eager to create a SARS virus with a furin cleavage site, exactly the type of virus we discovered when COVID-19 was sequenced. Virologist Simon Wain-Hobson described the DARPA proposal as basically a road map to a SARS-CoV-2-like virus.[11]

Realize that neither Fauci nor Daszak nor Baric volunteered to reveal or acknowledge this extremely relevant research proposal. But for the incredible tenacity of DRASTIC, the dangerous proposal might never have come to light. Alerted by a whistleblower, DRASTIC brought the proposal before the public. When it did, even scientists skeptical of the lab-leak theory began to reconsider.[12]

DRASTIC reported, "In other words, a branch of the federal government had already judged aspects of [EcoHealth Alliance's] research, and the corresponding shared research plan with the WIV, as falling under the definition of GOF, only for HHS to approve similar work without P3CO review in 2018 and 2019."[13]

When The Intercept released a trove of documents they gained via a federal court order (FOIA), its health and science reporter Sharon Lerner asked eleven "scientists who were either biologists or virology-adjacent experts on this, and seven of the eleven said this fits the NIH's own definition of gain-of-function research and nine said that it presented serious concerns about the safety and oversight of federally funded research."[14]

The lab-leak theory was no longer the conspiracy theory that Fauci and his yes-men would have us believe.

Congresswoman Cathy McMorris Rodgers sent a letter to Francis Collins, the head of the National Institutes of Health, a week after my exchange with Fauci on gain of function. In the letter, McMorris Rodgers notes that the Wuhan Institute of Virology had a "published record of conducting 'gain-of-function' research."[15]

Acting NIH deputy director Lawrence Tabak responded, "Neither NIH nor the National Institute of Allergy and Infectious Diseases has ever approved any grant that would have supported GOF research on coronaviruses that would have increased their transmissibility or lethality for humans."[16]

Tabak asserted that gain-of-function research is only regulated if "anticipated to enhance the *transmissibility* and/or *virulence* of potential pandemic pathogens, which could make them more dangerous to humans...."[17] So, as long as no one "anticipates" an increase in lethality, no harm, no foul.

By October 2021, though, there was a significant about-face from Tabak. In a letter to Representative James Comer, Tabak admitted that the Shi/Baric experiments adding the S protein from a newly discovered coronavirus to the backbone of the virus that causes SARS1 did make mice "sicker." He claimed that "this was an unexpected result of the research, as opposed to a result the researchers set out to do."[18] In the letter, Tabak admitted the research was gain of function without using that exact wording. If queried, I'm sure he would argue that no, no, it was not really gain of function because the gain of function was unplanned. According to this legerdemain, any research that didn't announce a plan to gain function was not gain-of-function research worthy of the scrutiny of the Pandemic (P3CO) Committee.

Tabak did admit that EcoHealth Alliance failed to notify NIH "right away" that their experiment showed gain of function and insisted NIH would follow up with them.[19] But the end result was that in 2022, the NIH sent new grant money to EcoHealth Alliance and continues to do so.[20]

So much for oversight.

CHAPTER 16

Fauci Confronted

Between May and July 2021, my distaste for Anthony Fauci's lies percolated. Every bit of evidence pointed toward the Wuhan research as being gain of function. On July 20, 2021, I got another chance to engage with Fauci.

The July 2021 HELP Committee Hearing was entitled "The Path Forward: A Federal Perspective on the COVID-19 Response." I didn't pull any punches but went straight for the jugular:

> **Senator Paul:** Dr. Fauci, as you are aware, it is a crime to lie to Congress.
>
> Section 1001 of the U.S. Criminal Code creates a felony and a five-year penalty for lying to Congress. On your last trip to our committee on May 11, you stated that the NIH

has not ever and does not now fund gain-of-function research in the Wuhan Institute of Virology. And yet gain-of-function research was done entirely in the Wuhan Institute by Dr. Shi and was funded by the NIH.

I would like to ask unanimous consent to insert into the record the Wuhan virology paper entitled "Discovery of a Rich Gene Pool of Bat SARS-Related Coronaviruses." Please deliver a copy of the journal article to Dr. Fauci. In this paper, Dr. Shi credits the NIH and lists the actual number of the grant that she was given by the NIH. In this paper, she took two bat coronavirus genes, spiked genes, and combined them with a SARS-related backbone to create new viruses that are not found in nature.

These lab-created viruses were then shown to replicate in human cells. The experiments combine genetic information from different coronaviruses that infect animals—but not humans—to create novel artificial viruses *able* to infect human cells. Viruses that in nature only infect animals were manipulated in the Wuhan lab to gain the function of infecting humans.

This research fits the definition of the research that the NIH said was subject to the pause in 2014–2017, a pause in funding of gain of function. But the NIH failed to recognize this research...and it never came under any scrutiny. Dr. Richard Ebright, a molecular biologist from Rutgers, described this research in Wuhan as "the Wuhan lab used NIH funding to construct novel chimeric SARS-related coronaviruses able to infect human cells and laboratory animals."[1]

This is high-risk research that creates new potential pandemic pathogens—potential pandemic pathogens that exist only in the lab, not in nature. In Dr. Ebright's words, "this research matches—indeed epitomizes—the definition of gain-of-function research" done entirely in Wuhan.[2] This is research for which there was supposed to be a federally mandated pause.

Dr. Fauci, knowing that it is a crime to lie to Congress, do you wish to retract your statement of May 11 where you claimed that the NIH never funded gain-of-function research in Wuhan?

Dr. Fauci: Senator Paul, I have never lied before the Congress, and I do not retract that statement! This paper that you were referring to was judged by qualified staff up and down the chain as not being gain of function.

Senator Paul: What does—

Dr. Fauci: Let me finish—

Senator Paul: You take an animal virus, and you increase its transmissibility to humans. You are saying that is *not* gain of function?

Dr. Fauci: That is correct. And, Senator Paul, you do not know what you are talking about, quite frankly. And I want to say that officially. You do not know what you are talking about. Okay, you get one person—can I answer your question?

Senator Paul: From the NIH definition of gain-of-function— this is your definition that you guys wrote. It says that scientific research that increases the transmissibility among mammals is a gain of function. They took animal viruses that only occur in animals, and they increased their transmissibility to humans. How you can say that is not gain-of-function—

Dr. Fauci: It is not.

Senator Paul: It is a dance, and you are dancing around this because you are trying to obscure responsibility for four million people dying around the world from a pandemic.

The Chairman: And let's let—Dr. Fauci.

Dr. Fauci: I have to—well, now you are getting into something. If the point that you are making is that the grant that was funded as a sub-award from EcoHealth to Wuhan created SARS-CoV-2—that is where you are getting. Let me finish.

Senator Paul: We don't know. We don't know if it did—but all the evidence is pointing that it came from the lab, and there will be responsibility for those who funded the lab, including yourself.

Dr. Fauci: I totally resent—

The Chairman: This committee will allow the witness to respond.

Dr. Fauci: I totally resent the lie that you are now propagating, Senator, because if you look at the viruses that were used in the experiments, that were given in the annual reports that were published in the literature, it is molecularly impossible—

Senator Paul: No one is saying those viruses caused it.

Dr. Fauci: It is molecularly—

Senator Paul: No one is alleging that those viruses caused the pandemic. What we are alleging is that the gain-of-function research was going on in that lab and NIH funded it.

Dr. Fauci: That is not—

Senator Paul: You can't get away from it. It meets your definition, and you are obfuscating the truth.

Dr. Fauci: I am not obfuscating the truth, you are the one.

The Chairman: Senator Paul, your time has expired, but I will allow the witness to—

Dr. Fauci: Let me just finish. I want everyone to understand that if you look at those viruses, and that is judged by qualified virologists and evolutionary biologists, those viruses are molecularly impossible to result in SARS-CoV-2.

Senator Paul: No one is saying they are. No one is saying those viruses caused the pandemic. We are saying they are gain-of-function viruses—

Dr. Fauci: They are not—

Senator Paul: Because they are animal viruses that became more transmissible in humans, and you funded it. Why won't you admit the truth?

Dr. Fauci: And you are implying—

The Chairman: Senator Paul, your time has expired, and I will allow witnesses who come before this committee to respond.

Dr. Fauci: And you are implying that what we did was responsible for the deaths of individual—I totally resent that—

Senator Paul: It could have.

Dr. Fauci: And if anybody is lying here, Senator, it is you.[3]

The Follow-Up Urging Prosecution

When liars are caught, dead-to-rights, a tactic is to misdirect and argue against a straw man, argue against something that your opponent is not suggesting. This was exactly the tactic used by Fauci in the committee exchange. He argued that none of the published super-viruses created by Dr. Shi in Wuhan are similar enough to COVID-19 to have been a precursor. He's right, but then again, exactly no one was making that argument. Proponents of the lab leak like myself were arguing that if COVID-19 leaked from the Wuhan lab, it came from a coronavirus or a recombinant coronavirus that has not yet been revealed by Dr. Shi. Shi's publications and Daszak's statements indicate there are literally hundreds of coronaviruses in their lab that have not been officially made public.[4] For example, Fauci's claim that the NIH did not fund gain-of-function research is directly contradicted by a 2016 email commenting on approval of a NIH/NIAID grant where grant recipient Peter Daszak exults, "This is terrific! We are very happy to hear that our Gain of Function funding pause has been lifted."[5]

There it is. The lie confirmed in black and white.

I don't make idle threats. So, true to my word, I fired off a criminal referral to Biden's attorney general, Merrick Garland.

The letter begins, "I write to urge the United States Department of Justice to open an investigation into testimony made to the United States Senate Committee on Health, Education, Labor, and Pensions by Dr. Anthony Fauci, Director of the National Institute of Allergy and Infectious Diseases."

I pointed out that Fauci testified that "the NIH has not ever and does not now fund gain-of-function research in the Wuhan Institute of Virology."

I referred Garland to a May 2016 National Science Advisory Board for Biosecurity report that defined gain-of-function research as referring "to changes resulting in the acquisition of new, or an enhancement of existing, biological phenotypes."[6]

In a paper entitled "Discovery of a Rich Gene Pool of Bat SARS-Related Coronaviruses Provides New Insights into the Origin of SARS Coronavirus," Dr. Shi Zhengli describes research conducted at the Wuhan Institute of Virology and funded under the NIAID Award R01AI110964 in which spike genes from two uncharacterized bat

SARS-related coronavirus strains, Rs4231 and Rs7327, were combined with the genomic backbone of another SARS-related coronavirus to create novel chimeric SARS-related viruses that showed cytoplasmic effects in primate epithelial cells and replication in human epithelial cells.[7] This research meets the definition of gain-of-function research.

I reminded Garland that under 18 U.S.C. § 1001, whoever makes "any materially false, fictitious, or fraudulent statement" to Congress "is subject to criminal fines and imprisonment up to five years."[8]

Needless to say, I'm not holding my breath waiting for the partisan Garland to begin a prosecution. But I do believe that a vast portion of Americans now know the devious nature of Anthony Fauci's COVID cover-up.

When Dr. Richard Ebright testified before Congress, he did not pull any punches. He said that Fauci's statement that NIH and NIAID didn't fund gain-of-function research was a lie.[9]

Lying to Congress is a felony punishable by up to five years. Biden's Justice Department has had no qualms about charging and trying Trump supporters for lying to Congress, but the DOJ has turned deaf ears to Fauci's fabrications.

Garland is, to say the least, not the most impartial of attorneys general we've ever had. A quick glance at the yearslong covering up of the Hunter Biden laptop gives an idea of Garland's partisanship. Some people propose that his anger over Republicans blocking him from the Supreme Court is reflected in his misuse of office. Whatever the case, we never received even a cursory response to our criminal referral of Anthony Fauci.

The Truth Spreads

I did begin to sense, though, that the tide was turning. The articles of Nicholas Wade, Nicholson Baker, and Katherine Eban had begun to open at least some minds.

Even the *Washington Post*—not famous for introspection and self-correction—reversed course, changing the headline on its story from 2020 that blasted Tom Cotton for having the temerity to argue that COVID-19 might have leaked from the Wuhan lab. The *Post* had smeared Cotton's suggestions as "conspiracy theory"[10]—the standard left-wing attack tactic where facts be damned and name-calling is sufficient. But something was brewing when this Democratic Party organ was shuffling through old stories and retroactively changing a headline. Now rather than the lab-leak theory being labeled "debunked," it was changed to "disputed."[11] Thank goodness for the remnant of honesty still left in journalism.

The awakening continued. Documents revealed that even Dr. Fauci's subordinates at NIAID warned him that the experiments in Wuhan were gain-of-function experiments. As early as May 2016, two of Fauci's staffers, Jenny Greer and Erik Stemmy, sent a letter to Daszak's EcoHealth seeking further explanation because their research in Wuhan "may include" gain-of-function research.[12]

Did this revelation prompt a review by the Pandemic P3CO Committee? Of course not. Anthony Fauci's NIAID merely asked the recipient of the money what he thought, and Daszak claimed that the Wuhan research was not gain of function.[13] That's like asking an NFL receiver if he had both feet in bounds on his sideline catch. To any objective observer, it would be crazy to ask the recipients of federal dollars to police themselves.

Fauci did not reveal this item voluntarily. Once again, we only know this because a federal judge required NIAID to reveal this information through a FOIA court order.[14]

When Professor Ebright viewed my exchange with Fauci and learned that Daszak had been allowed to police himself, Ebright was emphatic in his judgement that Fauci was "untruthful in his testimony to Congress" when Fauci stated "that NIH staff concluded up and down the line that the EcoHealth grant did not include gain of function research."[15]

The self-oversight legerdemain became even more ridiculous. It turned out that the NIH brokered a deal with Daszak's EcoHealth Alliance to *redefine* gain-of-function. Instead of defining it as viral recombination that increased the pathogenicity of a virus in humans, Fauci decided to arbitrarily redefine gain of function as experiments that increased viral growth by a factor of ten.[16]

Even accepting this arbitrarily created definition, Daszak's EcoHealth Alliance funded experiments by Baric/Shi that still qualified as gain of function because viral growth actually exceeded the arbitrary limit of tenfold growth.[17]

The Pandemic Committee didn't deliberate or decide on this new definition. It was concocted behind closed doors at the behest of a gain-of-function researcher.

In other words, the foxes were most definitely in charge of guarding the hen house.

By changing the definition of gain-of-function research, the Wuhan researchers had now exempted themselves from any oversight by the Pandemic P3CO Committee. When culpability finally attaches to Fauci for this worldwide disaster, he can't simply blame a bureaucratic or congressional committee.

Because Anthony Fauci, himself, neutered and destroyed the committee's ability to perform oversight.[18]

They Knew All Along

As early as February 1, 2020, Fauci and fellow NIH employees were privately acknowledging that the collaboration between Baric and Shi involved gain-of-function research. In an email to his assistant Hugh Auchincloss, Fauci lists in the subject heading "Baric, Shi et al—Nature medicine—SARS Gain of Function."[19] Privately, even Fauci was matter-of-factly acknowledging that the research was gain of function.

On January 27, 2020, another assistant had emailed Fauci talking points for a White House press conference which included the NIAID number for the Baric/Shi gain-of-function research.[20]

Without a doubt, Fauci and all his yes-men knew the risky game they were playing, and without great subterfuge, the entire world would discover that he had made the disastrous mistake of funding this dangerous type of research in Wuhan.

NIH Throws Fauci under the Bus

On October 20, 2021 (coincidently, my thirty-first wedding anniversary), an explosive admission came from an unexpected source— Lawrence Tabak, the acting deputy director of the NIH. The admission was unexpected since the NIH had resisted tooth and nail every request for information concerning gain-of-function research in Wuhan. Tabak's letter came as a response to a query by House Minority Oversight Committee ranking member James Comer (R-KY).

The letter concerned the NIH funding of the Wuhan lab research both during the so-called pause in funding and afterword during the years 2014–2019.

Tabak readily admitted that NIH had funded research in Wuhan via the conduit EcoHealth Alliance. He acknowledged that research in Wuhan created a novel chimeric SARS-related coronavirus, WIV1 SHC014 S, with a NIH grant. This laboratory-created virus does not exist in nature.[21]

According to Professor Richard Ebright, this virus "is one of at least three artificial, laboratory-constructed chimeric coronaviruses that were constructed by EcoHealth Alliance and its Wuhan partners using NIH funding and that were shown to infect human airway cells, to replicate in human airway cells, and to exhibit 10,000-fold higher viral growth and higher lethality than the parental natural coronavirus in infection studies in mice engineered to display human receptors on airway cells."[22]

The Tabak letter further revealed the deal NIH had cut with EcoHealth Alliance to continue gain-of-function research during the supposed pause in funding. The arrangement required that if any of the laboratory-created chimeric viruses grew greater than tenfold more than the parent virus, all experiments on the viruses must stop.

Even though EcoHealth Alliance was given special permission to continue gain-of-function research during the pause, they didn't even bother to adhere to the newly created, lax rules. According to Tabak's letter, they simply thumbed their noses at NIH and went on creating and growing viruses not found in nature.[23]

Ebright concludes that "the Tabak letter thus confirms that NIH funds supported gain-of-function research of concern and construction and characterization of an enhanced potential pandemic pathogen—a pathogen reasonably anticipated, indeed likely, to have enhanced trans-missibility and/or pathogenicity in humans—in Wuhan."[24] Yet, Tabak, like others before him, takes care to never use the words "gain of func-tion," despite acknowledging in detail that, yes, the laboratory-created viruses did gain function.

Tabak takes pains to state that the novel viruses created in Wuhan with NIH money are not COVID-19 and not likely to be a precursor of COVID-19. Once again, attacking a straw-man argument that no one was making while ignoring the real elephant in the room: What other novel viruses had the Chinese created during this period but had not yet published (and likely never would) because they were closely related to the virus that ultimately caused the pandemic?

The NIH continued to fund EcoHealth Alliance despite evidence that EcoHealth alliance was in defiance of the order to stop experiments if tenfold viral growth was detected, and despite EcoHealth repeatedly missing filing dates required by the NIH.[25]

Importantly, as Professor Ebright points out, EcoHealth's "proposed continuation of enhanced potential pandemic pathogen research—specifically proposing to construct and characterize additional novel chimeric SARS-related coronaviruses" was not forwarded to the Pandemic Review Committee as it should have because EcoHealth "falsely asserted that NIH funding had not supported gain-of-function research or enhanced potential pandemic pathogen research in Wuhan."[26]

Amidst these explosive admissions by the NIH, the mainstream media looked the other way instead of holding Fauci's feet to the fire. Their fawning coverage of "America's leading infectious disease expert" allowed Fauci to largely escape culpability for lying about gain-of-function research in Wuhan and then doing his best to cover up any notion that the pandemic started from a lab leak.

PART IV

Asserting the Truth

CHAPTER 17

Gain of Function and Fauci

B y the fall of 2021, a great deal was known about COVID. The
initial estimates that the death rate might exceed 3 percent were
tenfold higher than the actual death rate of approximately 0.3 percent.[1]

The public perception of the dangers of COVID was significantly
skewed, no doubt due to both media and government hype. A Gallup
poll of over three thousand Americans in the summer of 2021 revealed
that the public dramatically overestimated the risks of being hospitalized from COVID. The propensity of people to exaggerate the risks of
COVID-19 was most pronounced among Democrats. Forty-one percent
of Democrats believed that "at least 50% of unvaccinated people have
been hospitalized due to COVID-19." The actual percentage of unvaccinated people who were hospitalized because of COVID-19 was under

1 percent. Sixty-three percent of Democrats believed the hospitalization rate for the unvaccinated to be above 20 percent.[2]

Not only were Democrats misinformed on the severity of COVID, they were overwhelmingly in favor of using government force to punish anyone who disagreed with them. According to a Rasmussen poll, 55 percent of Democrats supported fines for anyone who refuses vaccination, 29 percent of Democrats approved of the government taking children away from unvaccinated parents, and 48 percent of Democrats favored fining and/or imprisoning those who "publicly question the efficacy of the existing COVID-19 vaccines."[3]

So much for "my body, my choice."

Amidst this lust for applied authoritarianism, a few showed great courage. Tennis player Novak Djokovic, who had been number one in the world for a record 353 weeks at the end of the 2021 season while winning twenty Grand Slam titles and nine Australian Open titles,[4] refused to be vaccinated even when it meant he had to forgo competing in the U.S. Open and Australian Open. When he was asked why he would give up so much, he responded, "Because the principles of decision-making on my body are more important than any title."[5]

Green Bay Packers quarterback Aaron Rodgers also took a stand against the authoritarians. In response to his critics, he said, "I am somebody who is a critical thinker, you guys know me." "I march to the beat of my own drum," Rodgers continued. "I believe strongly in bodily autonomy and the ability to make choices for your body. Not to have to acquiesce to some woke culture or crazed group of individuals who say you have to do something. Health is not a one size fits all for everybody."[6]

I couldn't have said it better. After my early and virtually asymptomatic bout with COVID-19, I made what I considered to be a rational decision. I decided to rely on my naturally acquired immunity—despite a daily dose of abuse from the left-wing media.

NBA star Jonathan Isaac, a power forward with the Orlando Magic, had this concise and intelligent response to why he refused the vaccine: "A lot went into my decision for not deciding to get the vaccine. For starters, I have had COVID in the past. I've come to understand…immunity by natural infection is robust and long-lasting…. With my current physical fitness level and my age group I don't feel I'm in a category of, you know, fear or of necessarily need right now to get the vaccine."[7]

Never before had the public reacted to a disease with such partisanship. Rasmussen polling also showed that 28 percent of Democrats believed that more than 10 percent of people infected with COVID will die.[8] The media breathlessly ran daily death counts that included the number of people dying from cancer, heart disease, and other illnesses as long as they also tested positive for COVID. No wonder the American public remained alarmed every minute of every day. The vast majority of Democrats receive their news from CNN and MSNBC, and a significant number of them came away believing that the COVID death rate is at least ten times higher than it actually is.[9] Perhaps the left-wing zealots hyped up to censor "misinformation" ought to begin by policing their own viewing habits.

The Foundation for Economic Education's Jon Miltimore tweeted out a possible answer to the negativity: "A new @nberpubs paper shows how US media created a climate of #COVID19 fear. 'Ninety one percent of stories by US major media outlets are negative in tone versus fifty four percent for non-U.S. major sources and sixty five percent for scientific journals,' the authors concluded."[10]

Even when COVID cases were actually, verifiably declining, the National Bureau of Economic Research found that "stories of increasing

COVID-19 cases outnumber stories of decreasing cases by a factor of 5.5 even during periods when new cases are declining."[11]

More Fauci Dissembling

Amid the continued hysteria being broadcast by CNN and MSNBC, Anthony Fauci returned to testify before the HELP Committee. The November 4, 2021, hearing was entitled "Next Steps: The Road Ahead for the COVID-19 Response."

A week before the committee hearing, internet sleuth Jeremy Redfern discovered that NIH had actually taken down their definition of gain of function—erased it from their website.

Redfern tweeted, "If anyone was wondering how I noticed—I was looking up the official definition of gain-of-function by the @NIH. I noticed the definition on the google archive of the link but not on the webpage. So, I decided to go into the wayback machine, and well... you know the rest."[12]

The term was completely memory-holed and replaced with some potential-pathogen wordplay intended to further absolve Fauci and the NIH from responsibility.

I couldn't help but pick up where I had left off with Fauci and his denials concerning funding gain-of-function research in Wuhan:

> **Senator Paul:** Dr. Fauci, I do not expect you today to admit that you approved of NIH funding for gain-of-function research in Wuhan, but your repeated denials have worn thin, and a majority of Americans, frankly, do not believe you.
>
> Even the NIH now admits that EcoHealth Alliance did perform experiments in Wuhan that created viruses not found in nature that actually did gain in lethality.

The facts are clear. The NIH did fund gain-of-function research in Wuhan, despite your protestations. You can deny it all you want, but even the Chinese authors of the paper, in their paper, admit that viruses not found in nature were created, and yes, they gained in infectivity. Your persistent denials, though, are not simply a stain on your reputation, but are a clear and present danger to the country and to the world.

As Professor Kevin Esvelt of MIT has written, gain-of-function research "looks like a gamble that civilization can't afford to risk,"[13] and yet, here we are again, with you steadfast in your denials.

Why does it matter? Because gain-of-function research with laboratory-created viruses not found in nature could cause a pandemic even worse the next time. We are suffering today from one that has a mortality of approximately 1 percent. They are experimenting with viruses that have mortalities of between 15 and 50 percent.[14]

Yes, our civilization could be at risk from one of these viruses. Experiments that combine unknown viruses with known pandemic-causing viruses are incredibly risky. Experiments that combine unknown viruses with coronaviruses that have as much as 50 percent mortality could endanger civilization as we know it. And here you sit, unwilling to accept any responsibility for the current pandemic, and unwilling to take any steps to prevent gain-of-function research from possibly unleashing an even more deadly virus.

You mislead the public by saying that the published viruses could not be COVID. Well, exactly no one is alleging that. No one is alleging that the published viruses by the Chinese are COVID.

What we are saying is that this was a risky type of research, gain-of-function research. It was risky to share this with the Chinese and that COVID may have been created from a not-yet-revealed virus.

We do not anticipate the Chinese are going to reveal the virus if it came from their lab. You know that, but you continue to mislead. You continue to support NIH money going to Wuhan. You continue to say you trust the Chinese scientists. You appear to have learned nothing from this pandemic.

Will you today finally take some responsibility for funding gain-of-function research in Wuhan?

Dr. Fauci: Senator, with all due respect, I disagree with so many of the things that you have said.

First of all, gain of function is a very nebulous term. We have spent—not us, but outside bodies—a considerable amount of effort to give a more precise definition to the type of research that is of concern, that might lead to a dangerous situation. You are aware of that. That is called P3CO.

Senator Paul: We are aware that you deleted gain of function from the NIH website.[15]

Dr. Fauci: Well, I can get back to that in a moment if we have time, but let's get back to the operating framework and guide rails of which we operate under, and you have ignored them.

The guidelines are very, very clear, that you have to be dealing with a pathogen that clearly is shown and very likely to be highly transmissible in an uncontrollable way in humans; and to have a high degree of morbidity and mortality; and that you do experiments to enhance that. Hence, the word EPPP, Enhanced Pathogens of Potential Pandemic.

Senator Paul: So when EcoHealth Alliance took the virus—

Dr. Fauci: Well, can I—I would love to finish.

Senator Paul: —SHC014 and combined it with WIV1 and caused a recombinant virus that does not exist in nature and it made mice sicker, mice that had humanized cells, you are saying that that is not gain-of-function research?

Dr. Fauci: According to the framework and guidelines of—

Senator Paul: So what you are doing is defining away gain-of-function.

Dr. Fauci: No.

Senator Paul: You are simply saying it does not exist because you changed the definition on the NIH website. This is terrible, and you are completely trying to escape the idea that we should do something about trying to prevent a pandemic from leaking from a lab.

The preponderance of evidence now points towards this coming from the lab, and what you have done is change the definition on your website to try to cover your ass, basically. That is what you have done. You have changed the website to try to have a new definition that does not include the risky research that is going on.

Until you admit that it is risky, we are not going to get anywhere. You have to admit that this research was risky.

The NIH has now rebuked them. Your own agency has rebuked them.

Dr. Fauci: That is—

Senator Paul: But, the thing is, you are still unwilling to admit that they gained in function when they say [the mice] became sicker. They gained in lethality. It is a new virus. That is not gain of function?

Dr. Fauci: According to the definition that is currently operable—

Senator Paul: (Laughter)

Dr. Fauci: You know, Senator, the new—let's make it clear for the people who are listening.

The current definition was done over a two-to-three-year period by outside bodies, including the NSABB, two conferences by the National Academies of Science, Engineering, and Medicine, on December 2014, March 2016. We commissioned external risk-benefit assessment.

And then, on January of 2017, the Office of Science and Technology Policy of the White House issued the current policy.

Senator Paul: And coincidentally—

Dr. Fauci: I have not changed—

Senator Paul: —the new definition appeared—

Dr. Fauci: —any definition.

Senator Paul: —on the same day the NIH said that yes, there was a gain of function in Wuhan. The same day the definition appeared, the new definition, to try to define away what is going on in Wuhan.[16]

Until you accept it, until you accept responsibility, we are not going to get anywhere close to trying to prevent another lab leak of this dangerous sort of experiment. You will not admit—

Dr. Fauci: Well—

Senator Paul: —that it is dangerous, and for that lack of judgment, I think it is time that you resign.

The Chairman: Thank you, Senator Paul, and I would like to give the time to Dr. Fauci.

Dr. Fauci: Yeah. Well, there were so many things that are egregious misrepresentation here, Madam Chair, that I do not think I would be able to refute all of them. But just a couple of them for the listeners to hear for.

You said that I am unwilling to take any responsibility for the current pandemic. I have no responsibility for the current pandemic. The current pandemic. Okay?

Number two. You said the overwhelming amount of evidence indicates that it is a lab leak. I believe most card-carrying viral phylogenists and molecular virologists would disagree with you; that it is much more likely—even though we leave open all possibilities—it is much more likely that this was a natural occurrence.

Third. You say we continue—

Senator Paul: They tested eighty thousand animals and no animals...

The Chairman: Senator Paul, please—

Senator Paul: —have been found with COVID.

The Chairman: Senator Paul, the time is for—

Dr. Fauci: And third.

The Chairman: —Dr. Fauci to respond.

Dr. Fauci: You made a statement just a moment ago that is completely incorrect when you say we continue to support research at the Wuhan Institute of Virology, which is completely—

Senator Paul: You approved it in August of last year.

Dr. Fauci: No, no. Your statement says, quote—I wrote it down as you were writing—"You continue to support research at the Wuhan Institute of Virology."

Senator Paul: You were in committee a month ago and said—

Dr. Fauci: Which—

The Chairman: Senator Paul.

Senator Paul: —you still trust the Chinese scientists and you still support the research over there. You said it a month ago in committee.

The Chairman: Senator Paul, I have allowed Dr. Fauci to respond. You have had your time. I am going to give him—

Senator Paul: If he is going—

The Chairman: —one more minute.

Senator Paul: —to be dishonest, he ought to be challenged.

The Chairman: Senator Paul, we will allow Dr. Fauci to respond after you have given accusations like that. Dr. Fauci?

Dr. Fauci: Well, I do not have any more to say except to say that, as usual—and I have a great deal of respect for this body of the Senate, and it makes me very uncomfortable to have to say something—but he is egregiously incorrect in what he says. Thank you.

The Chairman: Thank you.

Senator Paul: History will figure that out on its own…[17]

And history will ultimately not be kind to the prevaricator Anthony Fauci. It took more than a decade for us to discover that weaponized anthrax had accidentally leaked from a Soviet lab. We learned that only because a Soviet defector informed us.[18] I predict that the vast majority of scientists and the general public will ultimately conclude that COVID-19 came from a lab and they will judge Anthony Fauci harshly for funding this dangerous research in an authoritarian country with inadequate safety conditions.

We Must Stop This from Happening Again

On March 15, 2022, I introduced legislation to eliminate Anthony Fauci's position as titular head of NIAID and divide the position into three different positions that would require Senate confirmation. (Currently, Fauci's position has no time limit and is not Senate confirmed.)

My announcement read,

> We've learned a lot over the past two years, but one lesson in particular is that no one person should be deemed "dictator-in-chief."
>
> No one person should have unilateral authority to make decisions for millions of Americans.
>
> To ensure that ineffective, unscientific lockdowns and mandates are never foisted on the American people ever again, I've introduced this amendment to eliminate Dr. Anthony Fauci's position as Director of the National Institute of Allergy and Infectious Diseases, and divide his power into three separate new institutes.
>
> This will create accountability and oversight into a taxpayer funded position that has largely abused its power, and has been responsible for many failures and misinformation during the COVID-19 pandemic.

Fauci's position would be replaced with three new directors of the following new institutes:

1. National Institute of Allergic Diseases
2. National Institute of Infectious Diseases
3. National Institute of Immunologic Diseases

"Each of these three institutes will be led by a director who is appointed by the president and confirmed by the Senate for a 5-year term."[19]

As I spoke on the Senate floor in support of eliminating Fauci's position, I referred to the life of Galileo as a warning of what can occur when scientific inquiry becomes subordinate to government power.

"Advances in science often happen when we question conventional wisdom. History gives us too many examples of what happens when people in power make scientists bend to dogma. At the end of his life, Galileo was kept under lock and key simply for revealing truth that people in power—the government—didn't want to hear."[20]

My legislation brought an immediate response from Fauci. A *Newsweek* headline reported, "Dr. Fauci Hints He May Retire Soon as Rand Paul Works to Get Him Fired." *Newsweek* quoted Fauci as saying he "can't stay at this job forever." *Newsweek* implied that the legislation I had introduced a few days before may have prompted Fauci's discussion of retirement.[21] I hope so. To my mind, the only problem with Fauci's rumblings of resignation was that they came decades too late.

Fauci and J. Edgar Hoover, Soulmates
On March 28, 2023, I had this to say in an op-ed:

It took the death of J. Edgar Hoover for the public to finally discover the extent of his misdeeds. He'd been director of the Federal Bureau of Investigation for thirty-seven years. The government's civil rights abuses over that long period are now well known, but during Hoover's lifetime six presidents looked the other way. Hoover's FBI spied on groups from the NAACP to the ACLU and conducted domestic surveillance on almost any prominent figure who seemed politically threatening.

Albert Einstein, an early opponent of nuclear weapons, had an FBI file over 1,400 pages long by the time he died in 1955. John Lennon was put under surveillance after he met with anti-war activists in New York in 1971. The INS tried to deport him a year later. Perhaps most infamously, in 1964 Hoover's FBI sent an anonymous letter to Martin Luther King, Jr., attempting to blackmail him into committing suicide.

Many of the FBI's activities in those years were blatantly unconstitutional, but few were brave enough to speak out against them. It was too dangerous to cross Director Hoover. His influence was so strong that when he turned 70, President Lyndon Johnson issued an executive order granting him a special exemption from mandatory retirement under the Civil Service Retirement Act.

A decade later, public opinion began to shift. Six presidents had come and gone while Hoover remained at the top of the most formidable law enforcement agency the world had ever known. But when his abuses of office came to light, they sparked an outcry against one man holding the reins of power for so long. So, in 1976, Congress enacted a 10-year term limit for the FBI director.

It took the COVID lockdowns and abuse of civil and religious liberty to finally expose another power-hungry figure who outlasted *seven* presidents and oversaw his agency's transformation from a medical research institute into the foremost biodefense research agency on earth.

Despite this extraordinary accumulation of power over nearly four decades, the Senate never once voted to confirm Anthony Fauci. The law never required it. Congress never anticipated one person would stay so long and abuse power so much.

Anthony Fauci presided over the National Institute of Allergy and Infectious Diseases (NIAID) for nearly four decades. By the time he retired he was drawing the largest salary in the entire federal government.

His salary skyrocketed after 9/11, when the George W. Bush administration, at the behest of Vice President Dick Cheney, brought all biodefense research under the control of the NIAID director. This included projects that were previously overseen by military or intelligence agencies.

As Ashley Rindsberg reports at Unherd.com, "Far from being a public health expert, Fauci sits at the very top of America's biodefence infrastructure. And contrary to the notion that he is a Deep State string-puller of the Democratic party, it was George W. Bush and Dick Cheney who not only put Fauci there but created the very framework that the immunologist-physician commands."[22]

In the aftermath of the 9/11 attacks and the anthrax killings, the Bush administration rushed to create a powerful, centralized biodefense agency. As Rindsberg puts it, "With the stroke of Cheney's pen, all United States biodefence efforts, classified or unclassified, were placed under the aegis of Anthony Fauci [who].... went from being the director of one of the NIH's constituent 27 institutes to being the only one who really mattered."[23]

Within a few years, Fauci would oversee two billion dollars in biodefense funding, a total that was more than the government spent on breast cancer, stroke, tuberculosis, and lung cancer research. Bush would ultimately add billions more for development of vaccines.

Over the decades as Fauci's budget grew, so did his power. When the COVID pandemic hit, Fauci's power was at its zenith. He controlled billions of dollars in grants which, in turn, controlled the livelihoods of thousands of researchers. Fauci, over time, populated every position of authority in this military-science complex. Virtually no bureaucrat in the NIH held a position that was not a patronage of Fauci's largesse.

Like Hoover, Fauci developed hubris and narcissism over time. Like Hoover, Fauci created, with Francis Collins, an enemies list. In an email exchange that a federal judge forced him to release, Francis Collins pointedly tells Fauci to "take down" three internationally esteemed epidemiologists from Harvard, Stanford, and Oxford.

Unlike the abuses of Hoover that were ultimately and roundly condemned by the media and progressives, Fauci's excesses were coddled and glossed over by the Left. Submission of the population to mass edicts trumped any dispassionate critique of Fauci's abuse of power.

From atop his perch at the nation's biodefense research apparatus, Fauci felt safe outsourcing gain-of-function experiments on bat coronaviruses to China and bypassing the security protocol to screen out projects that posed too much risk.

J. Edgar Hoover and Anthony Fauci are two real-life examples of how too much power in too few hands creates an echo chamber where decisions cannot be questioned. But a free and open society depends upon questioning those in power. A people's trust in science depends upon it, too.

The American people deserve better. That's why I introduced the NIH Reform Act to divide the NIAID into three parts that align with its stated mission "to better understand, treat, and ultimately prevent infectious, immunologic, and allergic diseases."

As it's currently configured, the NIAID's jurisdiction covers everything from asthma to Ebola, from peanut allergies to the plague. My bill would replace it with three independent institutes: one for infectious diseases, one for immunologic diseases, and one for allergic diseases. The director of each new institute would be appointed by the president, confirmed by the Senate, and (in keeping with the 10-year precedent at the post-Hoover FBI) permitted to serve no more than two five-year terms.[24]

The Hacks React

In March of 2022, another victory for freedom of speech and debate occurred in what some might consider the unlikeliest of places, *Vanity Fair*. This is the same rag that just months before had this to say about me: "One of the loudest voices of misinformation and otherwise entirely unhelpful bullshit during the coronavirus pandemic has been Senator Rand Paul."[25]

So, it was with particular satisfaction that I discovered that even the worst of left-wing biased magazines, one that never seemed to print enough woke partisan blarney, was now open to the possibility that COVID-19 leaked from a lab. Hooray for the last remnants of journalism, however unrepentant and overdue.

Katherine Eban's article to the primarily left-leaning audience at *Vanity Fair* would continue to crumble Fauci's credibility. Eban discovered that Peter Daszak routinely schmoozed big-name bureaucrats with tony D.C. private soirées at the Cosmos Club. Daszak would routinely spend $8,000 on Brie, chardonnay, and who knows what for these cocktail parties intended to woo federal contracts.[26]

I couldn't resist a snarky retort on Twitter. I tweeted the link to Eban's article with this: "How did EcoHealth Alliance convince Fauci to give them over a $100 million? Well, an invitation to the Cosmos Club and this helpful tip from Fauci's staff: 'he normally says no to almost everything like this, unless ABC, NBC, CBS, and Fox are all there with cameras running.'"[27]

The Collusion of the Federal Bureaucracy

When Elon Musk purchased Twitter, America learned that it wasn't just the left-wing media pushing Fauci's narrative that the COVID pandemic could only have come from nature. The country discovered that spies from across the intelligence community were meeting with Twitter (that we know of) to censor any information that contradicted Fauci's opinions.[28]

The brave attorneys general of Louisiana and Missouri, Jeff Landry and Eric Schmitt, sued the federal government for using their offices to censor speech. They were successful in forcing Fauci to testify under oath. It turns out that "America's leading infectious disease expert" didn't seem to recall many details of his time atop the public health bureaucracy. It seems that making pronouncements was much more entertaining when he was receiving softball questions about baseball and football from obsequious broadcasters.

After the Fauci deposition, Landry tweeted, "Wow! It was amazing to spend 7 hours with Dr. Fauci. The man who single-handedly wrecked the U.S. economy based upon 'the science.' Only to discover that he can't recall practically anything dealing with his Covid response!"[29]

Landry summarized the case this way: "What we have in front of us is government actors then co-opting and coercing and colluding with private corporations—under which Americans utilize these corporations, these platforms, as basically a virtual public square—and having the government censor American speech."[30]

Bravo to attorneys general Landry and Schmitt for instigating this oversight action. The lawsuit is an important step for our country in reassessing the role of government in the public arena of speech.

Big Intel Aids and Abets the Cover-Up

The revelation that the FBI and other intel agencies were meeting with Twitter (and possibly other social media and tech concerns) and colluding with them to limit speech about vaccines, masks, and lockdowns of the economy and of schools should scare all defenders of the First Amendment.[31]

It shocks and concerns me that the Left, which once led the fight to end the FBI's trampling of the civil liberties of Vietnam War protestors and civil rights leaders, now largely is quiet or actually supportive of government censorship of so-called "misinformation."

It wasn't just government censoring contrary opinions on COVID. Pharmaceutical titans such as Pfizer jumped in to censor any opinions that might hurt vaccine sales. Scott Gottlieb was a former FDA commissioner before he became a well-compensated Pfizer board member ($365,000 from Pfizer in 2021 alone, according to Salary.com[32]). Gottlieb called his lobbyist to try to get Twitter to take down Brett Giroir, the former Trump associate secretary of the Department of Health and Human Services who had tweeted, "It's now clear #COVID19 natural immunity is superior to #vaccine immunity, by ALOT. There's no scientific justification for #vax proof if a person had prior infection."[33]

"This is the kind of stuff that's corrosive," Gottlieb told his Twitter lobbyist.

Who knew Pfizer board members had their own Twitter lobbyists?

Gottlieb went on to complain, "Here [Giroir] draws a sweeping conclusion off a single retrospective study in Israel that hasn't been peer reviewed. But this tweet will end up going viral and driving news coverage."[34]

And, of course, Gottlieb is not a disinterested party. His conflict likely runs into the millions of dollars he has or will receive from Pfizer. Time would also not be kind to Gottlieb's mercantile desire for censorship, as study after study would confirm that prior infection was indeed as good or better at preventing reinfection or illness with COVID-19.[35]

CHAPTER 18

Fauci and the COVID Booster for Children

A month later, Anthony Fauci was back before the U.S. Senate. On June 16, 2022, he and I squared off again. This time it was over his push to have every child in America given not one, not two, but *three* COVID vaccines. And while he would resist anyone charging that he wanted to mandate the vaccine for kids, it was common knowledge that his recommendation and the CDC's recommendation would have the cascading result of ultimately pushing states to mandate the COVID vaccine for children.

> **Senator Paul:** Dr. Fauci, the government recommends everybody take a booster over age five. Are you aware of any studies that show a reduction in hospitalization or death for children who take a booster?

Dr. Fauci: Right now, there is not enough data that has been accumulated, Senator Paul, to indicate that that is the case. I believe that the recommendation that was made was based on the assumption that if you look at the morbidity and mortality of children within each of the age groups, you know, zero to five, five to eleven—

Senator Paul: Right. So there are *no* studies—and Americans should all know this—there are no studies on children showing a reduction in hospitalization or death with taking a booster. The only studies that were permitted, the only studies that were presented, were antibody studies.

So they say if we give you a booster, you make antibodies. Now a lot of scientists would question whether or not that is proof of efficacy of a vaccine. If a patient is given ten mRNA vaccines and they make protein each time or they make antibody each time, does that prove that we should give ten boosters, Dr. Fauci?

Dr. Fauci: No, I think that is somewhat of an absurd exaggeration, Senator Paul.

Senator Paul: Well that is the proof that *you* use. Your committees use that. That is the only proof you have to tell children to take a booster so that they make antibodies. So it is not an absurdity. You are already at like five boosters for people. You have had, you know, two or three boosters. Where is the proof?

Now, I think there is probably some indication for older folks that have some risk factors. For younger folks, there is not. But here is the other thing. There are some risk factors for the vaccine. So the risk of myocarditis with a second dose for adolescent boys, twelve to twenty-four, is about eighty per one million.

This is both from the CDC and from the Israeli study. It is also in the VAERS study, remarkably similar, for boys, much higher for boys than girls, and much higher than the background. The background is about two per one million. So there is risk and there are risks. And you are telling everybody in America just blindly go out there because vaccines induce antibodies. So it is not an absurd corollary to say if you give ten vaccines [you'll create antibodies each time]. In fact, you probably make antibodies if you get a hundred boosters, all right. That is not science. That is conjecture. And we should not be making public policy on it.

Dr. Fauci: So, Senator Paul, if I might respond to that, we just heard, in his opening statement, Ranking Member Burr talk about his staff who went to Israel. And if you look at the data from Israel, the boosts, both the third-shot boost and the fourth-shot boost, were associated with a clear-cut clinical effect, mostly in elderly people, but also as they gathered more data, even in people in the forties and the fifties. So there is clinical data—

Senator Paul: But not in children. The thing is, you are not willing to be honest with the American people. So, for example, 75 percent of kids have had the disease. Why is the CDC not including this in the data? You can ask the question. You can do laboratory tests to find out who has had COVID and who hasn't had the disease.

What is the incidence of hospitalization and death for children who have been infected with COVID subsequently going to the hospital and dying? What is the possibility that if your kid has had COVID—which 75 percent of the country has)—what is the chance that my child is going to the hospital or dying?

Dr. Fauci: If you look at the number of deaths in pediatrics, Senator, you can see that there are more deaths—

I continued to ask Fauci how many children who had previously been infected had become reinfected and died, but he refused to provide a straightforward answer.

Dr. Fauci: Senator, we also know from other studies that the optimal degree of protection when you get infection is to get vaccinated after infection. And in fact, showing reinfection in the era of Omicron and the sub-lineages, that vaccinated—
Senator Paul: But you can't answer the question I asked. The question I asked is, how many kids are dying and how many kids are going to the hospital who have already had COVID? The answer may be zero, but you are not even giving us the data because you have so much wanted to protect everybody from all the data because [you believe] the public is not smart enough to look at the data.

When you released data earlier, when the CDC released the data, they left out the category of eighteen to forty-nine on whether or not there was a health benefit for adults eighteen to forty-nine. Why was it left out? When critics finally complained, it was finally included and it showed there was no health benefit from taking a booster [for those] between the [ages of] eighteen to forty-nine in the CDC study.

Another question for you: The NIH continues to refuse to voluntarily divulge the names of scientists who receive royalties and from which companies. Over the period of time from 2010 to 2016, twenty-seven thousand royalty payments were paid to eighteen hundred NIH employees. We know that not because you told us, but because we *forced* you to tell us through the Freedom of Information Act.

Over $193 million was given to these eighteen hundred employees.[1] Can you tell me that you have not received a royalty from any entity that you ever oversaw the distribution of money in research grants?

Dr. Fauci: Well, first of all, let's talk about royalties.

Senator Paul: That is the question. No, that is the question. Have you ever overseen or received a royalty payment from a company that you later oversaw money going to that company?

Dr. Fauci: You know, I don't know as a fact, but I doubt it.

Senator Paul: Why don't you let us know? Why don't you reveal how much you've gotten and from what entities? The NIH refuses.... We ask them whether or not, who got it, and how much—they refuse to tell us. They send it redacted. Here's what I want to know—it's not just about you, [it's about] everybody on the vaccine committee. Have any of them ever received money from the people who make vaccines? Can you tell me that? Can you tell me if anybody on the vaccine approval committees ever received any money from the people making the vaccines?[2]

Dr. Fauci: Are you going to let me answer a question? Sound bite number one. Are you going to let me answer a question? Okay. So let me give you some information. First of all, according to the regulations, people who receive royalties are not required to divulge them even on their financial statements, according to the Bayh-Dole Act.

So let me give you some example. From 2015 to 2020, I—the only royalties I have was my lab, and I made a monoclonal antibody for use in-vitro reagent that had nothing to do with patients. And during that period of time, my royalties ranged from $21 a year to $700 a year, and the average per year was $191.46.

Senator Paul: It is all redacted, and you can't get any information on the NIH—

The Chairman: Senator Paul, your time—

Senator Paul: So we want to know whether or not scientists received payments got from the people who manufacture vaccines...

The Chairman: Senator Paul, your time is long over expired. I gave you an additional two and a half minutes. The witness has responded. We are going to move on.[3]

The Biomedical Research Royalty Kickback Circus

Fauci's evasion from directly answering the vaccine-royalty questions leads inquiring minds to ask, *If you have nothing to hide, why the lack of transparency?* Stories abound of NIAID researchers "supplement[ing] their income with honoraria they earn by attending Pharma seminars and briefing pharmaceutical company personnel..."[4] A 2004 investigation by the Office of Government Ethics faulted Fauci for monetary arrangements between NIAID staff and Big Pharma. The investigation found that "two-thirds of NIAID's workers...were moonlighting in private industry."[5]

While Fauci himself hides behind legislation he claims allows government researchers to keep secret their royalties, his personal wealth has grown and grown. Fauci and his wife take home nearly $750,000 a year from their government jobs, not counting any royalties. Indeed, Fauci has grown rich in "the service of his country." Estimates are that his fortune doubled during the pandemic. OpenTheBooks reported that

Fauci's net worth "increased by $5 million between 2019 and 2021, and now exceeds $12.6 million." Somehow it is even legal for Fauci to take *foreign* money. During the pandemic, the Dan David Foundation based in Liechtenstein gave him nearly a million dollars for "speaking truth to power" and "defending science."[6] Who knew "science" could be so profitable?

Fauci referenced the Bayh-Dole Act when he claimed scientists working for the government don't have to divulge their royalties. My legislative team looked at the law and disagrees. According to my team, "The Bayh-Dole Act does specify that certain information deemed to be commercial and financial information provided to the federal agencies regarding the utilization of subject inventions is not subject to disclosure under FOIA without the permission of the contractor. It is not clear that royalty payments to NIH employees should be covered under this prohibition."

We sent an appeal to the Government Accountability Office to try to force the NIH to adhere to the law, not make up the law.

In addition, several other Senators and I sent a letter to the NIH demanding information. We wrote the following:

> Each year, NIH awards tens of billions of dollars in the form of federal grants, and under §401.10 of the Patent and Trademark Law Amendments (Bayh-Dole) Act, federal agencies and employees may receive royalty payments for products and inventions when listed as an inventor or "co-inventor" on a product's patent.
>
> A 2020 study conducted by the Government Accountability Office showed that, in total, 93 NIH patents contributed to 34 FDA-approved prescription drugs, generating roughly $2 billion in royalty payments to the agency between 1991–2019. In 2004 alone, some 900 NIH scientists earned approximately

$8.9 million in royalties for drugs and inventions they discovered while working for the government.

In 2005, the National Institutes of Health (NIH) implemented a policy requiring its employees to disclose these royalty payments on the consent forms for clinical trial participants; however, the agency has taken no action to disclose such payments to the public at large. In fact, even after the nonprofit organization Open the Books submitted a Freedom of Information Act (FOIA) request to disclose royalty payments made between 2009 and 2020, the agency only provided the names of the employees receiving the payments and the number of payments they received between 2009 and 2014; the amounts of the individual payments, the innovation in question, and the names of the third-party payers were redacted by NIH. These FOIA redactions contradict a 2005 statement by an NIH spokesman that an entity "would have to make a request via the Freedom of Information Act to find out royalty payments to individual researchers."

We request [from the NIH] . . . royalty payments made by third parties to [NIH] employees between January 1, 2009, and December 31, 2021 . . . [including]:

1. The amount and date of each individual royalty payment made by third-party payers to employees and administrators of the National Institutes of Health, [including] the names, official employment titles, and pay grades of the recipients, as well as the names of the third-party payers.
2. The aggregate amount each NIH employee/administrator received in royalty payments.

3. Regarding royalty payments made by pharmaceutical companies to employees of the National Institutes of Health between January 1, 2018, to March 1, 2022, please provide...the following:

4. The dollar amount and date of each individual royalty payment made by pharmaceutical companies [with companies identified] to employees and administrators of the National Institutes of Health....

5. As required by the criminal conflicts of interest law at 18 U.S.C. § 208(a), Federal employees may not participate personally and substantially in any particular matter in which they know they have a financial interest unless they first obtain a written waiver or qualify for a regulatory exemption.

6. Have all NIH employees receiving royalty payments by pharmaceutical companies completed this written waiver or qualified for regulatory exemption? If not, please explain why.[7]

The NIH responded with a nonresponse. None of the questions were answered. The NIH basically said, "Sorry, not sorry. We don't have to tell you anything." NIH did not give us the information we requested and justified that by stating that the royalties are not subject to disclosure as privileged and confidential information. Their letter also argues that royalties are considered income by the government, which is also not required to be reported.

The NIH responded to their allies in the press, "Royalty payments to NIH inventors are considered income and NIH does not track how individual employee incomes are spent, beyond what falls under federal financial disclosure requirements."[8]

OpenTheBooks, a nonprofit watchdog group, revealed that "between fiscal years 2010 and 2020, more than $350 million in royalties were paid by third-parties to the agency and NIH scientists—who are credited as co-inventors." These royalties are largely from pharmaceutical companies.

The NIH under the forty-year tutelage of Anthony Fauci dispenses about $30 billion in grants to over fifty thousand scientists, and NIH scientists receive back hundreds of millions of dollars with no transparency.

As OpenTheBooks stated, "Because those payments enrich the agency and its scientists, each and every royalty payment could be a potential conflict of interest and needs disclosure."[9]

OpenTheBooks discovered these royalty payments only after suing the NIH in federal court. OpenTheBooks commented on how difficult it was to obtain this supposedly public information: "Since the NIH documents are heavily redacted, we can only see how many payments each scientist received, and, separately, the aggregate dollars per NIH agency. This is a gatekeeping at odds with the spirit and perhaps the letter of open-records laws."

OpenTheBooks describes how, at every turn, those at the NIH did whatever they could to hide the information. In addition to resisting the Freedom of Information Act, the NIH "used expensive taxpayer-funded litigation to slow-walk royalty disclosures (releasing the oldest royalties first). Although the agency admits to holding 3,000 pages, it will take ten months to produce them (300 pages per month)."[10]

Even when a federal judge forced the NIH to comply, they "heavily redacted key information on the royalty payments. For example, the agency erased...the payment amount, and...who paid it! This makes the court-mandated production virtually worthless, despite our use of the latest forensic auditing tools."[11]

The "sainted" Dr. Fauci apparently is no stranger to using lawyers and tax dollars to do everything he can to rule his fiefdom in secrecy.

In late 2022, Moderna inked a deal to share profits with NIH since NIH had partially funded the research and held some of the patents used in the process.[12] A first payment of $400 million dollars was sent to NIH in the spring of 2023.[13] Talk about conflict of interest. The same public officials promoting vaccine mandates were now receiving over $400 million from the vaccine manufacturers. That money would ultimately end up in the pockets of these same scientists in the form of salaries and grants.

We immediately asked which individuals received the money and whether any of these individuals create or influence policy on vaccine mandates, which would of course be a huge conflict of interest.

Bernie Sanders complained to me that Moderna signed the deal before he became chairman of the HELP Committee, trying to evade his oversight.[14] He's likely correct.

In March of 2023, Senator Sanders announced he would bring the CEO of Moderna before our committee. A few days before the testimony, the Moderna president, a fellow physician, came to my office for a private chat. The conversation was relaxed and nonconfrontational. The Moderna president was quite open and honest about the vaccine-induced risks of myocarditis in adolescent boys.[15] I was shocked when I asked the same questions of Moderna's CEO in a public hearing and got what sounded to me like wildly different answers.

CHAPTER 19

Will the Real Fauci Please Stand Up...

The internet erupted when some sleuth discovered a C-SPAN interview with Dr. Fauci from 2004. I thought it might be interesting to confront him with his own words, indeed, with his own televised words.

So when Fauci appeared once again before the HELP Committee on September 14, 2022, I decided to play the forty-second video of the C-SPAN interview. The problem was that Patty Murray, the far-left senator from Washington State, had created a rule banning video—unless, of course, it was *her* video. My staff warned me she might try to sabotage my presentation.

I decided the best plan was to ask for forgiveness, not permission. My strategy was to start the video before beginning my remarks. I had my staff put my iPad on the desktop in front of me, direct the microphone toward it, and push play. My hope was that the video would be finished before the Democrats complained. As luck would have it, Murray had stepped out, and Bob Casey from Pennsylvania was filling in—and not fast enough on the trigger to stop me.

Casey recognized me for my questions. My staff immediately set the iPad down and hit play.

The C-SPAN video clip began playing:

News Anchor: But she has had the flu for fourteen days. Should she get a flu shot?
Dr. Fauci: Well, no. If she got the flu for fourteen days, she is as protected as anybody can be, because the best vaccination is to get infected yourself.
News Anchor: And—
Dr. Fauci: If she really has the flu, if she really has the flu, she definitely doesn't need a flu vaccine—if she really has the flu.
News Anchor: She should not get it again?
Dr. Fauci: She doesn't need it, because it is the best—it is the most potent vaccination is getting infected yourself. [End of video clip.][1]
Senator Paul: This is an ongoing question. And, you know, we have had ever-evolving opinions from you, Dr. Fauci. Currently, antibody surveys show that 80 percent of children, approximately 80 percent of children have had COVID.

And yet there are no guidelines coming from you or anybody in the government to take into account their naturally acquired immunity. You seemed quite certain of yourself in 2004, but in 2022 there is a lot less certainty. One of the things that we also know, after looking at this for two to three years, is that the mortality from COVID is very similar, if not less than influenza.

So when we look at this, we wonder, you know, why you seemed to really embrace basic immunology back in 2004, and why you seem to reject it now.

Dr. Fauci: Well, I don't reject basic immunology, Senator, and I have never denied that there is importance of the protection following infection.

However, as we have said many times, and as has been validated by the authorization of the—by the FDA through their committee and the recommendation by the CDC through their committee, that a vaccination following infection gives an added extra boost. And that film that you showed is really taken out of context.

I believe that was when someone called in who had had a reaction to a vaccine and asked me through a telephone in the interview if they should get vaccinated again. So it was in the context of someone who had a reaction.

And as a matter of fact, Reuters fact-check looked at that and said [that] Fauci's 2004 comments do not contradict his pandemic stance.

Senator Paul: Actually, words don't lie. If you look at the words behind me, we can go over them a little bit at a time. [You said and I repeat]: "She doesn't need it because the most potent vaccination is getting infected yourself."

Dr. Fauci: It is true. It is true, Senator. It is a very potent way to protect.

Senator Paul: So when you are trying to tell us that kids need a third or a fourth vaccine, are you including the variable of previous infection in the studies? No, you are not. Because the committees that have approved the COVID vaccine for children don't report anything on hospitalization or death or transmission.[2]

They only report the fact that if you give them the jab, they will make antibodies. And you can give kids hundreds of jabs and they will make antibodies every time, but that does not prove efficacy. So what you are doing is denying the very fundamental premise of immunology, that previous infection does provide some sort of immunity. It is not in any of your studies.

Almost none of your studies from the CDC or from the government have the variable of whether or not you have been previously infected. So let's look at adults [who have] had three injections. Should they get a fourth one?

If you are going to measure whether you get a fourth one, you need a category that has a fourth one in it, and you need one that has nothing in it: no vaccine versus the fourth vaccine. But you also need to know whether the individual has been previously infected. If you ignore whether they have been infected, you are essentially ignoring a vaccine, you are ignoring a variable.

So when you decry and people decry "vaccine hesitancy," realize it is a result of the gobbledygook that you give us. You are not paying attention to the science; the very basic science is that previous infection provides a level of immunity.

If you ignore that in your studies, if you don't present that in your committees, you are not being truthful or honest with us.

Dr. Fauci: Senator, if I might respond, I have never, ever denied fundamental immunology. In fact, I wrote the chapter in the textbook of medicine on fundamental immunology. You know—

[I should have asked him to re-read it, as his pronouncements showed no evidence of his having written or read his own chapter.]

Senator Paul: Do any of the government guidelines for vaccines factor in previous infection in the determination of whether to vaccinate or not? Do any of the guidelines consider previous infection? Because you neglected to consider previous infection in the guidelines, you can conveniently ignore and discount important medical choices for patients. And furthermore, we have been asking—and you refuse to answer—whether anybody on the vaccine committees gets royalties from the pharmaceutical companies.[3]

I asked you last time, and what was your response? "We don't have to tell you."

We have demanded an answer through the Freedom of Information Act, and what have you said? "We are not going to tell you."

But I tell you this, when [the Republicans regain control of Congress], we are going to change the rules, and you will have to divulge where you get your royalties from, from what companies—and if anybody in the committee has a conflict of interest, we are going to learn about it, I promise you that.[4]

Dr. Fauci: Mr. Chair, can I respond to that, please?

Senator Casey: You may.

Dr. Fauci: Okay. There are two aspects for what you said. You keep saying, "You approve, you do this, you do that." The committees that give the approval are FDA, through their advisory committee.

The committees that recommend are CDC through their advisory committee. And you keep saying I am the one that is approving a vaccine based on certain data. So I don't really understand, with all due respect, Senator—

Senator Paul: You are the one that said you would not reveal—you would not reveal what company gave you royalties or what company gave the other scientists royalties—

At this point, Senator Casey wrapped up my question time, but couldn't resist a moment of chastising me over the video I played: "Senator Paul, you are over. Everyone is over a little bit. I just want to make sure we keep on time here. For the record, I know Chair Murray and previous chairs of this committee of both parties, both parties, have found videos to be out of order, and I will note for the record, the video is out of order."[5]

Ending the Royalty Racket

It certainly was out of order, but worth every second of it to watch Fauci squirm and try to weasel out of his own words. Pathetic.

In a Fox News interview the same day, I reiterated my call for transparency with regard to royalty payments to members of the vaccine-approval committees, but really for *all* of the U.S. government's scientific bureaucracy. I repeatedly asked what reason could possibly justify withholding this information.

Members of Congress must publicly disclose all sources of income in order to reduce conflicts of interest and ensure transparency. Why shouldn't the same rules be applied to government scientists entrusted with making billion-dollar decisions regarding drug approval? Doesn't the American public deserve to know if the scientist *approving* vaccines is benefitting from the very companies *manufacturing* the vaccines?

It continues to disturb me that the mainstream media lets Fauci and the rest get away with not divulging their royalties. Imagine if a local school board member voted to award a textbook contract to a book company but did not reveal that he or she owned the book company. There would be hell to pay.

But eighteen hundred scientists collected $193 million in royalties, and not a peep from most of the fourth estate as to whether those royalties might present a conflict of interest.[6]

CHAPTER 20

Exposing the Gain-of-Function Shell Game

For over two years, I lobbied without success to get chairmen Gary Peters (D-MI) and Bernie Sanders (I-VT) to hold hearings on the origins of COVID-19. They stonewalled me every step of the way. This should disturb every American, whether you are a Republican, a Democrat, or an Independent.

Why were these entrenched chairmen so opposed to investigating the source of the COVID pandemic that killed millions? Why was there a concerted effort to cover up and obscure the origins of the virus?

Finally, as election season began to heat up in the summer of 2022, Maggie Hassan (D-NH) agreed to allow me to hold a hearing via her subcommittee of Homeland Security. I titled the hearing "Revisiting Gain-of-Function Research: What the Pandemic Taught Us and Where Do We Go from Here?"[1]

Shamefully, Democrats largely boycotted the hearing. Meanwhile, CNN and MSNBC continued to complain that the debate had become politicized. But who exactly was politicizing the debate? The hearing I organized included three prominent scientists, none of whom were known to be partisan.

The hearing opened with only Republicans present. Jon Ossoff (D-GA) popped in momentarily, but seeing no Democrat colleagues, he left without listening to testimony or asking questions. Subcommittee chair Hassan didn't bother to show up at all, breaking with tradition and proffering an insult at the same time—not to me, but to the American people.

On August 3, 2022, I offered this opening statement:

> Good afternoon and welcome to each of our panelists. Thank you for joining us. The purpose of this hearing by the Subcommittee on Emerging Threats and Spending Oversight is to discuss, as our name implies, the emerging threat posed by gain-of-function research.
>
> We will hear from a panel of three witnesses, all of whom are extraordinarily accomplished experts in the scientific community. We are grateful for that work, and we are grateful to each of you for taking the time to appear here with us this afternoon.
>
> Gain-of-function research is a controversial scientific research method involving the manipulation of pathogens to give them a new aspect or ability, such as making viruses more transmissible or dangerous to humans. Despite all we have learned about the potential risks of this particular method of research, this is the first congressional hearing on the subject.

Today we will discuss 1.) what gain-of-function research entails, 2.) how gain-of-function research is defined, and 3.) whether the definition of gain-of-function research is applied consistently by the Department of Health and Human Services P3CO Review Committee, which is responsible for evaluating the risks & benefits of such research.

We'll also discuss how this Potential Pandemic Pathogen Care and Oversight Committee (P3CO) operates. The P3CO approves or denies projects [to receive or not receive] federal funding based on whether the pathogen is considered to be a "credible source of a potential future human pandemic," and if "the potential risks as compared to the potential benefits to society are justified." In other words, a project is not gain-of-function if the review committee is unsure if a recombinant virus will create a future pandemic. Such a broad criterion gives one sole committee, comprised of an unknown group of bureaucrats, the power to spend millions of taxpayer dollars on a single preemptive guess—with potentially devastating consequences.

Today we will also consider whether gain-of-function research was being performed at the Wuhan Institute of Virology. First, no one—not myself or anyone I'm aware of—argues that a recombinant super-virus that has been published in scientific journals is COVID-19 or a close relative. If COVID-19 leaked from the Wuhan lab, it would be a laboratory-created virus that the Wuhan scientists have not yet, and are unlikely to ever, reveal.

I maintain that the techniques that the NIH funded in Wuhan to create enhanced pathogens may also have been used to create COVID-19. The American people deserve to know how this pandemic started, and to know whether NIH-funded research caused this pandemic.

Gain-of-function research has the potential to unleash a global pandemic that threatens the lives of millions, yet this is only the first time the issue has been discussed in a congressional committee. I am sure each member of this committee as well as the full Senate can agree that we need stronger government oversight of how our tax dollars are being used to finance experimenting with mutating fatal diseases with outstandingly high mortality rates.

Again, I thank each of our distinguished witnesses for being here today, and I thank Senator Hassan for working with me to convene this hearing.[2]

Finally, Testimony from Scientists

In the August 3, 2022, U.S. Senate Homeland Security and Governmental Affairs Committee hearing, my expert witnesses included esteemed scientists with hundreds of peer-reviewed journal articles between them. Their testimonies were created individually and without cooperation between them, but they came up with remarkably similar ideas for preventing future pandemic pathogens from escaping laboratory settings.

One of the witnesses was molecular biologist Dr. Richard Ebright, Ph.D. He is the Board of Governors Professor of Chemistry and Chemical Biology at Rutgers and Laboratory Director at the Waksman Institute of Microbiology. Dr. Ebright serves as project leader on two National Institutes of Health (NIH) research grants. His research involves both priority public health bacterial pathogens, such as staph infections, strep infections, and tuberculosis, and priority biodefense bacterial pathogens, such as pathogens responsible for anthrax, plague, and tularemia. Ebright is also a member of the Institutional Biosafety Committee of Rutgers University and has been a member of the Working Group on Pathogen Security of the state of New Jersey, the Controlling Dangerous Pathogens Project of the Center for International Security Studies, and the Biosecurity Advisory Board of the Center for Civilian Biodefense.

Our second expert witness was Dr. Steven Quay, M.D., Ph.D. Quay is a biotech entrepreneur and founder of Atossa Therapeutics. He received his M.D. and Ph.D. in biochemistry from the University of Michigan. Quay did a postdoctoral fellowship at MIT with Nobel laureate H. Gobind Khorana, was a resident at Harvard Mass General Hospital, and was on the faculty of Stanford University School of Medicine. He has invented seven FDA-approved drugs, holds ninety-three patents, and is coauthor of the book *The Origin of the Virus: The Hidden Truths behind the Microbe That Killed Millions of People.*[3]

Our third expert, Dr. Kevin Esvelt of MIT, came to my attention when he published an op-ed on October 6, 2021, in the *Washington Post.* The *Post* describes Esvelt as "an evolutionary and ecological engineer and an assistant professor at MIT and an inventor of CRISPR-based gene technology." Simply the fact that the mainstay and flagship of liberalism, the *Washington Post*, chose to print a reasoned, insightful look at the risks of gain of function was an amazing step forward. Especially when you consider that for a year and a half Fauci and his yes-men had been throwing the entire weight of the billion-dollar medical industrial complex at anyone who dared to question the party line.

Esvelt's op-ed entitled "Manipulating Viruses and Risking Pandemics Is Too Dangerous. It's Time to Stop" was a long-awaited breath of fresh air, and so important that I've reprinted it in its entirety:

> For 20 years, taxpayer-funded research programs have sought to identify or create pandemic-causing viruses, all

with surprisingly little transparency. The latest evidence of the problem surfaced on Sept. 21 when a group of online snoops released purportedly leaked documents revealing a 2018 grant proposal. The proposal, which went unfunded, sought $14.2 million for a project to discover, combine and engineer highly infectious SARS-like coronaviruses.

Much of the attention stirred by the revelation focused on the proposal's inclusion of preliminary data from the Wuhan Institute of Virology—a Chinese lab under scrutiny as a possible source of the covid-19 pandemic.

Questions about public oversight, accident risks and pandemic origins are all legitimate. But perhaps the biggest question of all isn't being asked insistently enough: Why is anyone trying to teach the world how to make viruses that could kill millions of people?

Like nuclear physics, with its potential for global catastrophe when put to destructive ends, the proliferation of pandemic biology ought to be considered a matter of international security.

Making a nuclear weapon requires the resources of a nation-state, but many individuals can now single-handedly build and edit viruses. Some fearmongers about biotechnology claim that anyone could do this in a garage. That's mistaken; such bioengineering requires years of training. Still, the number of people who can build a virus from synthetic DNA is not small. In my own laboratory at MIT alone, five people have that capability.

So why search for new pandemic viruses? The enticing idea: If researchers could learn which of the estimated 500,000 animal viruses that could spill over into humans might actually cause the next pandemic, then we may be able to prepare defenses against the most threatening ones.

But to credibly identify a single virus as capable of causing a pandemic is to give thousands the power to wield it as a weapon. To discover many dangerous viruses, or learn to enhance weaker ones, is to share the blueprints for an arsenal of plagues.

Good people advocate for such research, and the world needs someone to make the case—it's always possible that the benefits of the knowledge will be worth it. Perhaps the likelihood of virus misuse and accidents is tiny, natural spillovers are more common than history suggests, and studying nature's killers would save even more lives.

But before we discover viruses that might rival nuclear weapons in lethality, we should be aware that the consequences of misuse could be worse than if any of those pathogens spilled over naturally. A malevolent individual could introduce multiple pandemic viruses in different locations around the world—say, at half a dozen major airports—making containment nearly impossible.

Thankfully, we don't yet know of any animal viruses expected to cause a pandemic if deliberately released. That won't last if gain-of-function research projects succeed in engineering or evolving ones that can. Even more alarmingly, multiple health agencies around the world are actively funding efforts to find, study and rank-order the animal viruses most likely to cause a new pandemic.

These projects are the work of well-meaning scientists doing their best to save us from natural plagues. But they are biomedical researchers and epidemiologists, not defense experts; security and nonproliferation issues aren't part of their training or mandate. Once we consider the possibility of misuse, let alone creative misuse, such research looks like a gamble that civilization can't afford to risk.

Many physicists who contributed to the Manhattan Project lived to see nuclear proliferation threaten the world. For pandemics, the critical experiments have not yet been performed. I implore every scientist, funder and nation working in this field: Please stop. No more trying to discover or make pandemic-capable viruses, enhance their virulence, or assemble them more easily. No more attempting to learn which components allow viruses to efficiently infect or replicate within human cells, or to devise inheritable ways to evade immunity. No more experiments likely to disseminate blueprints for plagues.

There are few commercial or strategic incentives to attempt any of these things, and even if some nation-states continued experimenting in defiance of nonproliferation agreements, at least the work would go far more slowly than if the scientific community led the way.

Instead, health and security agencies should work together, ideally with considerably more than the $65 billion requested by the White House, to build adequate defenses against future pandemics. We need sequencing-based early-warning networks to detect anything becoming exponentially more common in airport wastewater or clinical samples, millions of diagnostic tests and vaccine doses made available within weeks of a threat identification and comfortable powered respirators for every essential worker.

Natural pandemics may be inevitable. Synthetic ones, constructed with full knowledge of society's vulnerabilities, are not. Let's not learn to make pandemics until we can reliably defend against them.[4]

Esvelt, Ebright, and Quay all testified to the dangers of gain-of-function research. In fact, all three were on the record previously as labeling the EcoHealth Alliance's research in Wuhan as gain of function. In the spring of 2021, Esvelt commented that the research performed in Wuhan funded by EcoHealth used "certain techniques that...seemed to meet the definition of gain-of-function research."[5]

Ebright also has been quite clear about the research the NIH and NIAID funded in Wuhan: "The EcoHealth/Wuhan lab research 'was—unequivocally—gain-of-function research.'"[6]

Dr. Ebright's testimony focused initially on what gain-of-function research is and why it is dangerous: "Gain-of-function research of concern is defined as research activities reasonably anticipated to increase a potential pandemic pathogen's transmissibility, pathogenesis, ability to overcome immune response, or ability to overcome a vaccine or drug. Some definitions also include research activities reasonably anticipated to reconstruct an extinct or eradicated potential pandemic pathogen."[7]

Dr. Quay defined gain of function "as making artificial changes to a microbe in a laboratory, seeing what new properties it acquires by those changes, and then often performing additional research to find vaccines or therapeutics that can stop this synthetic virus. So create something that doesn't exist in nature and see if you can kill it."[8]

Ebright explained that gain-of-function research "involves the creation of *new health threats*—health threats that did not exist previously and that might not come to exist by natural means for tens, hundreds, thousands, or tens of thousands of years. Most gain-of-function research of concern to date has been performed in the US with US funding or overseas with US funding."[9]

Fauci and the advocates of gain-of-function research argue that it would be a mistake to let government regulate science, but the truth is that government has an obligation to oversee where and how tax dollars are spent. Besides, the debate over regulating gain-of-function research is really a debate over a small niche in a wide ocean of scientific research.

As Ebright explained, "Gain-of-function research of concern is a small part of biomedical research (less than 0.1% of all biomedical research and less than 1% of virology)."[10]

Quay agreed that the dangerous research we were discussing was only "a tiny sliver of all the research funded by NIH. Specifically, there were over 36,000 RO1 grants funded by NIH in 2020, the latest year with statistics. Of these, the self-described 'gain-of-function on potential pathogens' research grants numbered only twenty-one in the latest funding year. Even expanding this by tenfold with a less stringent definition of gain-of-function would mean we are talking about less than 1% of all NIH research funding."[11]

Even though gain-of-function research comprises a small portion of government-funded research, the danger is so disproportionately high that our government is inviting tragedy by ignoring these risks.

Professor Ebright explained why the risks of this type of research are potentially catastrophic: "Gain-of-function research of concern poses *material risks* by creating new or enhanced potential pandemic pathogens. If a resulting new potential pandemic pathogen is released into humans, either by accident or deliberately, this can cause a pandemic."[12]

To those critics who argue that the research could be safeguarded, Ebright responded that "the risks posed by gain-of-function research of concern are *inherent* risks. In some cases, the risks can be mitigated, but in no case can the risks be eliminated."

As to the benefits of this type of research, Ebright was skeptical that the benefits would outweigh the risks. According to Ebright, "gain-of-function research of concern has no civilian practical applications. In particular, gain-of-function research of concern is not needed for, and does not contribute to, the development of vaccines and drugs. (Companies develop vaccines and drugs against pathogens that exist and circulate in humans. Not against pathogens that do not yet exist and do not yet circulate in humans.)"

Ebright was quite convicted that "Gain-of-function research of concern is performed because it is easy and fast (much faster and much easier than vaccine or drug development) and because, it is fundable and publishable. Not because it is needed."[13]

Dr. Quay's testimony agreed with Ebright's assessment. Quay began by asking, "Has gain-of-function research been useful to the COVID19 response or other public health infectious disease emergencies?"

In Quay's analysis, "[T]he collected gain-of-function research over approximately two decades... [did not show] findings that could reasonably be considered to have helped in either the COVID pandemic or other smaller epidemics."[14]

The historical argument had been that since vaccines can take years to develop, wouldn't it be wiser to try to identify pathogens *before* they cause a pandemic and make the vaccine in advance? The problem with this argument is that after a decade or two, no such vaccine was ever designed in advance, largely because it was impossible to predict what pathogens would cross over from the animal kingdom to the human sphere.

Now with the advent of mRNA technology, as Quay pointed out in his testimony, "we know that an mRNA vaccine can be designed within literally days of a new outbreak once the pathogen is sequenced, and large-scale manufacturing can begin soon thereafter. This capability has now been fully road tested and provides, in my opinion, the best defensive capability against future microbes."[15]

Was COVID-19 the Result of Gain of Function Gone Awry?

To understand how and why scientists might have altered COVID-19 (SARS-CoV-2) in the lab, Quay explained how COVID-19 infects human cells. The process of the virus entering the cell is "governed by the two-step verification system.... Step one is the handshake between the receptor binding domain and the human ACE2 receptor on the surface of the human respiratory system. Step two is the spike protein cleavage site, in CoV-2 the so-called furin cleavage site, which puts a cut in the spike protein. At that point the virus injects its genetic material into the cell and begins the 12 hour or so process of replicating. This ends with the cell dissolving and thousands of new viruses being released."

To Quay, it was extraordinary that "in SARS-CoV-2, the receptor binding domain was largely perfected for human infection. Specifically, the first virus to infect humans had only 17 mutations it could make out of 4,000 that would improve the ACE2 handshake." In other words, the vast majority of mutations needed to allow COVID-19 to interact with human ACE2 receptors had already occurred when the very first person was infected with COVID-19. COVID-19 showed up with a 99.5 percent fit. Whereas, as Quay points out, when SARS1 began infecting people, the virus "had only 15% of the mutations needed for the epidemic."[16]

The Australian professor Nikolai Petrovsky was also fascinated by the pre-adapted nature of COVID to almost perfectly fit the human ACE2 receptor. Petrovsky is the director of endocrinology at Flinders University.

In a unique experiment, Professor Petrovsky used Oracle's supercomputer to run a model asking the question of which animal host receptors are best adapted to interact with COVID-19, the hypothesis being that the animal whose receptors best fit COVID-19 would be the likely source of the virus.

Petrovsky wanted to see which animals were best able to bind COVID-19 to a cell-surface receptor called ACE2. Animals have these receptors also, but they are different in each species. One of the reasons COVID-19 is so infectious is that it binds very well to human ACE2 receptors. In fact, COVID-19 binds to human ACE2 receptors at least ten times better than the original SARS1 virus. Petrovsky loaded all the information for ACE2 receptors for many different possible animal hosts and then asked the supercomputer to predict from which animal COVID-19 most likely made the leap. Petrovsky had the result in March of 2020.

The answer was extraordinary. The animal best able to bind COVID-19 was…humans! As journalist Sharri Markson reported in her book, "Normally with a new pandemic virus, whatever species that virus came from would be the best fit and the virus would initially half fit the human lock but then mutate over time to try and become a better fit."[17]

Petrovsky described this in his published paper: "This finding is particularly surprising as, typically, a virus, would be expected to have the highest affinity for the receptor in its original host species, e.g. bat, with a lower initial binding affinity for the receptor of the new host, e.g. humans."[18]

Petrovsky's experiment throws shade on Fauci's contention that COVID-19 came naturally from animals. Not surprisingly, the medical establishment tried to blackball and delay publication of Petrovsky's study. Initially, the study was submitted to pre-print servers for peer review but was rejected. Only Petrovsky's perseverance enabled the paper to finally get published.

The whole experience left Petrovsky wondering if ". . . only research suggesting a natural origin [would] be allowed to see the light of day."[19]

The evidence was stacking up. COVID-19 presented with almost all of the adaptations necessary to be readily transmissible among humans, whereas SARS1 started out with only 15 percent of the mutations needed to transmit among humans and took a significant period of time to obtain enough mutations to be infectious among humans. In fact, SARS1 never adapted enough to become nearly as transmissible as COVID-19 was from the very beginning.

Risk-Benefit Ratio for Gain of Function

Dr. Ebright argued that "because gain-of function research of concern poses high—potentially existential—risks and provides limited benefits, the risk-benefit ratio for the research almost always is unfavorable and in many cases is extremely unfavorable. Therefore, it is imperative that gain-of function research of concern be subject to national- or international-level oversight to ensure that, before the research is started, risk-benefit assessment is performed, risk-benefit profiles are acceptable, and mitigable risks are mitigated."[20]

Likewise, Dr. Esvelt's testimony agreed that the risk of gain-of-function research greatly outweighed any perceived benefits. Esvelt concisely put the potential disaster of pandemics in perspective: "A million Americans have lost their lives to COVID-19, more than have perished in combat in all of our nation's foreign wars. A pandemic virus can demonstrably kill more people than any single operational nuclear weapon."[21]

Comparing gain-of-function research to nuclear weapons was an apt analogy. Americans are aware of the dangers of nuclear weapons or WMD (weapons of mass destruction) falling into the hands of terrorists. But few Americans understand that the creation of novel viruses in the lab rivals the danger of nuclear weapons.

Esvelt pointed out, "For 75 years, the United States has successfully kept nuclear capabilities out of the hands of terrorists. Due to recent technological advances that have made it easy to assemble viruses from synthetic DNA, pandemics now represent a considerably greater challenge for nonproliferation, not least because they are wrongly viewed as a problem for health agencies that largely lack security expertise."

To make matters worse, the Fauci-led scientific bureaucracy was hellbent on publishing the DNA or RNA sequences of all viruses in the world. Fauci and his consiglieres were spending hundreds of millions of taxpayer dollars basically publishing a how-to list of deadly viruses for potential terrorists or rogue nations to exploit.[22]

Esvelt made clear the unintended danger if "pandemic-capable viruses are credibly identified and their genome sequences are shared with the world—as is the goal of well-meaning programs operated by the U.S. National Institutes of Health and the U.S. Agency for International Development—individual terrorists will gain the ability to unleash more pandemics at once than would naturally occur in a century."[23]

Ebright agreed: "Gain-of-function research of concern poses *information risks* by providing information on the construction and properties of new potential pandemic pathogens. Publication of the research provides instructions—step-by-step 'recipes'—that can be used by a rogue nation, organization, or individual to construct a new potential pandemic pathogen and release it to cause a pandemic. With current biotechnology, the technical means to do this are within the reach of most nations. With improvements in biotechnology in the next decade, the technical means to do this likely also will be within the reach of most sub-state organizations and individuals."[24]

Esvelt drove the point home: "As a practicing biotechnologist who specializes in harnessing evolution using viruses as tools and inventing methods of editing laboratory organisms that will controllably spread in the wild, I am reasonably confident that pandemic virus identification represents a greater near-term threat to national security than anything else in the life sciences—and a more severe proliferation threat than nuclear has ever posed."[25]

Could virus identification allow us to create vaccines for all of the world's viruses so as to be prepared for any and all pandemics, natural or lab-created? Hardly. Esvelt explained how even if we had a "proven vaccine...already stockpiled in large numbers near major cities," it would be impossible to stop a pandemic virus that is "deliberately released." Looking at the lightning speed that propelled the Omicron variant around the globe, Esvelt reminded everyone that "the omicron variant spread from a single point of origin to infect 26% of Americans on the other side of the world within 100 days of detection."

Esvelt particularly warned of the possibility of terrorists getting hold of pandemic viruses: "If many pandemic-capable viruses become known—even if each has only a moderate chance of causing a pandemic—a terrorist could assemble and release them all, potentially unleashing more and faster-spreading pandemics at the same time than would naturally occur in a century."

Esvelt argued against the universal identification of all viruses as proposed by Daszak, Bill Gates, and others. Esvelt maintained, "Successful pandemic virus identification will immediately cause widespread proliferation.... Twenty years ago, the only way to obtain physical virus samples was from clinical specimens or laboratory stocks. Today, thousands of individuals can assemble many types of viruses from commercially available synthetic DNA and virus assembly instructions, often called 'reverse genetics' protocols."[26]

Anthony Fauci Evades the Gain-of-Function Pause

In 2008, it's not as if everyone in government turned a blind eye to the dangers of gain-of-function research. When Dr. Ron Fouchier mutated an avian flu virus to allow it to spread via aerosol, a spirited debate about the inherent risks occurred, and ultimately the government instituted the so-called pause of gain-of-function research from 2014 to 2017. Before 2014, there was effectively no federal oversight of gain-of-function research.

The pause applied to selected gain-of-function research involving influenza, MERS, and SARS viruses. The government stated that this research funding pause would be effective until a robust and broad deliberative process was completed, resulting in adoption of a new gain-of-function research policy. Scientists were encouraged to voluntarily pause any research that had already been started.

During the period of the pause, eighteen projects were put on hold. However, according to Ebright's testimony, "at least 7 of the 18 projects that were paused were allowed to re-start almost immediately (based on a certification by the NIH Director that the projects were 'urgently necessary to protect the public health or national security')."[27]

Who allowed the dangerous experiments to continue, despite the moratorium?

Well, none other than the ever-present Tony Fauci.

How did he do this? Well, he simply claimed that adding gain of function to bat viruses was not really gain of function. And when confronted with the fact that some of these bat viruses being mutated in Wuhan were also deadly human viruses, Fauci simply claimed the experiments did not create enough gain *in* function to be gain of function.[28] Is that perfectly clear? Of course not.

Fauci's obfuscations, denials, and outright lies are nothing more than subterfuge. As a result, dangerous experiments with MERS (death rate approximately 30 percent) and SARS1 (death rate about 10 percent)[29] were not paused and continued uninterrupted in Wuhan, the United States, and around the world.

And if defining away any real definition of gain of function were not enough, Fauci fashioned the rules of the so-called pause to specifically allow the head of the funding agency to grant an exemption if he or she determined that the research is "urgently necessary to protect the public health or national security."

Of course, Anthony Fauci made certain he had the power to evade the entire regulatory regime of the pause. EcoHealth's gain-of-function research proceeded blithely on uninterrupted. Both EcoHealth and NIH now claim they weren't given an exemption—because their experiments never involved gain-of-function research at all.

Their emails, obtained under duress by order of a federal judge, disagree.

These emails show NIAID staffers questioning the gain-of-function aspect of the Wuhan research but then being placated by EcoHealth claiming the research was allowable as long as the gain of function was not more than tenfold.[30] As Ebright would ultimately testify, the gain of function in viral growth was actually ten thousand–fold.[31] EcoHealth failed to report it and was never disciplined.[32] Until recently, at least $1.4 million in taxpayer dollars flowed via EcoHealth Alliance to the Wuhan Institute of Virology post-pandemic.[33]

The pause in funding gain-of-function research was to end when the government adopted its final policy on gain-of-function research. Very quietly, without any briefings that high-ranking Trump administration officials can recall, the pause was lifted not long after the election that would swear in Trump.[34] To date, I have sent over thirty letters to eight government agencies requesting documents concerning grants during the pause and after—to no avail. Subpoenas from the new GOP majority in the House will, perhaps, reveal that there was fraud during the years of our alleged national pause in gain-of-function research.

Like many so-called government reforms, there was a lot of smoke and mirrors without true reform. Ultimately the pause was replaced with a new oversight regime, the P3CO framework, which required the researchers to "self-declare" if their research met the criteria for gain-of-function, a situation unlikely to happen among researchers hungry for the millions of government dollars dangled before them.

The End of the Pause (2017) and P3CO Framework

After Fauci quietly lifted the gain-of-function pause, he replaced it with the Health and Human Services framework for research involving potential pandemic pathogens, or P3CO. The P3CO Committee was to evaluate proposed research that is *reasonably anticipated to create, transfer, or use enhanced PPPs*. Pathogens to be scrutinized included any disease-causing organism that is "likely highly transmissible and likely capable of wide and uncontrollable spread in human populations" and "likely highly virulent and likely to cause significant morbidity and/ or mortality in humans."

Also to be scrutinized were any enhanced potential pandemic pathogens resulting "from the enhancement of the transmissibility and/ or virulence of a pathogen." Naturally occurring viruses were exempt from the protocol even if considered to be dangerous.[35]

As Ebright explains, "Under the P3CO Framework, covered projects are to be identified and flagged by HHS funding agencies (i.e., the NIH and the CDC), and covered projects are to be reviewed by a committee appointed by the HHS Secretary (i.e., the HHS P3CO Committee)."

The P3CO framework was intended to scrutinize research proposals *before* the study's onset, using the standard of whether gain of function or pathogenic risk was "reasonably anticipated."

To Ebright, the policy's intentions are crystal clear: "They are as clear as in any US statute or rule having a 'reasonable person' standard. The policy covers research activities reasonably anticipated to increase the transmissibility or the pathogenicity of a potential pandemic pathogen, including research activities in which neither the pathogen to be modified nor the enhanced pathogen to be generated is known to infect humans."[36]

Ebright is quite specific: "The research at the Wuhan Institute of Virology included activities that met the definition of 'selected gain-of-function research' in the US policy in effect in 2014–2017 and that met the definition of 'enhanced potential pandemic pathogen research' in the US policy in effect in 2018–present."[37]

U.S. government funding allowed the researchers at the Wuhan Institute of Virology to recombine portions of different coronaviruses to create novel viruses not found in nature. Dr. Shi and her fellow researchers then showed that these novel hybrid viruses, or chimeric viruses, could infect human cells.

According to Dr. Ebright, the newly lab-created viruses "exhibited up to 10,000-fold enhancement of viral growth in lungs, and up to 4-fold enhancement of lethality, in mice engineered to display human receptors on airway cells ('humanized mice')."[38]

No serious scientist not on Fauci's payroll would argue that this research doesn't meet the definition of gain-of-function research. As Ebright points out, the policy in effect at the time ordered "immediate cessation of work" if the experiments showed viral growth that "exceeded—by more than three orders of magnitude—the threshold set by the NIH for enhancement of viral growth...."[39]

Not only did the NIH fail to stop this gain-of-function research, they didn't indicate that the experiments were even covered by the gain-of-function policy. This would be a recurring theme of mischief as EcoHealth Alliance, Dr. Shi, and Dr. Baric would simply argue that the research didn't need to be reviewed because it wasn't "gain-of-function" research. But that was precisely what the review was supposed to determine. Any legislative reform to regulate these dangerous experiments would have to allow the review committee to determine which experiments to review, not the funders, or even worse, the experimenters themselves.

Ebright maintains that even after the pause expired and was replaced with the P3CO framework for identifying risky gain-of-function research, the experiments in Wuhan still met the definition of risky research and should have been scrutinized by the committee. They weren't.

Ebright concluded, "Although the research also met the definition of enhanced potential pandemic pathogen research in the US policy in effect in 2018–present (the P3CO Framework), and although the NIH was informed of project objectives and results in a proposal for renewal of the grant for 2019–2024, the NIH failed to identify the project as being covered by the policy, and failed to forward the proposal to the HHS P3CO Committee for the risk-benefit assessment required by the policy."[40]

This failure, alone, should have been enough to result in the firing of Anthony Fauci and Francis Collins.

Problems with the P3CO Framework

However well-intended, the P3CO framework to regulate gain-of-function research was an abject failure. It is debatable whether the regulations were *designed* to fail by advocates of gain of function, but either way, fail they did. As Ebright describes it, "In principle, the P3CO Framework provides for risk-benefit assessment and risk-mitigation review for gain-of-function research of concern. *However, in practice, the P3CO Framework largely has existed only on paper.* In the four-and-one-half years since the policy was announced, *only three projects have been reviewed*: two projects that had been carried over from the Pause, and one new project."

The problem was less about pandemic regulations than about the complete evasion and exemption to the regulation. As Ebright points out, "Most covered projects—including the project on engineering of SARS- and MERS-related coronaviruses by EcoHealth Alliance and the Wuhan Institute of Virology—were not reviewed, due to a failure by the NIH to identify covered projects, flag them, and forward them to the HHS P3CO Committee for review. In addition, the HHS P3CO Committee has operated with complete non-transparency and complete unaccountability. The names and agency affiliations of its members have not been disclosed, its proceedings have not been disclosed, and even its decisions have not been disclosed."[41]

And yet, no one admitted the basic fact that the P3CO framework failed to stop the funding of dangerous research in Wuhan. The framework failed for many reasons, but reason number one was that Fauci and his apparatchiks allowed the Wuhan funding to continue without ever sending it before the very committee intended to provide the safety and security analysis.

Perhaps even worse than Fauci evading his own agency's regulatory protections that might have prevented this research and the ensuing pandemic from happening, congressional Democrats didn't even bother to show up for this extremely revelatory and informative hearing. If the hearing had been about an oil company or an auto company failing to adhere to regulations, Democrats would have been all over it. If the hearing had been about "a lack of diversity in professional hockey," Democrats would have lined up to attend.

And yet, when clear evidence was provided that dangerous research was funded by the government in defiance of the law, Democrats looked the other way. Over a million Americans died either from or with COVID-19, and Democrats did not lift a finger to investigate if our tax dollars actually funded the catastrophic accident that led to a worldwide pandemic.

CHAPTER 21

Origins of SARS-CoV-2

As the first committee hearing on gain-of-function research pro-
gressed, it was inevitable that the discussion would turn to the
possible origins of COVID-19.

Steven Quay spent the greater part of his testimony discussing
the lab-leak hypothesis. Dr. Quay, like Jeffrey Sachs, concluded
after two years of investigation that the pandemic began with a
laboratory-acquired infection.

To support his hypothesis, Quay testified that the virus had multiple
"genomic regions that have the signature of synthetic biology, that is,
gain-of-function research."[1]

Quay, like Bob Kadlec (who spent eighteen months investigating
the origins of COVID for the Senate HELP Committee) and others
who examined the research conditions in Wuhan, concluded that the

safety levels were inadequate to perform "synthetic biology research at the Wuhan Institute of Virology...in low level, BSL 2/3 facilities."[2] This type of dangerous research demanded more secure facilities, such as a BSL-4 lab. Inadequate safety in Wuhan was for many observers the initial clue in supporting the notion that COVID-19 might have leaked from a lab.

Even though Fauci had tried to push Kadlec into the yes-men cabal with that 3:00 a.m. email on February 1, 2020,[3] Kadlec did not succumb. In the fall of 2022, Kadlec would ultimately show his independence after spending eighteen months investigating the origin of the COVID virus. As a summary of his investigation concludes, "SARS-CoV-2 and the resulting COVID-19 global pandemic was, more likely than not, the result of a research-related incident associated with coronavirus research in Wuhan, China."[4]

Professor Richard Ebright, a longtime critic of gain-of-function research, was also open to the theory that COVID-19 came to infect humans as a result of "a research-related accident" and that "the genome sequence of SARS-CoV-2 indicates that its progenitor was a bat coronavirus."

Ebright acknowledged that bat coronaviruses have been documented in various parts of China and that "the first human infection could have occurred as a natural accident, with a virus passing from a bat to a human, possibly through another animal. There is clear precedent for this. The first entry of the SARS virus into the human population occurred as a natural accident in a rural part of Guangdong province in 2002."[5]

The Collapse of the "Wet-Market" Theory

But Ebright testified that equal weight should be afforded the lab-leak hypothesis, knowing that "bat coronaviruses also are collected and studied by laboratories in multiple parts of China, including the Wuhan Institute of Virology. Therefore, the first human infection also could have occurred as a research-related accident, with a virus accidentally infecting a field-collection staffer or a laboratory staffer, followed by transmission from the staffer to the public."[6]

Unlike Fauci's yes-men, Ebright is truly an objective scientist. He did not smear any scientist who argued that COVID-19 came naturally from animals. In fact, Ebright was very clear that "at this point in time, there is no scientific or other secure basis to assign relative probabilities to the natural-accident hypothesis and the research-related-accident hypothesis."

Ebright did, however, describe three lines of circumstantial evidence that should be noted:

> First, the outbreak occurred in Wuhan, a city of 11 million persons that is more than 800 miles from, and outside the flight range of, known bat colonies with SARS-related coronaviruses.
>
> Second, the outbreak occurred in Wuhan, on the doorstep of the laboratory that conducts the world's largest research project on bat viruses, that has the world's largest collection of bat viruses.... The laboratory actively searched for new bat viruses in bat colonies in caves in remote rural areas in Yunnan province, brought those new bat viruses to Wuhan, and then mass-produced, genetically manipulated, and studied those new bat viruses, year-round, inside Wuhan.
>
> Third, the bat-SARS-related-coronavirus projects at the Wuhan Institute of Virology...[were performed using] personal protective equipment (usually just gloves; sometimes not even gloves) and biosafety standards (usually just biosafety level 2) that would pose high risk of infection of field-collection or laboratory staff....[7]

Epidemiology investigations are pieced together as a detective would, painstakingly connecting evidence and clues. In his quest to discover the origins of COVID-19, Dr. Quay looked into every detail of the locations of the first COVID-19 patients in Wuhan:

> The competing hypotheses are a natural spillover at the Huanan Seafood market in Wuhan China and a laboratory-acquired infection, most likely at the Wuhan Institute of Virology or WIV. Before December 2019, the WIV had published over 65% of all coronavirus scientific papers in the world. Until it was removed from the WIV website at 2 am local time, September 19, 2019, they maintained a database of over 21,000 viruses collected over two decades, in part with NIH funding. To my knowledge, no western scientist or organization has had access to this database since the pandemic began.[8]

So, proponents of a natural spillover event allowing COVID-19 to jump from animals to humans have a thorny "proximity" problem: How to explain a coronavirus pandemic beginning just miles away from the largest depository of coronaviruses in the world.

For investigators, the ability to examine the databases that recorded the genetic sequences of coronaviruses for a nearly identical precursor virus that Chinese scientists may have been manipulating in the lab would be like finding the holy grail. Finding a precursor would be a key to solving the origin of the virus.

The Chinese databases that existed before the pandemic may hold the answer. This should become the focus of the new House GOP majority as they look for evidence of a valid precursor to COVID-19 that may have been uploaded into the database that Shi may have taken down in September 2019.

To Quay, it is telling that "no animal has ever been found to be infected with CoV-2. Hundreds from the market were tested and over 80,000 throughout China were all negative," which suggests strongly that COVID-19 leaked from a lab. The opposite was true when the SARS1 epidemic occurred in 2002–2003. The intermediate animal was discovered within months, and nearly all of the animals tested were positive for previous or current SARS1.[9]

The WHO investigative team did find COVID-19 genetic sequences at the market, but found that the sequences were identical. This is a key difference from SARS1 and other animal precursors. If multiple animals were infected with COVID-19, one would expect a variety of genetic sequences, not just one. As Quay concludes, "All environmental specimens from the market were the result of human infection, not animal infection."[10] If the infections were originating from animals, there should be a variety of genetic sequences that differed from the genetic sequences found in COVID patients. No such diversity was found.

Chinese reports on early cases, according to Quay, "suppress cases from the eastern side on the Yangtze River, near the WIV, for no apparent reason," even though these early cases near the WIV were identified by the WHO investigation.[11] Why were cases from the eastern side of the Yangtze River downplayed? Perhaps because they didn't support the theory of the origin being the wet market.

Quay points out that "the most ancestral version of CoV-2 that infected humans, named Lineage A, did not infect any patient from the market." So, the earliest isolated COVID-19 genetic sequence, Lineage A, was actually found in patients who had not been to the wet market but *did* live or work in close proximity to the Wuhan Institute of Virology.[12] Instead of the wet market being the original source of COVID-19, many scientists now suspect that the marketplace was the site for a human super-spreader event unrelated to the animals on sale.

In fact, even the official government line in China ultimately settled on the fact that the wet market was likely not where COVID-19 originated.

Likely very few mainstream reporters have any clue that China's version of the CDC admitted in the spring of 2020 that the wet market was not the original source of COVID-19.[13]

Quay, like many investigators, became interested in the exact location of the earliest infections. Quay's investigation "identified the earliest cluster of hospitalized patients with both the Lineage A and Lineage B virus at the People's Liberation Army Hospital in Wuhan...." This particular hospital is only a few kilometers from the Wuhan Institute of Virology and, as Quay notes, is "along Line 2 of the Wuhan subway system." Quay's research also showed that "all early cases were along this same subway line, one of nine in Wuhan, and that the probability this was by chance is one in 68,000."[14]

The "Line 2 COVID Conduit," as Quay called it, provides transit between "the PLA Hospital, the WIV, the market, and...the international airport." As Quay pithily puts it, "You can literally walk down into the subway system [with your] next exit in the world in London, Paris, Dubai, and New York City, all before having any symptoms. In the fall of 2019 one million people a day used Line 2 and modelling by others suggested the pandemic could not have occurred without the spreading impact of Line 2."[15]

As Elaine Dewar writes in her book *On the Origin of the Deadliest Pandemic in 100 Years: An Investigation*, "of the early cases, 44.6% had no history of market exposure."[16] Also arguing against the market being the origin of the pandemic was a retrospective analysis of blood specimens from the first week in 2020 showing COVID-19-positive patients in "six different districts of Wuhan, indicating that the virus had already spread widely by the first week in January."[17]

If COVID-19 originated in the wet market, one would expect the people who worked in the market to be more likely to have antibodies to COVID-19 than the average citizen of Wuhan. This was true of the first SARS1 epidemic. People who worked at the market where the infected animals were sold showed a significantly higher percentage of previous infection than the general public.

Quay describes how this previous epidemic manifested: "In the SARS1 epidemic, once an antibody test was available to identify people who had been infected, stored blood samples were tested for previous, undiagnosed infections. Workers in the market had a 20% positivity, while in the general population you could find about 1% of people who were infected. These people were the training ground on which SARS1 learned to infect humans and learn to support human-to-human spread."

With COVID-19 no such "similar training ground in stored human specimens from Wuhan before the pandemic" has been found. Quay pointed out that "36,000 blood specimens were tested, and none were positive [for COVID-19]. If [COVID-19] was like SARS1 we would have expected at least 360 positive stored specimens."[18]

When viruses jump from animals to humans, they are clumsy at first and don't transmit well among humans. It took months for the SARS1 virus to mutate enough for human transmission. For COVID-19? It showed up already primed and ready to go.

Quay asked, "Where could [COVID-19] have 'learned' to infect humans?" He went on to explain, as other scientists have, that "replicating a virus in human cell cultures, that is, a test tube would do it. So would passing the virus in mice genetically modified to contain human lung tissue, so-called humanized mice. And we know that a US coronavirus researcher, funded by the NIH, provided the WIV with his laboratory's humanized mice for doing this type of research."[19] That researcher was, of course, Ralph Baric of UNC.

The Telltale Furin Cleavage Site

Quay testified that another aspect of COVID-19 that hinted at its originating as a lab construct was the furin cleavage site which "contributed to infectivity and pathogenicity." Viruses need an enzyme to cleave a protein on the surface of the cell to gain entry to the interior of the cell. Throughout the human system, the enzyme furin is abundant, and any virus that could utilize furin would have extraordinary powers of infectivity. Researchers have known this fact for some time, as Quay explained: "[P]utting a synthetic furin cleavage site is a common go-to 'gain-of-function' exercise. In fact, since 1992, at least 14 publications have described adding a furin cleavage site to a virus that didn't have one, including a study from the WIV." In each experiment, the insertion of a furin cleavage site made the recombinant virus more dangerous to humans.[20]

In fact, it was the discovery that COVID-19 had a furin cleavage site that initially set off the alarm bells with Fauci's yes-men, Kristian Andersen, Bob Garry, and Eddie Holmes. Quay in his testimony pointed out that Drs. Shi and Baric had actually requested U.S. funds in 2018 for "synthetically inserting a 'human specific furin cleavage site' into a bat virus."[21] Jamie Metzl, a WHO advisory board member, put it this way to *Vanity Fair*: "If I applied for funding to paint Central Park purple and was denied, but then a year later we woke up to find Central Park painted purple, I'd be a prime suspect."[22]

Fauci's yes-men might argue that since the DARPA gain-of-function grant was denied, there was "no harm, no foul." But many scientists who previously doubted the lab-leak hypothesis became much more suspicious once they were aware that Shi, Daszak, and Baric had applied for U.S. tax dollars to add a furin cleavage site to a SARS-like coronavirus in 2018, and then, lo and behold, in 2020 a coronavirus originates in Wuhan with the first-ever-recorded furin cleavage site. This does not merely seem suspicious. It seems damning in its implications.

Quay pointed out, as had Sachs and Harrison, the unlikeliness of "finding the exact furin cleavage site in SARS2 that is also found naturally in an important human lung protein, ENAC, that controls water flow into the lung."[23]

Fauci's yes-men might argue that other coronaviruses had furin cleavage sites, but they would fail to mention that the other coronaviruses with furin cleavage sites were quite distinct evolutionarily from COVID-19, and not likely to exchange information. If the furin cleavage site came about through natural recombination, you would expect COVID-19 to be still able to infect some animals easily. Instead, as Quay points out, COVID-19 "is so adapted to the human host that it can no longer infect bat cells in culture."

According to Quay, COVID-19 is an unusual virus for two reasons: "First, in 1,000 years since the SARS2-related viruses separated from the other related beta coronaviruses, there has never been a virus with a furin cleavage site." So, none of the viruses among COVID's close relatives have a furin cleavage site. The discovery of the furin cleavage site in COVID's genetic sequence is really what set off alarm bells in virtually every researcher to evaluate COVID's genome. Quay also found COVID unusual because COVID "uses a rare genetic sequence that has also never been used by these related viruses in nature. The sequence is a common genetic sequence used in the lab when gene jocks juice up viruses."[24] So, in other words, not only was the furin cleavage site an astonishing finding, but the particular genetic sequence used to code the furin site was a sequence much more commonly found in lab experiments than in animals.

Quay explained to our Senate subcommittee that "the furin cleavage site in SARS2 also explains why this virus but not SARS1 can infect the brain, heart, lungs, kidneys, and other organs. This is because these organs also have the furin enzyme on their surface."[25] The original SARS1 from the 2002–2003 epidemic, like most closely related coronaviruses, did not have a furin cleavage site.

The ORF8 Smoking Gun

Many scientists have described the unusual aspect of COVID having a furin cleavage site, but Dr. Quay was the first to point out another area of COVID's genetic sequence that seems inconsistent with a natural origin—ORF8, or "Open Reading Frame 8." To understand what an open reading frame is, it is helpful to review a little of how RNA, DNA, and viruses interact.

RNA is the messenger molecule of the cell. It takes instructions from the DNA in the nucleus to other cellular bodies that generate proteins and various components of life. When a virus invades, it takes over these information-transfer functions and forces the cell to manufacture more copies of itself, eventually killing the cell. In such cells, examining RNA is a way to examine the genetic coding of the virus. RNA contains "stop" and "go" instructions called reading frames. Open reading frames (ORFs) are typically long sequences of RNA that do not have "stop" signals to interrupt translation, so ORFs often are the coding sequence for proteins, which are very large molecules and must be generated by one large instruction.[26]

Quay makes a case for another part of COVID-19's genetic code possibly being the result of gain-of-function research. He points out that RNA Open Reading Frame 8, found in infected cells, explains some of the reasons for asymptomatic cases of COVID, and conversely may also account for some of the severe outcomes of COVID-19.

Quay points out that COVID-19 genetically instructs its host to make "a protein called ORF8, so named because it is the eighth protein in the SARS2 genome. It is one of the only proteins that is not part of the finished virus or is involved in taking over the cellular machinery that makes new viruses. ORF8 is diabolical. It is made early after an infection, before other viral proteins begin to be synthesized. At this point, the cell is largely unaware it is infected and hasn't mounted any defenses. ORF8 enters the blood stream and interacts with the immune system" blocking the production of interferon.[27]

Interferons are signaling proteins also known as cytokines that upgrade the immune system to fight infection, particularly viral infection. Interferon is produced by T cells, monocytes, and fibroblasts.

As Quay puts it, interferon "is a blunt weapon against infections that is used early by the body to slow down an infection, allowing time for antibodies to be produced and T-cells to respond. And second, it produces the familiar symptoms of an infection: fever, chills, sweating, red skin. The symptoms of an infection are not directly from the microbe itself but are from the body's response to the presence of a microbe. Take interferon away and you have asymptomatic spread." That is, the virus breeds inside the body but produces no outward signs at first that it is spreading.

To Quay, it is suspicious that COVID-19 has an asymptomatic infection rate of 30–40 percent. If one were to design a virus that would escape detection and containment, one would work for a virus that can spread asymptomatically. It is not proof of laboratory manipulation but, to Quay, it is suspicious. He states that he is "aware of no other new respiratory virus that is asymptomatic when it first entered the human population."

In addition to blocking production of interferon, ORF8 also, according to Quay, "interferes with the immune system's process of making antibodies and teaching T-cells about the virus. This so-called MHC antigen presentation system is important for fighting infections. The AIDS virus is the poster child of viruses that become chronic infections because, among other things, it inhibits the normal immune system response. No one knew about ORF8 and these features when the [COVID] vaccine target was being selected and so immunity [via] vaccination does not include inhibiting ORF8. Interestingly, in a natural infection, your body recognizes ORF8 as a highly foreign protein and actually makes more antibodies against it than any other protein."[28]

As researchers at Columbia University Medical Center reported, COVID-19 "utilizes its ORF8 protein as a unique mechanism to alter the expression of surface MHC-I expression to evade immune surveillance."[29]

If one were to design a bioweapon, creating a pathogen that can evade the immune system would be at the top of the list.

A study from the Mayo Clinic links the ORF8 protein to severe COVID-19 infection and points to it as a possible culprit for the so-called cytokine storm. Clinicians taking care of COVID-19 patients describe a crisis they call a cytokine storm that occurs in the severely ill when one's bodily fluids leak into the airspaces of the lungs. The study showed high levels of ORF8 in patients with this severe form of the disease. Researchers also found a "selective inhibitor" of this inflammatory cascade suggesting a possible therapeutic for severely ill COVID patients.[30]

To summarize, COVID-19 makes the protein ORF8. ORF8 disrupts the normal cooperation between T cells and antibodies, making detection by the patient's immune system more difficult. It also exacerbates inflammation making the disease more severe.

According to Quay, there's more than circumstantial evidence to suggest Wuhan researchers might have wanted to optimize "the ORF8 gene and its function and . . . [create] a synthetic biology pathway for manipulating this protein and putting it in viruses in the laboratory."[31]

The amazing internet sleuths who call themselves DRASTIC discovered two unpublished master theses from WIV students written in Mandarin that describe gain-of-function research with ORF8.

In an interview with *Vanity Fair*, one member of DRASTIC, Gilles Demaneuf, a data scientist from New Zealand, concluded, "I cannot be sure that [COVID-19 originated from] a research-related accident or infection from a sampling trip. But I am 100% sure there was a massive cover-up."[32]

Quay scoured the scientific literature and "found no western virolo-gist that was doing research on ORF8 before the pandemic."

Quay laments that we didn't know sooner about the dynamics of ORF8. In his committee testimony, he argues that the vaccines might have been more effective if they had included "immunizing against ORF8."[33]

The Nipah Virus Nightmare

In Quay's quest to discover the origin of COVID-19, he made the bombshell discovery that researchers in Wuhan were working on the Nipah virus—which has a 60 percent mortality for the infected. Quay had examined the raw data that Shi made available from her December 2019 coronavirus research and discovered snippets of genetic material consistent with the Nipah virus. Constructing the sequence of a virus involves painstakingly putting short sequences of RNA or DNA together to create the final sequence. The raw data shows these snippets of RNA that may have been used in the generation of COVID-19. But there also appear short snippets of RNA likely left over from other experiments run on that particular DNA/RNA sequencer. These remains suggest possible genetic engineering work done on Nipah sequences. Quay described the evidence that Shi was working with Nipah as "the most dangerous research I have ever encountered."

According to Dr. Quay, "The Nipah virus is a smaller virus than SARS2 and is much less transmissible. But it is one of the deadliest viruses, with a [greater than] 60% lethality. This is 60-times deadlier than SARS2. The lab where the human specimens were processed is not the highest level biosafety lab, BSL-4, but was in the BSL-2 or -3 facility."[34] If Quay is right, our worries about COVID-19 are only the tip of the iceberg.

CHAPTER 22

Gain-of-Function Research and Bioterrorism

As our committee delved into gain-of-function research, I continued to hold Anthony Fauci accountable. Reports of his resignation were in the news. I tweeted, "Fauci's resignation will not prevent a full-throated investigation into the origins of the pandemic. He will be asked to testify under oath concerning any discussions he participated in concerning the lab leak."[1] As our subcommittee continued to explore the dangers of gain-of-function research, I never for a moment let up on holding Fauci—whom I believe to be the one person ultimately responsible for this pandemic—accountable.

Our committee was finally hearing not only about the dangers of gain-of-function research, but we were also learning about the possible ways to protect the world from this menace. It is my hope that this discussion will ultimately lead to a bipartisan bill to regulate U.S. taxpayer funding of this dangerous research.

Congress's first hearing on COVID's origin also led to a discussion of how this dangerous research could be used by terrorists. To Dr. Kevin Esvelt of MIT, the national security implication of identifying pandemic pathogens were the most alarming of all possible scenarios.[2] For years, Peter Daszak, Fauci, Bill Gates, and others had pushed for billions of dollars to be spent on the identification of all the viruses in the world. Consider what that involves: literally digging the viruses out of caves where humans might never encounter them and transporting these rare viruses to major metropolitan areas.

The risk-benefit ratio doesn't add up. Esvelt concludes that "deliberate pandemics" will kill "many more people than identification could save." Esvelt estimates "the chance that any given identified virus will be released by a terrorist [at no] less than 1% per year... meaning each identified virus would be released within a century. Because a virus deliberately introduced at multiple sites would spread more rapidly than if the same virus were to cause a natural pandemic, successfully identifying a new equivalent of SARS-CoV-2 and sharing its genome with the world is expected to cost well over a million American lives."[3]

Proponents of identifying the world's viruses argue that, once we classify them, scientists will be able to create cures in advance of pandemics. But Esvelt warned that "even if identifying a pandemic-capable virus in nature allowed us to perfectly prevent that virus from causing a natural pandemic, and we could do so with zero risk of accidents, we should expect terrorists to use the same virus to kill a hundred times as many Americans as would be saved."[4]

Scientists in favor of identifying all viruses argue that if we don't do it, the terrorists will.

Esvelt disagrees and argues that "malicious actors are exceedingly unlikely to identify pandemic-capable viruses if health agencies decline to do so." He argues that while terrorists would likely try to construct pandemic viruses with published sequences, terrorists are unlikely to take the painstaking steps of basic science to sift through enough bat guano to find these viruses.[5]

Indeed, worldwide government agencies have put hundreds of millions of dollars into identifying the world's viruses, and so far they have not found a credible threat. It is much more likely that terrorists would use the cookbook chemistry already published to assemble a known pathogen rather than do the meticulous, yearslong field research of retrieving and identifying viruses in the wild.

The modern era of warfare, particularly during the Cold War, saw ostensibly civilized countries stockpiling chemical weapons, nerve gases, and biological weapons. The United States ultimately came to the conclusion that these weapons of mass destruction were uncivilized, and we've spent the last few decades destroying most of our arsenal. We have signed international treaties and encouraged the world to follow.

In order to convince other countries to dismantle or not assemble these weapons, our goal should be the international prevention of state-sponsored biological warfare with pandemic pathogens. As Esvelt stresses, we should persuade other countries

> that pandemic virus identification is not in their strategic interest. Pandemic-class agents kill indiscriminately and cannot currently be engineered to spare one's own population. Large nations that attempt to vaccinate their own populations in advance would likely be discovered by foreign intelligence agencies, and even if population-specific targeting became possible, its use by a nation-state would be so obvious that it would invite mass retaliation. Therefore, pandemic-capable viruses offer little if any strategic utility

to powerful nation-states; indeed, quite the opposite. The
United States, China, and even Russia have a shared interest
in joining forces to prevent rogue actors and terrorist zealots
from gaining access to pandemic-capable viruses.[6]

For decades now, the United States has been the top international
funder of pandemic virus identification. Esvelt believes that if the United
States were to end support for the virus ID program, the rest of the
world could be influenced to do the same. Our goal should be one of
de-escalation, just as it is in nuclear arms control.

Esvelt demonstrated how easy it would be for a terrorist to get
started. Since "2002, [when] the poliovirus was successfully assembled
from chemically synthesized DNA.... the cost of synthetic genes has
fallen by a factor of a thousand." Synthetic DNA has become so inex-
pensive that you can order it online.[7]

Voluntarily, corporations involved in producing synthetic DNA have
come together to form the International Gene Synthesis Consortium,
an organization that screens DNA orders.[8] By screening orders, the
consortium aims to prevent gene sequences that are components of
pandemic pathogens from being sold. In addition, the screening is
designed to identify rogue actors or potential terrorists before they can
make a purchase. The consortium membership includes 80 percent of
the market. The U.S. government also has regulations, but in Esvelt's
opinion, they are currently inadequate, and "despite the best efforts of
the International Gene Synthesis Consortium, it is currently easy to
obtain unscreened synthetic DNA."[9]

Increasingly large numbers of individuals have the technical skills
to put genetic sequences together to create viruses. According to
Esvelt, "The U.S. grants 125 doctoral degrees in virology each year,
accounting for one-third of the total worldwide. At least four times as
many individuals with degrees in related fields—such as my own PhD

in biochemistry—possess similar skills. If we assume a 20-year active career, approximately 30,000 individuals are capable of assembling any influenza virus for which a genome sequence is publicly available."

If that wasn't bad enough, scientists have essentially put online the "how-to" instructions to build most viruses that could easily be codified by bad actors. In fact, as Esvelt points out, scientists have actually published instructions enabling people with basic technological training to utilize reverse genetics to create coronaviruses like SARS1 and COVID-19.[10]

Esvelt's warnings are not new, but the COVID-19 pandemic has made these warnings more relevant.

For over a decade, biosecurity experts have been warning of the dangers of synthetic biology and gain-of-function research. Homeland Security News Wire reported back in 2010 that "scientists have been engineering genetic sequences for decades and commercial gene sequencing has been around for years—but this year, researchers for the first time were able to design and produce cells that do not exist in nature without using pre-existing biological matter...."[11]

Yet, despite the current pandemic, not one Democrat-led hearing into the dangers of gain-of-function research was conducted in the first two years of the COVID-19 pandemic.

PREDICT was funded for a decade by USAID (U.S. Agency for International Development) with the goal of identifying the world's viruses. According to Elaine Dewar, who authored a book on COVID-19's origin, PREDICT failed to live up to its name and predict any pandemics and, in fact, was a key funder of the gain-of-function research in Wuhan that may have led to the COVID-19 pandemic.[12]

Esvelt, along with many other scientists, agrees: "Without action by Congress, the first highly credible pandemic viruses might be publicly identified and their complete genomes irreversibly shared by well-meaning scientists funded by USAID, NIH, or other agencies as soon as this coming year. We need to keep the risk window closed for as long as possible."[13]

Kelsey Piper at *Vox* writes that "some experts are raising another, even sharper question: What if viral discovery is not just an ineffective tactic but a terrible idea, one that might not only fail to prevent the next pandemic but potentially even make it more likely?"

Piper quotes Andy Weber, "an assistant secretary of defense for nuclear, chemical, and biological defense programs under the Obama administration": "Do you really want to be going into these bat caves to collect and then catalogue which ones are most dangerous to humans?"

According to Piper, Weber's "concern isn't just that we're looking for a needle in a haystack that we may never find. It's that if we did discover a virus that would devastate the world if it crossed over into humans, someone might expose themselves accidentally while researching it, as has happened with smallpox and with influenzas. Worse, finding a virus and infecting animals with it in a lab could open the door to accidental release or intentional use. Success, in other words, could be worse than failure."[14]

Advocates for identifying the world's viruses argue that the knowledge gained will aid in developing vaccines. But, after decades of virus identification, *no human vaccine has been developed in advance of a human epidemic.*

Andy Weber agrees that little evidence exists that these vast efforts to identify the world's viruses have helped. Weber concludes, "After having done this work for 15 years, I think there's little to show for it. As the intelligence community concluded, it's plausible that it actually caused this pandemic, and to me that's enough.... We don't have to be sure what caused this pandemic to reduce the risk of the next pandemic. It was of zero help in preventing this pandemic or even predicting this pandemic."[15]

In our gain-of-function hearing, Esvelt worried that "for 75 years, the United States has successfully kept nuclear capabilities out of the hands of terrorists. Today, we're on the verge of irreversibly handing them blueprints for viruses as lethal as nuclear weapons—all in the name of public health. Let's not."[16]

Sometimes the best of intentions backfire. Upon learning that scientists want to protect us by identifying every virus in the world, it's easy to react, as Bill Gates did, by opening your checkbook. But good intentions don't always guarantee good policy.

As part of identifying the world's viruses, scientists test the ability of the discovered viruses to infect human cells. But the experiments don't stop there. Some scientists feel compelled to mix and match genes from the different viruses they find to discover whether a "recombined virus" is capable of producing a pandemic.

Much of the research that was being done by Shi in Wuhan was funded by dollars intended to identify the world's viruses. The money came from NIH, USAID, PREDICT, and an alphabet soup of U.S. defense biowarfare agencies. In other words, from the U.S. taxpayer.

As Esvelt told our committee, it's not that these scientists simply search out and identify viruses, they actually work "to enhance the transmissibility of especially lethal animal viruses, like the bird flu...." Taking a virus, like the bird flu, and adapting it in the lab to make it transmissible by aerosol is foolish in the extreme. Even if it's all done to estimate whether a virus might someday naturally mutate to become a pandemic pathogen, in Esvelt's opinion, "These pandemic virus identification experiments are the virological equivalent of nuclear testing."[17]

Advocates for identifying the world's viruses argue that if you can identify a pandemic virus before humans become infected, then a vaccine could be developed. But after a decade, and millions of dollars spent, it's appropriate to emphasize once again this basic fact: no such vaccine has resulted from the virus collection and identification program. Zero. Zilch.

Ironically, even many pro-gain-of-function scientists like Fauci's yes-men—in this case, Holmes, Rambaut, and Andersen—actually do not support efforts to identify all the world's viruses to predict pandemics.[18] According to Esvelt, "many of the most vocal proponents of a natural origin for SARS-CoV-2 have vociferously argued that it will do neither [that is, prevent spillover or accelerate vaccine development]. These scientists fully support the other aspects of the One Health program for spillover prevention that are backed by USAID, but they view pandemic virus identification as a wasteful diversion of resources that would be better spent monitoring high-risk populations at the animal-human interface and helping those communities contain outbreaks."[19]

Despite the fact that Rambaut was an early member of the "nothing to see here" crowd—those calling anyone considering the lab-leak hypothesis a conspiracy theorist—he was quite forthright when it came to criticizing the idea of gathering and identifying all the world's viruses: "The more we look, the more new viruses we find. The problem is that we have no way of knowing which may be important or which may emerge. There is basically nothing we can do with that information to prevent or mitigate epidemics."[20]

According to Esvelt, in order to determine if "virus identification is worth the risk, we need low and high estimates of the benefits from early therapeutic development and improved spillover prevention, the likelihood of accidents that lead to outbreaks and then pandemics, and the probability of deliberate pandemics caused by terrorists who release one or many candidate viruses across multiple sites."[21]

Pandemic Virus Identification Will Not Significantly Accelerate Vaccine Development

Another reason why many scientists now believe we don't need to harvest viruses from every bat cave in the world and transport them to labs in metropolitan areas is that mRNA technology has transformed and dramatically shortened the time period necessary to develop vaccines.

According to Esvelt, "Moderna's SARS-CoV-2 vaccine was designed in less than two days. With suitable manufacturing facilities, we can produce enough doses in a week to run combined [clinical trials]...."[22] The technological advances in mRNA vaccines have essentially made moot the arguments for virus identification as a means to create vaccines.

In addition, it's never been likely or probable that out of the millions of viruses in nature, we could identify in advance a virus destined to create the next pandemic. We have no way of knowing which of these viruses would ever come in contact with humans or spill over to cause human disease. Esvelt makes the point: "Pandemic virus identification may help prevent spillover—*if* the virus would have spilled over.... [But] the risk of an accidental pandemic may or may not outweigh the benefits of identification."[23]

In the case of COVID-19, estimates of worldwide deaths range from six million to eighteen million. If COVID-19 originated as a lab accident related to the desire to identify the world's viruses, we must ask, is the risk worth it? Has the world project to identify viruses allowed us to create vaccines or avoid pandemics? Has the virus identification project been able to predict which pathogens will create pandemics?

My answer is an emphatic no, but others might disagree. Instead, all we get is silence.

You would think at least some Democrats would be interested in this issue. How did we get to a point in our country where not one Democrat-controlled committee has even seen fit to debate whether it is a good idea to venture to the farthest recesses of the planet in search of deadly viruses?

Despite the fact that it was boycotted by Democrats, I am hopeful that our Senate minority committee hearing on gain-of-function research is just the beginning and holds the promise of future bipartisan legislation to regulate this dangerous research, and in that goal I will not waver.

PART V

Holding Deceit Accountable

Chapter 23

Protecting America and the World from
Gain-of-Function Research

In December of 2022, Congress passed a 4,155-page spending bill, appropriately called an "omni"—since everything but the kitchen sink was thrown into the bill. The price tag was $1.7 trillion, with over a trillion dollars of that to be borrowed. On page 3,354, though, a bit of welcome oversight was included. The text reads, "Beginning not later than 60 days after the date of the enactment of this ACT, the Secretary of Health and Human Services shall not fund research conducted by a foreign entity at a facility located in a country of concern...involving pathogens of pandemic potential or biological agents or toxins."[1]

While those words are a welcome attempt to stop the funding of dangerous research around the world, especially in Wuhan, we the people need to watch carefully to see if the bureaucrats actually enforce the provision or if they attempt to evade them.

Just before the omni passed (over my strenuous objection, I might add) I met, for the first time with Dr. Bob Kadlec. He had been the Assistant Secretary for Preparedness in the Trump administration and the head of the Pandemic Committee, P3CO, tasked with reviewing dangerous research. I was astonished to learn that the Wuhan research had never been referred to his committee for evaluation. It was also alarming to learn the reason. *The committee itself was not given the power to choose which research needed scrutiny.* And finally, hearing him explain how he also had no power to restrict funds to laboratories and research that his committee *might* deem dangerous was downright appalling.[2]

I came away from my meeting with Dr. Kadlec convinced that much more is needed to control gain-of-function research. During our August 2022 committee hearing, I asked each of our experts to outline what steps would be necessary for legislation to effectively regulate this out-of-control, dangerous practice.

Dr. Richard Ebright detailed three aspects of effective oversight. "First, research proposals that include gain-of function research of concern must be identified. Second, a risk-benefit assessment and a risk-mitigation review must be performed…. Third, compliance with the decision from the risk-benefit assessment and risk-mitigation review must be mandated, monitored, and enforced."[3]

In addition to our expert witnesses, thirty-four prominent scientists put together a series of reforms to "strengthen the US government's enhanced potential pandemic pathogen framework." Included on the list were many of the scientists who have figured prominently in the theories put forward on COVID-19's origin. These include Drs. Jesse Bloom, Kevin Esvelt, Lynn Klotz, Marc Lipsitch, and David Relman. Referred to hereafter as the Gain-of-Function Reform Group (GoF Reform Group), the group's recommendations mirrored many of the suggestions of our committee witnesses.

The Gain-of-Function Reform Group recommends that gain-of-function experiments that confer "efficient human transmissibility" on a pathogen should be regulated.[4] Adopting this standard would explicitly stop Anthony Fauci, and others, from dancing around the gain-of-function definition and looking the other way as researchers create viruses that spread more easily in humans. Current regulations allow Fauci and other apologists for this dangerous research to simply argue, *Well, the increased lethality was unexpected...*

Fauci's quibbling over the definition of gain of function is reminiscent of Bill Clinton's response to a question during the Starr investigation: "Is that correct [that you had sexual relations with Ms. Lewinsky]?" To which Clinton replied, "It depends on what the meaning of the word 'is'—is."[5]

The GoF Reform Group also recommended that regulations not be limited to pathogens already recognized "because the risk of creating an EPPP [pandemic pathogen] does not depend on the starting point, but rather on the end-product."[6] For example, COVID-19 might not be much of a pathogen without the furin cleavage site. Even with the site, the overall mortality likely will end up being less than 1 percent. Yet COVID-19 still killed millions of people worldwide, and any research to mix and match unknown S proteins to SARS-like viral backbones should absolutely be regulated, if not prohibited.

Because current regulations allow gain-of-function research to occur if the research is said to be concerned with "developing or producing" a vaccine, that exception could allow exemptions for virtually every known gain-of-function experiment, since that is their purported intent. The Gain-of-Function Reform Group proposed that any creation of chimeric viruses (recombined viruses) to assess transmissibility or virulence, even if ostensibly in the pursuit of a vaccine, still be regulated by pandemic regulations and not exempted.[7]

Fixing the P3CO

Drs. Richard Ebright, Kevin Esvelt, and Steven Quay all recommended that any congressional reform of gain-of-function research require clear separation of the oversight and approval of research from the funding of such research. Under our current lax guidelines, there exists a clear conflict of interest wherein researchers can essentially approve of their own grants as long as they toe the line. Consider the particularly egregious example of Kristian Andersen receiving a million-dollar grant just months after abruptly switching his scientific opinion on COVID's origin from a likely lab leak to "natural spillover."[8] There are far too many incestuous relationships throughout the world of government-funded research. We need checks and balances, especially in light of the inherent dangers of virus research.

The GoF Reform Group called for regulators to "recuse any individual whose agency is funding or participating in the proposed [gain-of-function research] from decision making in the [pandemic] review process." Reviewers "should be subject to conflict of interest rules...."

The GoF Reform Group also recommended an idea that I had previously introduced to include "representatives of civil society" in the review of potential pandemic pathogens.[9] For several years, I have been proposing something similar for all grants funded by the federal government.

In fact, even before I became aware of the extent of Fauci's abusive reign, I had introduced this idea as legislation to reform science grant–funding committees. I called the bill the "BASIC Research Act."[10]

My reform would add at least one scientist to each funding committee from a major field of research that has more unanimity of support, such as heart disease, diabetes hypertension, cancer, or Alzheimer's. The goal is to create more debate on the best use of limited government research funds. I would also add a taxpayer advocate to all funding committees. Perhaps then we would start to question some of the absurd "scientific" research grants such as the $2.3 million the NIH spent injecting beagle puppies with cocaine, or the $3 million NIH grant to watch hamsters on steroids fight.[11] Perhaps if we had scientists representing other specialties on these committees, they would recognize such absurdity and could direct these funds to cancer research instead.

Government research funds should—at the very least—pass the common-sense smell test. I think most Americans would conclude that spending $700,000 of autism money to study what Neil Armstrong said when he first walked on the moon—was it "One small step for man" or "One small step for *a* man?"—is a waste of money.[12] These are funds that could be better spent on actual autism research.

In addition to adding two new representatives to each federal panel that approves grants, my legislation would disallow grant applicants from requesting their own friends for funding review. I would also make all federal grant applications public.[13]

Every year, I publish a government waste report filled with crazy behavioral studies such as the study that spent half a million dollars examining whether taking a selfie of yourself smiling and reviewing the photo later in the day will make you happier.[14] Or the study to determine if the mating calls for Panamanian tree frogs differ for country frogs and urban frogs.[15] Or several hundred thousand dollars spent to investigate whether Japanese quail are more sexually promiscuous when you give them cocaine.[16] The National Science Foundation actually

spent taxpayer dollars to study whether the comic book character
Thanos could snap his fingers when wearing his "infinity gauntlet."[17]

Who approves this crap? The answer is always the same: a small
group of researchers in the behavioral sciences who then the following
week approve their buddy's research to verify that kids love their pets.
Or something of the sort.

No, I'm not making this up, exaggerating, or distorting it.

The easiest way to eliminate this waste would be to give the
agencies less money to waste, particularly the National Science
Foundation—which, of course, was also funding gain-of-function
research in Wuhan. But even the mention of spending cuts, or even
a halt in the built-in automatic spending increases, results in media
hysteria and fearmongering. Nothing is ever cut. In fact, Republicans
and Democrats recently passed a computer chip subsidy bill that also
nearly doubles the budget for the National Science Foundation (NSF).[18]

It is appalling.

I'm sure former senator William Proxmire, now deceased, would
be aghast. He was a vocal foe of wasteful spending, particularly at the
NSF, and awarded them many "Golden Fleece" awards. One memo-
rable Golden Fleece award was for a $50,000 study to discover what
makes people fall in love.[19] The studies aren't any less dumb today, just
more expensive.

We must get control of this wasteful and dangerous lack of oversight of federally funded science grants, especially in regard to research
on potential pandemic pathogens.

Professor Ebright proposed that "responsibility for US oversight
of gain-of-function research of concern should be assigned to *a single,
independent federal agency that does not perform research and does
not fund research*. The oversight of research on fissionable materials
by the Nuclear Regulatory Commission provides a precedent and a
model" [emphasis mine].[20] Quay echoed the belief that reform should

use "the model [of] atomic energy research, which is funded by the Department of Defense, but which is overseen by the Atomic Energy Commission."[21]

Ebright, like the GoF Reform Group, also recommended that U.S. oversight of gain-of-function research "should cover all US and US-funded research, irrespective of funding source, classification status, and research location" and "should be codified in regulations with force of law and should be mandated, monitored, and enforced—in the same manner that US oversight of human-subjects research and vertebrate-animals research is codified in regulation.... and is mandated, monitored, and enforced."[22]

Esvelt agreed that Congress should "require external security oversight of life sciences research. At present, health agencies and funding recipients are instructed to regulate themselves with respect to security issues.... No funding agency or recipient can be expected to oversee itself; that is the definition of a conflict of interest."

Similar to my idea for more diversity of thought on funding committees, Esvelt argued that Congress should "establish a panel of experts from security agencies to provide oversight for life sciences research funded by the U.S. government, including reviewing and approving all requests for proposals before they are released. Members should be required to recuse themselves from oversight of proposals from their own agencies."[23]

Current regulations don't adequately assess the national security risk of gain-of-function research. Scientists tend to preoccupy themselves with the possible good without spending enough time contemplating the possible nightmares that might unfold if a pandemic pathogen gets into the hands of terrorists.

Since the beginning of government, there has been the awareness that recipients of federal dollars might try to game the system. Conflict of interest regulations are littered throughout the federal code. One would think recusal for conflict of interest would be the standard fallback procedure for all federal science funding. Yet when I questioned Fauci about whether any of the scientists on the vaccine-approval boards also received royalties from the drug companies that make the vaccines, Fauci responded that he did not have to inform Congress of any royalty payments. This is an insult to the American taxpayer.

We should not allow such a conflict of interest. Yet here we are at the highest levels of our federal government with a forty-year bureaucrat, Fauci, haughtily letting us know that royalty payments for vaccine board members are none of the people's business! Disgusting.

In order to more completely regulate gain-of-function research, the GoF Reform Group also recommended that all U.S. government agencies be bound by the new pandemic pathogen regulation.[24] Current regulations only apply to HHS, but a significant amount of the funding for gain-of-function research actually comes from defense agencies.

Quay, to be honest, said he could "find no actual benefit of gain-of-function research." He felt "efforts to ban it, given the vested interests of literally the entire virology community, and maybe others, [are] a hill too steep to climb." Quay stated that an achievable reform would be to place gain-of-function research under the purview of institutional review boards, which already exist and could be given this extra task.

Quay, like Esvelt, advocated expanding the review committees to include "unaffiliated lay people and community members [who] could place guardrails on the field and eliminate the most dangerous research." The standard argument against expanding the review committee, albeit an elitist argument, is that the common man is unable to comprehend and intelligently judge complicated research. Quay countered that "the argument that the research is too complex to explain to non-scientists fails when you point out that chimeric antigen receptor genetic engineering of the human immune system to fight cancer is routinely placed within the oversight of the IRB [Internal Review Board] system [where ordinary citizens are members]. This research is arguably more complex than gain-of-function work. In addition, the IRB system is an international standard that is used everywhere, including in China."[25]

We Need a New System of International Controls

Because we truly live in a global world of trade and science, reform must include international rules. "The US should call for an additional, international-level layer of oversight for the highest-risk, highest-consequence subset of gain-of-function research of concern," Ebright suggested. "The oversight of research on smallpox virus by the World Health Organization Advisory Committee on Variola Virus Research provides a precedent and a model."[26]

The United States, using its leadership status, could bring together the civilized nations of the world to agree to heightened oversight and regulation of dangerous gain-of-function research.

Similarly, Esvelt called for leveraging "shared strategic interests to prevent pandemic proliferation globally. The nature of many emerging technologies places the U.S. and China at loggerheads, but our strategic interests are nearly perfectly aligned when it comes to the proliferation of access to pandemic viruses: both nations have little to gain and much to lose."

One idea that Congress and the president should immediately accept is bringing this debate to the "Biological Weapons Convention (BWC), which prohibits 'the development, stockpiling, acquisition, retention and production of biological agents' while 'permitting the fullest possible exchange of equipment, materials, and information for peaceful purposes.'"[27]

Esvelt warned that "today, it's impossible to identify a credible pandemic-capable virus from most families, including corona-, influenza- and paramyxoviruses, without immediately giving thousands of individuals the ability to assemble infectious samples."[28] The GoF Reform Group agrees that publishing the genetic sequences of pandemic pathogens could essentially become a blueprint for terrorists.[29] Therefore, the pandemic pathogen regulations must control the public release of sequencing information.

Esvelt suggested that "Congress…instruct the State Department to begin negotiating a Pandemic Test-Ban Treaty that would narrowly forbid pandemic virus identification experiments, defined as those that could substantially increase our confidence that an animal virus or an engineered virus could cause a new pandemic."[30]

All of these commonsense ideas are reasonable and should not inspire partisan rancor. Yet, to date, no Democrat has stepped forward and pledged to place controls on gain-of-function research. Indeed, for nearly three years Democrats have blocked and boycotted all of my efforts.

We Need Export Controls on the Research Technology Itself

In addition to international agreements to limit dangerous gain-of-function research, Quay and Esvelt both felt that Congress should create "export controls and monitoring" on the technology used in gain-of-function research such as DNA synthesizers, genetic sequencers, and DNA sequences for sale. Quay suggested, "There are ways to build into these systems a forensic and law enforcement capability…."[31]

One large area for reform involves more of a philosophical consideration than bureaucratic regulatory change. Public policy must come to grips with the understanding that sometimes a policy that sounds great at first blush turns out to be quite dangerous.

We have blindly accepted the positions of Bill Gates, Peter Daszak, and others that it is a good idea to identify the world's viruses in order to study deadly pathogens that could possibly leap from the animal kingdom to humans. Their argument is that we could preemptively create vaccines for potential future outbreaks. But it turns out that going to deep, dark recesses of caves seeking viruses that likely never would have seen the light of day and transporting them to major metropolitan areas is not a risk-free endeavor—as anyone who acknowledges the likely possibility of the Wuhan lab leak—or a lab leak anywhere, at any time—will admit.

Esvelt recommends that Congress "stop funding pandemic virus identification experiments."[32] Nearly all of these virus ID programs are funded by our government. It is within the power of Congress to stop this dangerous research simply by cutting the revenue stream.

Despite Fauci's repeated denials, Esvelt acknowledges that the NIH "has a long history of funding projects aiming to enhance the transmissibility of viruses, including but not limited to lethal pathogens such as H5N1 and MERS. Many of these projects, which have been compiled and summarized by reporters from the *Washington Post*, were not covered by the moratorium on 'gain-of-function' research *due to disputes over what exactly is meant by that term.* Congress can resolve the confusion over definitions by blocking federal funding of pandemic virus identification experiments, defined as those that could substantially increase our confidence that a virus would cause a pandemic if repeatedly introduced" [emphasis mine].

To those scientists that argue that we need to find and identify the world's viruses to defend against potential pandemics, Esvelt responds that "our best current defense against pandemic weapons of mass destruction is to keep them from being developed in the first place."[33]

Congress Can Update the Federal Select Agent Program
Esvelt suggests that a regulatory program should do the following:

1. Automatically list a virus as soon as a single result from a pandemic virus identification experiment suggests that it may be pandemic-capable
2. Regulate any DNA construct that was generated from pieces of regulated Select Agents
3. Give the program the power to immediately lift all restrictions on any Select Agent confirmed to be actively spreading in order to accelerate research on countermeasures[34]

Fauci has repeatedly danced around the definition of "gain of function" to disingenuously maintain that he didn't fund the dangerous research in Wuhan. To eliminate gamesmanship over definitions, Esvelt suggests defining a virus as "a credible pandemic threat if it:"

- Can grow in relevant human tissues or be transmitted between relevant animal models nearly as well [as] an endemic human virus of the same family
- Is poorly recognized by the immune systems of most humans relative to endemic human viruses of the same family.[35]

Esvelt pointed out that modifications of the select agent list are not uncommon.[36] In the past few years, the U.S. government, specifically the CDC, has begun regulating synthetically created DNA. There is no reason why the federal government can't do more by identifying and adding more agents to the select list.

Finland senior officer of Welfare and Health, Marko Ahteensuu, echoes Esvelt's arguments in a peer-reviewed paper in *Science and*

Engineering Ethics, when he warns of "(1) a spread of the required know-how, (2) improved availability of the techniques, instruments and biological parts, and (3) new technical possibilities such as 'resurrecting' disappeared pathogens."[37]

None of these suggested reforms are radical or unwarranted, but Washington has become consumed by a Congress with very little scientific education and a blind willingness to let the so-called experts make these decisions. The problem is that although a significant number of experts do seek reform, the powers that be are monolithic and have been controlled by one man for four decades—that man is Anthony Fauci. One can only hope that once Fauci's hegemony ends, rational debate will resurface.

Regulate the Sale of Synthetic DNA

According to Esvelt, we should "require DNA synthesis screening matching or exceeding the industry standard." Many researchers around the world can utilize standard virus assembly protocols to create viruses, but they cannot synthesize the needed DNA or RNA on their own. So, laws limiting the ability to order DNA or RNA would decrease the number of technicians actually able to create viruses *de novo*. In fact, as Esvelt points out, "California's legislature passed a bill that would require all providers of synthetic DNA and manufacturers of synthesis machines to screen orders at least as well as the International Gene Synthesis Consortium, but it was vetoed on the grounds that federal legislation is needed to avoid a regulatory patchwork."[38]

While I'm not a big fan of federal laws for every malady, I do believe there is a national security risk at stake here. Just as we regulate who can and cannot enrich uranium, I see no reason why we shouldn't do the same for limiting the sale of synthetic DNA.

Synthetic DNA

If ever there was an Icarus moment, it had to be when scientists created the first virus from nothing but its organic components. Literally, man was now able to pluck components out of the primordial ooze and create life. That story should spark awe from even the most jaded of observers. Imagine the potential. Imagine creating viruses or bacteria that feed on methane and could transform a moon like Titan into a place habitable by humans. Already, scientists are able to introduce genes in bacteria or yeast to co-opt their cellular machinery to make synthetic insulin. So it's easy to visualize and appreciate what gene slicing and dicing can do.

But it's also easy to imagine what might happen if this technology gets into the wrong hands.

The question is how to regulate DNA synthesis without tipping off bad actors as to what genetic sequences are dangerous. As Dr. Esvelt points out, "New algorithms are making it possible to automatically screen all DNA synthesis without revealing which sequences are considered hazardous, reducing unauthorized access to pandemic-class threats by a hundredfold and nudging scientists away from publicly disclosing them in the first place."[39]

Our Department of Defense is aware of the risks of synthetic DNA. The DOD report "Biodefense in the Age of Synthetic Biology," completed by the National Academies of Sciences, Engineering, and Medicine, details how DNA synthesis might be used to create biological weapons. The report explains the very real risks of creating biological weapons by synthesizing known pathogens.

Michael J. Imperiale, a scientist at the University of Michigan Medical School and the lead author of the report, emphasized, "Synthetic biology has the potential to enable new types of weapons."[40] The report listed Ebola, SARS, and smallpox as pathogens that might be used as bioterrorism weapons. This report was published in 2018, well before the current COVID pandemic.

Another author of the report, Patrick Boyle, a design specialist at Ginkgo Bioworks, warned that synthetic biology could be used to create microbes that produce toxins.

Boyle warns that "the effects could resemble a chemical weapon or food poisoning."[41] It would be extremely difficult to discover the unnatural origin of such a weapon.

Synthetic biologists recently created a pathogen, horse pox, closely related to smallpox, demonstrating that scientists now have the knowledge to re-create horrors such as smallpox. Gregory Koblentz, an associate professor of biodefense at George Mason University, laments, "Safeguards against the misuse of those tools are weak and fragmented."[42]

Any hope for preventing man-made pandemic pathogens must confront the wide availability of synthetic DNA and regulate this technology the same way we treat items such as centrifuges that enrich uranium.

Liability for Pandemics

Another idea Esvelt has for trying to prevent pandemics is to implement catastrophe liability and require insurance coverage. I have my doubts as to the congressional will to enact this reform, but it's worth examining. The argument is that if the business community were required to assess the risk of potential pandemics, it would provide a strong incentive to seek out and prevent potential sources of pandemics.

Esvelt believes, "Not only is it entirely reasonable to hold responsible anyone whose actions are subsequently shown—through the due process of law—to be instrumental in the genesis of such catastrophes, but requiring general liability insurance to cover that liability would effectively require professional risk analysts to evaluate the likelihood and set rates accordingly. That is, such a law would induce the market to impose costs upon institutions proportional to the available information concerning the likelihood that their current and planned actions will, at even very low probabilities, lead to extreme catastrophe."[43]

Recent history over the past few decades, though, has seen Congress reject the benefits of risk evaluation for catastrophes. When my father, Ron Paul, was first elected in a special election in April of 1976, reports of a swine flu epidemic consumed the news. Two days after he was sworn into office, the House Appropriations Committee voted $135 million for swine flu containment.[44] My father ended up becoming one of two votes against the spending bill.

The swine flu H1N1 was in the influenza A family responsible for the 1918 worldwide flu pandemic that likely killed more than fifty million people. Naturally, public health doctors were on edge when reports emerged of an H1N1 influenza outbreak at Fort Dix, New Jersey. One soldier died, and thirteen others were hospitalized. A frenzy began to vaccinate everyone in the United States, and in August my father voted with eighty-two other congressmen against giving vaccine liability protection to the vaccine makers. In the rush to vaccinate, and with liability protection, it turned out that the influenza epidemic at Fort Dix was largely contained. The only death from the swine flu had been that first young soldier.[45] Yet twenty-five people ended up dying from the swine flu vaccine, and several hundred suffered from Guillain-Barré syndrome, which injured and paralyzed hundreds.

Instead of the vaccine makers paying for the individuals injured by their vaccine, the U.S. government paid 439 patients and the heirs of the twenty-three deceased $365 million in compensation, or about $831,435 each.[46]

In 2002, Congress passed legislation requiring the taxpayer to assume the risk for acts of terrorism. That law, the Terrorism Risk Insurance Act of 2002, was intended to protect the insurance industry from being bankrupted by the large financial payments required by a terrorist act such as the 9/11 destruction of the twin World Trade Center towers in NYC.

Critics of this type of protectionist legislation argue that the liability should not be taken over completely by government but shared with private insurers, who should be required to cover damage up to a certain deductible before the taxpayer funds kick in.

The argument can be made that when the federal government shields insurance companies from liability, it also removes the incentive to develop innovations to protect against terrorism, such as security screening for entering buildings. From the point of view of the insurance companies, it is easy to understand their perspective. They have little ability to protect skyscrapers from jet aircraft. Nevertheless, any innovations in that regard, even building smaller, less conspicuous, or less accessible targets, are stifled by liability protection.

These same arguments are part and parcel of the debate over liability waivers for vaccine manufacturers. The drug companies that make the vaccines argue that the FDA has approved them, and many governments then follow with mandates to use the vaccines. Shouldn't government itself then be the ultimate payer for damages or side effects of vaccines?

The argument against liability protection for vaccine manufacturers is that, once exempt from liability, the companies have insufficient incentive to warn of risks or remove dangerous vaccines from the market. Since no individual in government assumes any personal financial risk, less oversight occurs.

The problem with this debate is that the unintended consequences of liability protection are never fully comprehended: namely that liability protection often leads to less caution among participants because the ultimate payer will be someone else—namely the U.S. taxpayer. The mob that is often the majority in Congress typically takes the easy road of liability protection.

The idea of encouraging the private marketplace to assess the risks of bioterrorism from synthetic biology and gain-of-function research may be a good one, but if history serves as precedent, Congress is more likely to protect the insurance companies rather than acknowledge that liability could serve to force companies selling DNA synthesis to take protective measures against the possibility of their services falling into the hands of terrorists.[47]

Conclusions from the Historic Gain-of-Function Hearing

Fox News asked me to summarize our breakthrough, first-ever hearing on the origins of COVID-19 and the dangers of gain-of-function research. I responded, "Throughout this pandemic, I have led the effort to uncover the origins of this virus that has killed over six million people worldwide.

"Shockingly, with over one million Americans killed and trillions of dollars spent, last Wednesday was the first congressional hearing on the dangerous, virus-enhancing research known as gain-of-function and its relation to the origins of the COVID-19 pandemic."[48]

As Dr. Richard Ebright said in the hearing, "Gain-of-function research of concern involves the creation of *new health threats*—health threats that did not exist previously and that might not come to exist by natural means for tens, hundreds, or thousands of years."[49]

Why in the world would we willingly create a more transmissible or more dangerous virus that has the potential to unleash a global pandemic that threatens the lives of millions?

As Dr. Steven Quay observed, the Global Virome Project's goal is to "collect the estimated 500,000 unknown viruses that are capable of infecting humans and bring them back to a laboratory near you. What could go wrong?"[50]

During the hearing, Dr. Kevin Esvelt explained precisely what might go wrong, noting that scientists "never considered that these advances in technology...would allow a single skilled terrorist to unleash more pandemics at once than would naturally occur in a century."[51]

We also learned during the hearing confirmation that President Biden's chief medical advisor, Anthony Fauci, has been lying—shocking, I know.

The three elite scientists all agreed that the research in Wuhan was dangerous research. Two of the three "absolutely said it was gain of function," I explained in an interview with Fox News. "The third said it was dangerous research and should have gone before a committee."[52]

Nevertheless, Fauci persisted in saying that the NIH has never funded gain-of-function research in Wuhan. The evidence argued otherwise. The only reason the Wuhan research was not caught early and rejected was because Fauci allowed it to evade review by the Potential Pandemic Pathogen Care and Oversight Committee (P3CO). As a consequence, the Wuhan gain-of-function research never received the proper scrutiny.

These facts became readily apparent during the hearing, but no Democrats would be the wiser, since they all boycotted the hearing. We learned a lot of things from this hearing, but it's only the start.

We reconfirmed that Fauci is not being honest with us. Yes, the NIH funded gain-of-function research. Yes, it was dangerous. Even worse, no duly instituted regulatory body looked over or reviewed the research.

While there still seems to be a significant lack of curiosity on the part of Democrats, I am sure each member of Congress can agree that we need stronger government oversight of how our tax dollars are being used to create viruses capable of causing pandemics.

I find it ironic that Democrats, who regularly accuse Republicans of not wanting to regulate enough, turn a blind eye to the necessary due diligence and oversight of government-funded research that has the capability of killing millions.

We may never know with absolute certainty whether the pandemic arose from a lab in Wuhan or occurred naturally, but the emergence of COVID-19 serves as a reminder that dangerous research conducted in a secretive and totalitarian country is simply too risky to fund, and greater oversight must take place.

CHAPTER 24

The Tide Turns toward Truth

In the fall of 2022, Biden announced that the COVID pandemic was over. Of course, the pandemic was over and had been over for some time, but now our Chief Hysteric, the man who campaigned from his basement, the man who had required that people sit in their cars at his events—*this* man was finally admitting the pandemic was over.

Only he really wasn't. As with so many Biden revelations, he wasn't authorized to say what he had just said, and it would be quickly walked back.[1] Consider his repeated reference to getting cancer from a local oil refinery when he was a kid or his statement that he was sending troops to Ukraine.[2] Isn't it surreal how everyone just accepts that he has no idea what he is saying and ignores his nonsensical claims?

A few weeks later, the Biden administration's HHS renewed the government's emergency declaration.[3] Ninety days later, in January

2023, the Biden administration renewed the emergency order again.[4] Even CNN had made a start at tamping down on the hysteria by drastically reducing their use of their death ticker, which was only loosely, at best, connected to actual COVID deaths.[5] Finally, in mid-November 2022, an extraordinary shift occurred. A dozen Senate Democrats voted with every Senate Republican to end the COVID emergency. Under the emergency, the administration issued executive powers "to suspend the payment deadlines for student loans, close ports of entry and extend customs deadlines." This was the first time that any significant number of Democrats had broken party lines to oppose the emergency mandates. Unfortunately, Nancy Pelosi's lame-duck House refused to hold a vote on ending the COVID emergency.[6]

Emergency Presidential Powers

Few members of Congress and, for that matter, few members of state legislatures were aware of the extraordinary powers governors and presidents could assume during an emergency. Most legislators had never really concerned themselves with these powers, because they assumed these powers would be brief and only used in times of natural disasters such as tornados, hurricanes, or floods. But some of us remembered that governments of all stripes and persuasions have long aspired to vast emergency powers. The lessons of 9/11 emergency orders and the excesses of the PATRIOT Act should have had everyone on full alert.

President Trump initiated the COVID federal emergency on March 13, 2020. Virtually no one would have guessed the emergency would still be in force till May of 2023. While I question the constitutionality of such powers, Congress has acquiesced over the decades to allow presidents extraordinary powers—but never so sweeping as those utilized during the COVID "emergency."

According to a press release from Senator Roger Marshall's office, "The National Emergencies Act (NEA)...allows the President to make available robust powers to deal with crises other than war or natural disaster.... Under the NEA, Congress is mandated to determine whether the emergency should continue, a process Congress has not fully enforced, ceding power to the executive." Congress can restore constitutional law at any point. In fact, "a provision in the NEA grants Congress termination review of national emergencies, stating that after six months, and every six months after the emergency continues, 'each House of Congress shall meet to consider a vote on a joint resolution to determine whether the emergency shall be terminated.' However, Congressional interpretation of this law has determined that the absence of a resolution introduced by any member signals unanimous consent for continuation. In failing to meet, debate, and vote on an emergency, Congress is effectively ceding more unchecked emergency powers to the executive similar to its failure to enforce War Powers provisions." As a consequence, many emergencies remain active and are never terminated. "There are currently 31 national emergencies in effect dating back to the Carter Administration, highlighting the failure of Congress to consider termination of emergencies declared by the President. Only six termination resolutions have been submitted over the history of the NEA."[7]

COVID-19 Emergency Powers Invoked

The press release also noted that "the NEA does not assign specific powers but allows the executive to call up powers outlined in other statutes."[8] Actions taken by the executive under the COVID national emergency declaration include activation of the Ready Reserve and the Coast Guard, closure of international borders, suspension of student loans, as well as commandeering of U.S. industry through the Defense Production Act.

In one particularly egregious use of emergency powers, President Trump defied the law and congressional instructions to take money intended for another purpose and spend it on border wall construction.[9] Though I support additional security at our southern border, I and several principled constitutionalists voted against allowing Trump to gut Congress' power of the purse.

Our Constitution never envisioned rule by emergency or martial law. In fact, the one exception when the Constitution allows for the suspension of basic civil liberty is during a "rebellion or invasion." Even then, the Supreme Court has held that the "privilege of the Writ of Habeas Corpus" cannot be validly suspended by the president alone but must be approved by Congress.[10]

As Aaron Kheriaty points out in *The New Abnormal*, "When the president declares a national emergency, he gains access to an additional 136 statutory emergency powers."[11] The law provides a variety of powers to the president to respond to an emergency. These powers include the authority to seize property, organize and control the means of production, seize commodities, assign military forces abroad, institute martial law, seize control of all transportation and communication, regulate the operation of private enterprise, restrict travel, and so forth. So, when that Pandora's box of powers is opened, a great deal of mischief is potentially unleashed.

Well before the COVID emergency, I became very worried about the growing use of emergency powers. I considered Trump's ploy to circumvent congressional approval of appropriations a grave threat to the principle of the separation of powers that brought the United States yet another step closer to autocracy.

The debate over emergency presidential powers led me to introduce the REPUBLIC Act, which would limit any presidential emergency to seventy-two hours. Current law leaves a presidential emergency in place unless Congress votes to end the emergency. My bill would make any congressionally approved emergency automatically expire in ninety days unless Congress voted affirmatively to continue the emergency. The REPUBLIC Act would also make a motion to end a presidential emergency a privileged motion, meaning that any senator could call for a vote.

In addition, the REPUBLIC Act would repeal what some have referred to as the "Internet kill switch," a Depression-era bill that allows a president to unilaterally control all communications, which with today's technology would now include the internet, cell phone service, and television/radio broadcasts.[12]

My view didn't change no matter whether a Republican or a Democrat occupied the White House. I opposed Donald Trump's usurpation of power and continued to oppose Joe Biden's abuse of emergency powers.

The Senate finally began to show a spine and grow restless about granting so much unchecked power to the president in November 2022 by voting 62–36 to end the emergency.[13] Nancy Pelosi's House refused to take up the measure. Ultimately, in March 2023, the Senate again voted to end the emergency, this time 68–23. This time a Republican House took up the measure and voted 229–197 to end the emergency and, despite grumblings from Biden, he agreed to sign the bill.[14]

House Unclassified Report on COVID Origins

I met with the incoming chairman of the House Intelligence Committee Michael Turner (R-LA) in mid-December 2022, the day before his Republican minority released their interim report on the origin of COVID-19. Often members of the intelligence committees are standoffish and jealously guard their turf. For years, my father and other libertarians had complained that the intel committees lacked adequate oversight as their budgets were classified and much of the intel information was blocked from the view of most members of Congress. In fact, the elite eight (majority and minority leaders of both houses and their respective intel committees) are typically the only ones who have real ability to oversee our surveillance. There is no other accountability. Pelosi once infamously claimed she was not briefed on the CIA torture program even though attendance records indicate she was.[15] The public is misled to believe that all of Congress is privy to important classified material when in reality only eight members of Congress are granted any meaningful access, and apparently even those "elite eight" are not always paying attention.

U.S. Government Funded Chinese Military Research

In October of 2022, a bombshell intelligence report on the origins of COVID-19 was released by House Republicans with the explosive discovery that the U.S. government has been funding genetic manipulation of coronaviruses not only at the Wuhan Institute of Virology but at a Chinese military research facility.[16]

While the United States routinely—and rightly—lectures China on being more transparent and cooperating more on the COVID investigation, we don't expect much. Admitting mistakes or failure under a totalitarian regime often has terminal consequences.

But we do expect much more in the land of the free and the home of the brave. We expect that the intelligence community works *for* the democratic republic. Much ballyhoo has been broadcast about "threats to our democracy," but having an intelligence community that refuses requests from Congress is the true threat to our Constitution, our freedom, and everything America stands for.

The most powerful threat to democracy is secrecy. A major check and balance on government agencies is Congress's ability to ask questions. The cover-up of COVID's origins, the veil of secrecy, the refusal to divulge commonplace records—all create an atmosphere of fear and distrust.

Despite repeated attempts, the U.S. intelligence community refuses to reveal the names of scientific experts they employed to review the Chinese gain-of-function experiments. Why is this important? Well, one so-called scientific expert is Peter Daszak, whose organization is also the conduit for carrying NIH cash to Wuhan. Daszak is the very definition of conflict of interest. If he's one of the experts, you can understand why the CIA might be doing a little CYA.

It never ceases to amaze me that real news—absolutely vital information behind the deaths of over six million COVID victims—is ignored and sloughed over while we are treated to ad nauseam reports on the January 6 hullabaloo, the so-called "day democracy died."

House Republicans have released a document that reveals the U.S. government funded a Chinese military research institute where a coronavirus scientist and general by the name of Zhou Yusen announced on February 24, 2020, that he'd already developed a COVID vaccine.[17]

By May 2020, less than three months after he filed a patent for a COVID-19 vaccine, Zhou was dead. Either he jumped from a window or was pushed. In China, the truth often remains murky.[18]

Vanity Fair published a report that three scientists they consulted felt that General Zhou would have had to have the genetic sequence in November to possibly develop a vaccine so fast. The official date China admitted to knowing the COVID sequence was January 11, 2020.

It boggles the mind that General Zhou and Dr. Shi collaborated and were together awarded at least three NIH grants. The U.S. government literally funded a bioweapons military expert in China.[19]

Zhou's wife, Lanying Du, also worked for the Academy of Military Medical Science in Beijing and, like her husband, has spent a great deal of time in the United States, first at the New York Blood Center and now at Georgia State doing coronavirus research supported by NIH.[20] When

Georgia State received a request from Homeland Security to interview her, university officials acted as if they had no idea she was married to a prominent member of the People's Liberation Army of China. In fact, she claimed she rarely discussed her research with him, despite the fact that they both did research in the field of coronaviruses.[21]

More Strange Ties to China

One of the many loudmouths supporting vaccine mandates and denigrating naturally acquired immunity is Peter Hotez, M.D., dean of the National School of Tropical Medicine at Baylor College of Medicine and codirector of the Texas Children's Hospital Center for Vaccine Development. Hotez acknowledges working with General Zhou's widow on coronaviruses for more than a decade.[22] Small world...

Because Hotez spends so much time being a Twitter troll attacking anyone who puts forth evidence of the lab-leak hypothesis, he's not found time to reveal the $6.1 million NIH grant he shared with Dr. Shi.[23] Interestingly, the grant's stated mission included study to cope with "accidental release from a laboratory."[24]

Clearly political gamesmanship infects the high-finance world of the medical-pharmaceutical complex.

When I dueled with Fauci over his ridiculous wearing of two masks in committee, Hotez sided with Fauci (who coincidentally oversees Hotez's funding; no conflict of interest here, according to the left-wing media). Hotez maintained after a year of COVID that it was too early to consider not wearing masks, even for people who were vaccinated or had already survived it.[25] Needless to say, the vast majority of his fellow Texans paid him no heed and were already living their lives proudly showing their faces wherever they went.

The public knew better. In spite of constant misinformation from Fauci and the media, people understood that most masks have no effect on aerosolized transmission because the viral particles are more than six hundred times smaller than the mask pores.[26]

The Turner Report

House Republicans, including intel chair Mike Turner, have told the director of national intelligence that they will withhold funds if the intel community doesn't come clean. This story isn't over—and neither is the story of the COVID cover-up.

The one million Americans who died during the pandemic deserve better.

When Turner released his unclassified "Interim Report on the Origins of the COVID-19 Pandemic," he artfully told us much of what likely is in the classified version without technically revealing the so-called "state secrets."

Turner reminded everyone of "the long history of coronavirus collaboration between scientists from the Chinese People's Liberation Army (PLA) Fifth Institute of the Academy of Military Medical Sciences and scientists at the Wuhan Institute of Virology."

China in the 1990s "officially declared the Fifth Institute as part of its defensive biological weapons program...." But, as Turner points out, "In 2005, the U.S. State Department publicly stated the U.S. assessment that China also operates an offensive biological weapons program...."

Turner complained that Biden's report on the pandemic "failed to address [the Fifth Institute's] publicly stated interest in the development of engineered coronaviruses for biological weapons...."[27]

Turner's unclassified interim intel report summarizes a plausible hypothesis: "General Zhou's team of Fifth Institute researchers already possessed SARS-CoV-2 prior to the pandemic as part of bioweapons research; [Zhou] was working on vaccine-related experiments involving the virus at the WIV in 2019; and that a safety incident at the WIV led to its release into the world (presumably amplified by a super-spreader event at the Huanan Wet Market)."

Instead of saying, *We know this to be true because we have classified intelligence that says so*, the report cleverly states, "The Committee is aware of key classified intelligence relevant to this hypothesis."[28] What a world—our own intelligence agencies over-classify everything and the only way the truth can be revealed is by describing a hypothesis and then explaining that the intelligence community has information "relevant" to the hypothesis.

If ever there was a need to revisit Senator Frank Church's commission that investigated FBI abuses, the time is now. Not only is the intelligence community hiding documents that implicate China in the origins of the pandemic, they are now directing social media companies to restrict speech across America.

PART VI

The Aftermath of Deception

CHAPTER 25

Zhou Yusen and China's Zero-COVID Policy

After ten people, including a three-year-old, died in Urumqi, China, protesters gathered, questioning whether China's insane zero-COVID policy may have hindered the response of emergency personnel or prevented apartment renters from being able to flee. Spontaneous protests arose around the country. Not an insignificant event given the historical consequences for protest in China, from the murderous madness of the Cultural Revolution to the killing of demonstrators in Tiananmen Square.[1]

As the protesters gathered, some were heard singing a familiar song—"Farewell," from a century ago:

Outside the long pavilion, along the ancient route, fragrant green grass joins the sky,

I ask of you, as you go this time, when are you to return?
When it's time to come please don't hesitate.[2]

The lament takes on new meaning when a permanent farewell might be necessary any time a friend is detained for participating in what the Chinese government describes as "gathering crowds to disrupt public order." Cao Zhixin, a twenty-something book editor, had the audacity not only to gather in public to sing but to record a YouTube testimonial before her impending arrest. For this "crime," she was ultimately charged with "picking quarrels and provoking trouble," which can carry a sentence of ten years in prison. Ms. Cao, whose hobbies include bird watching and ukulele playing, is now considered an enemy of the state in authoritarian China.[3]

World Democracies Disappoint

China's response to COVID is unfortunately not surprising. What surprised even the most jaded of observers were the authoritarian responses of so-called liberal democracies like Australia, New Zealand, Canada, and America. What many had thought was a sincere liberal belief in bodily autonomy apparently did not include opposition to forced inoculations.

So-called liberals looked away when Novak Djokovic, the world's top tennis player, was expelled from Australia and denied entry into the United States. While Democrats demanded banning, they were perfectly fine with unmasked, unvaxxed migrants flooding in.

Meanwhile, in Australia, the police fired rubber bullets at protesters angry with government stay-at-home orders.[4] Practically everyone positive for COVID was forcibly detained and carted off to government detention camps. Even individuals with negative tests were sometimes captured and taken away if they had simply been exposed.[5]

In the Netherlands, police fired upon citizens protesting COVID restrictions.[6]

In New Zealand, police clad in riot gear rounded up and arrested dozens of protesters. As Jon Miltimore described it in the *Washington Examiner*, "This kind of head-busting of protesters is typically something found more in banana republics than liberal democracies, but it helps explain why [New Zealand's prime minister] Ardern sees firearms as necessary only for the state—'for things like peace control and biodiversity.' And it fits with her larger track record of authoritarianism."[7]

In Canada, Trudeau took the unprecedented action of invoking the Emergencies Act to freeze the bank accounts of truckers peacefully protesting in the capital. The Canadian Civil Liberties Association warned that the action "threatens our democracy and civil liberties."[8]

American Democrat Hysteria Continues

And even here at home in America, Democrat pundits called for involuntary detention and stripping of rights from anyone audacious enough to assert their prerogative to make their own medical decisions. When we consider how Americans were subjected to a daily media barrage of misinformation that created fear and distrust between friends and families, is it really surprising that nearly half of Democrats supported fining or imprisoning their fellow citizens for the crime of questioning the efficacy of the COVID vaccine? The unvaccinated were ostracized as selfish, hateful, or conspiracy theorists. People were attacked for not wearing a mask in public.

CNN's omnipresent Leana Wen lectured that "we can't trust the unvaccinated,"[9] and therefore they should not be allowed to leave their homes.[10] CNN's Don Lemon inflamed the worst instincts in people with his demands that "it's time to start shaming" the unvaccinated.[11] Howard Stern responded with a typical lowbrow attack on anyone daring to make their own medical decisions with the eloquent "Fuck them, Fuck their freedom."[12] Former California governor Arnold Schwarzenegger recorded himself snarling, "Screw your freedom.... You're a schmuck for not wearing a mask."[13] Biden ominously threatened that "our patience is wearing thin."[14]

Americans internalized the constant fear and shame propaganda and began turning against their own friends and family members who dared to question the authorities. People proudly recorded their anger and disgust with neighbors, coworkers, and relatives. The virtue-signaling went into overdrive on social media as people sanctimoniously posted the number of vaccines they had received and pictures of themselves wearing their "Believe Science" masks, along with angry exhortations to "Wear a Damn Mask!"

I found it astonishing that merely reminding people of COVID's 99 percent survival rate caused them to react with anger rather than relief. There was no room for context, perspective, or objective risk analysis. For millions of people, mostly left-leaning but certainly not all, the response to the pandemic became quasi-religious in its fervor. In their anxious desire to be safe and therefore controlled, they developed a zealous need to punish any who refused to comply. The response to COVID revealed this truth: totalitarianism does not require a dictator to enforce compliance—just groupthink.

And Democrat governors across the country capitalized on this fear. In Kentucky, Governor Andy Beshear passed martial edicts banning travel and assembly that were nearly all struck down by the courts. One constitutionalist judge from Northern Kentucky, Richard Brueggemann, wrote of Beshear's edicts that the judicial question was not about politics but rather about "whether the constitution applies during a virus."

"Under our constitutions, government may not uproot liberty on a hope that it can hide society from pathogens," Brueggemann went on to write. "Individuals, not government, should decide if the risk of walking out their front door is worth the potential reward."[15]

A federal judge in Kentucky, Justin Walker, responded dramatically to similar restrictions by Louisville's Democrat mayor Greg Fischer, writing, "On Holy Thursday, an American mayor criminalized the communal celebration of Easter. That sentence is one that this Court never expected to see outside the pages of a dystopian novel, or perhaps the pages of The Onion." Fischer commanded "Christians not to attend Sunday services, even if they remained in their cars to worship—and even though it's Easter." Walker concluded that "the Mayor's decision is stunning. And it is, 'beyond all reason,' unconstitutional."[16]

Governor Beshear threatened churchgoers that the state police would record the license plate numbers of any cars seen at services and the owner would be forced to go into quarantine.[17] Such impulse to authoritarianism should not surprise any students of history, but it was concerning how many people meekly and quickly submitted to edicts reminiscent of martial law over a virus with a 99 percent survival rate. Fortunately, our judicial system still has a significant number of constitutionalists still on the bench.

CHAPTER 26

As the new Congress was sworn in in January of 2023, I had great hopes of finally beginning a real investigation into the origins of the COVID pandemic. With Republicans in charge of the House and the threat of subpoenas, surely we'd overcome the Democrats' resistance to revealing our government records on the funding of gain-of-function research.

Already, the dialogue had changed in tenor. Martin Kulldorff, the Harvard epidemiologist, brilliantly testified before a new GOP-led House committee: "We knew about [infection-acquired immunity] since 430 BC, since the Athenian plague, until 2020—and then we didn't know about it for three years, and now we know about it again."[1]

Perhaps the tide had truly shifted.

The COVID Twitter Files

Elon Musk's historic release of behind-the-scenes collusion between the federal government and Twitter added fuel to the desire for truth. Matt Taibbi revealed that the FBI was not only paying Twitter to take down information of questionable validity but also paying them to take down "stories of true vaccine side effects." According to Taibbi "six major Internet platforms were 'onboarded.... daily sending millions of items for review," or, in other words, censorship. The project was called the Virality Project and, as Taibbi reported, "knowingly targeted true material and legitimated political opinion, while often being factually wrong itself."

Taibbi concluded that "as Orwellian proof-of-concept, the Virality Project was a smash success. Government, academia, and an oligopoly of would-be corporate competitors organized quickly behind a secret, unified effort to control political messaging."

Furthermore, the effort, according to Taibbi, "accelerated the evolution of digital censorship, moving it from judging truth/untruth to a new, scarier model, openly focused on political narrative at the expense of fact."[2] The Virality Project policed internet platforms with the warning that even "true stories that could fuel [vaccine] hesitancy" should be considered "misinformation."[3]

Our government actively suppressed the truth if it hurt its efforts to push the vaccine into every American arm, regardless of age or risk factor. This concerted propaganda campaign is unparalleled in its scope and audacity. In a sane world, those government bureaucrats responsible would be criminally charged.

Fauci's Folly Continues

And what of the man behind this subversion of truth and abuse of power? Even though 2023 found Anthony Fauci allegedly gone, he really wasn't. Rumors were he was still coming to the office a few days a week, keeping himself on the federal payroll so he could get free twenty-four-hour security.[4] Some speculated that Fauci also intended to utilize government lawyers if he was indicted for lying to Congress or hiding official communications.

Fauci intended to milk the position for as long as he could.

In late August 2023, it was announced that Fauci had joined the faculty of Georgetown University.

Before that, while Fauci officially remained on the government rolls, he had simultaneously earned $100,000 a speech in the private sector and was no longer available for routine questioning.[5]

I had to target my questions to those left guarding the secrets.

The Quest for Truth Goes On

On February 9, 2023, that target became Deputy Secretary of State Wendy Sherman. I began my five minutes of questioning with this line of inquiry:

> **Senator Paul:** Ms. Sherman, it's estimated that between five million and eighteen million people died from COVID-19 worldwide. To a significant number of scientists, the evidence suggests that this originated from a lab leak in Wuhan. Does the State Department fund coronavirus research in China?
> **Ms. Sherman:** Do we fund coronavirus? I don't believe so, but I don't know. I'll double-check, and we will get back to you on that, Senator.
> **Senator Paul:** The answer is yes, you do, and it has been going on for more than a decade, and it is done through a program called PREDICT and then the Global Virome Project. [These programs may be connected to COVID-19.]

Over a million Americans died, and we really haven't had any discussion of this. No hearings. Nothing. People are unaware that [our own government is funding this risky research].

We found out recently through the House unclassified report that money was going from the NIH to American universities to the Academy of Military Medical Sciences Research in China. We are subcontracting money and sending it over, but millions is coming from the State Department.

So the idea is this: We will identify all the viruses in the world. We will be safer because we identified them. But here is the question: Are we safer to have some guy or some woman crawling down a cave ten hours away from Wuhan, coming up with bat guano, coming up with viruses, and bringing it to a city of fifteen million like Wuhan?

This is what has been going on for a decade. It is a setup for an accident, it's a setup for a mistake, and nobody is doing anything about it. We continue to fund it.

The main group that has been getting this money is EcoHealth Alliance, over $100 million dollars, a lot of it through the State Department. They continue to get money. They've failed to file their reports on time. They promised to stop their experiments if dangerous gain of function occurred, but they did not stop their experiments. And yet [the NIH, the State Department, the Defense Department continue to] reward them with more money.

Fifteen million people died, and we have not done a thing about it. Nobody seems to care.... [Many in the government continue to deny or are not even sure we fund gain-of-function research.] The State Department is a big funder of this project. It is a multi-decade-long project. But there are scientists as we speak from Stanford, from MIT, from prestigious universities around the country—these are not partisans, most of them are not Republicans—who stand up and say, *Oh, my God, what are we doing, bringing these viruses from remote bat caves to major metropolitan areas and with no controls over this?*

We have been asking for information from the State Department because we want to know more about this. U.S. Right to Know has been sending FOIA requests for two and a half years, and [the government sends them heavily redacted records].

So, Mr. Chairman, I have sent two letters—some of them are six months old now—and...[the Biden administration continues to conceal records related to coronavirus research].

What I would hope for is that we could have—people always talk about bipartisanship—could we not get bipartisan support for records? This is not partisan. We want to know what the U.S. State Department is funding. NIH resists our requests on their funds.

Two things that we know for certain have led us to believe this came from the lab. One was the leaked DARPA grant request. Chinese researchers wanted DARPA money to create a virus, that, guess what, looks [very much] like COVID-19. They asked for it in 2018. DARPA turned them down. Fortunately, the U.S. government did the right thing for once. We turned them down. But that doesn't mean they didn't do the research.

And so many scientists had an aha moment. They saw this and they said, *Oh, my goodness, the Chinese asked for money to create something that looks almost exactly like COVID-19.*

So, in nature you do not have coronaviruses that infect people that have what is called a furin cleavage site. The Chinese scientists said, "Give us money! We are going to stick a furin cleavage site [on a coronavirus] to see if it infects humans more [readily]."

We discovered this DARPA grant request, "but not because anyone in government let us know," I noted. "They still resist." The entire government claims everything is top secret. Everything is classified. "This is the whole problem of classification," I argued. "But over-classification can also be used to cover up things." As a prime example, I detailed how Congress and the public knew nothing about the 2018 Wuhan DARPA grant request until an illegal leak occurred. A brave whistleblower revealed that in 2018 the Wuhan lab "wanted to create a virus just like COVID-19."[6]

The other thing we know is that three researchers in the Wuhan Institute of Virology got very sick with flu-like symptoms similar to COVID in November.[7] We only know that, though, because the Trump administration declassified it on the way out.

So, we have to get over all the classification. We also have to be more forthcoming, and I am hoping the chairman will consider looking at our request. These are not partisan.

We want to know all the information about funding of research in China. We want to know the interactions. There were cables going back and forth between the State Department saying, "Holy cow, they are not even wearing gloves! They do not wear masks in [handling potentially deadly viruses]! They are doing this [risky research] in what is called a BSL-2 as opposed to a BSL-4."[8]

Most of the research that we think escaped was not done in the appropriate lab, and the State Department knew about it, but we have had no hearings about this. They refuse to give us information. Fifteen million people died, a million Americans died, and you won't give us information.

So, what I would ask is for you to look at our request. This isn't partisan. This should be about discovering the origins of COVID-19. The scientific community is about 50/50 now [on the origins of COVID]. We suspect the Chinese of not being honest and withholding information—but it is sad that the U.S. government is also withholding information from its representatives.

Ms. Sherman: I will take back your request. Again, Senator, I would urge a briefing, perhaps in a SCIF, with the intelligence community on this because, as you know, there is not a single view about this particular set of issues. But I understand your desire to understand what occurred.

Senator Paul: We are asking you for unclassified information that you hold, not intel.

Ms. Sherman: I understand that.[9]

The Follow-Up

A few weeks after Deputy Secretary Sherman's testimony, I was finally allowed access to classified documents that acknowledged that the Department of Energy had received new information and now concluded that COVID originated from a lab leak in Wuhan. The problem was that this information was classified and I was forbidden from talking publicly about it.

Why in the world would the government classify a conclusion that doesn't reveal sources or techniques? Your guess is as good as mine.

It does illustrate the farce of the classification racket that serves to obstruct oversight. How can I develop the arguments for regulating dangerous lab experiments if the government won't reveal how dangerous those experiments truly are?

Every scrap of paper that comes from the intel community seems to be classified. This over-classification problem led to the imbroglio concerning Trump, Biden, and Pence all having classified documents at home. Instead of wasting time and millions of dollars hiring special counsels, it would be wiser to put forth legislation to end the over-classification regime.

I didn't have to wait long before the revelation that DOE now believed that COVID came from a Wuhan lab leaked into the media. A few weeks later virtually everything was leaked to the *Wall Street Journal*.[10]

DOE's change of mind was significant because they had concluded otherwise when Biden asked the entire intel community to reassess the origins debate in 2021. Now we had both DOE and the FBI concluding that the evidence indicated a leak from the Wuhan lab.[11]

Some of us had wondered why it took this long for DOE to come around. Another classified report from Lawrence Livermore scientists—a report that I still can't discuss publicly—had been leaked more than a year before. It was reported to conclude that a lab leak was plausible and should be investigated further.[12]

Months before these new conclusions by the DOE were leaked to the press, my office had requested a meeting with the Lawrence Livermore scientists. The DOE leak threatened to derail efforts to get other publicity-shy intel agencies from cooperating.

Luckily, we did finally get to sit down with the scientists. Unfortunately, this was yet another classified briefing. Their arguments for their conclusion that COVID-19 leaked from the lab are still classified, but the media has reported that the DOE scientists' conclusion "drew on genomic analysis of the SARS-COV-2 virus."[13]

In other words, an analysis similar to the many unclassified sources that cited features such as a lack of genetic diversity of the original strains of COVID, the pre-adapted nature of COVID's binding site, and, of course, the unusual furin cleavage site.

The Deep State Continues Its Obstruction

For more than two years now, I'd been fighting obstructionism from Democrats and over-classification from the intel community. I had sent literally dozens of requests to the alphabet soup of agencies either doing bioweapons research or ostensibly doing research to protect us against bioweapons.

And yet, consider this disturbing fact. As a sitting U.S. senator who spent two years trying to investigate the origins of the pandemic, I only learned about the request for DARPA to fund the insertion of a furin cleavage site into a coronavirus from a leak to the media. In addition to the leaks, the investigation was greatly aided by U.S. Right to Know, which more than any other group has doggedly pursued and sued under FOIA in order to shed sunlight on this cover-up.

One of the agencies that we requested information from was DTRA (Defense Threat Reduction Agency). They stonewalled us. A federal judge did force them to give some records to U.S. Right to Know, including records of an internal review of EcoHealth grants. One of DTRA's conclusions was that "the possibility exists that they (EcoHealth) may be expending some grant funds on efforts beyond the purposes specified in the grant agreement."[14]

In an interesting email exchange, the director of Cooperative Threat Reduction, Robert S. Pope, Ph.D., writes that the disparaging quote should be removed from the assessment because "If this letter gets FOIA'd someday, DOD doesn't need to deal with explaining this sentence...."[15] These spooks seem to spend quite a bit of time trying to make sure the truth is well hidden from oversight.

On September 22, 2022, internal emails from DTRA leadership begin to discuss my requests for records. DTRA leadership made sure to expressly describe my requests as "sent from Senator Paul's personal member office not the Homeland Security Permanent Subcommittee on Investigations."[16] The implication being, of course, that they could ignore an individual member of the Senate but maybe not a committee request.

Reassuring each other as they tried to justify their cover-up, the directors argued, "The information in question was redacted for permissible reasons; Members of Congress and their staff are not legally bound to hold unclassified information in confidence...." They seemed to fear that the unclassified documents might have "negative implications" or be "misconstrued, misrepresented."[17] So, in their capacity as overlords protecting "The Homeland," they concluded that they could ignore the requests of a sitting U.S. senator. When pundits decry the deep state, this is exactly what they are talking about.

The email exchanges continued over about a week's time until one correspondent on September 26 opined, "I think we need a strategy at this point,"[18] presumably a strategy to block my requests and to explain, if need be, why they blocked the requests of a senator. Another anxious DTRA director responded, "Even if we were to answer Senator Paul's question...[we] should ensure it is in line with their other responses."[19] In other words, make sure the lies you feed Senator Paul are consistent with the lies you've already told U.S. Right to Know. The deep state is alive and well, and it should terrify every American who believes in representative government and due process of law.

How concerned is the deep state about the truth leaking out? Well, we know from the FOIA emails that they follow closely any stories in the media concerning DTRA funding of EcoHealth Alliance. In private, they maintain that none of their "funding [is] tied to the Wuhan Lab."[20] But the questions we have are much more extensive. Does DTRA fund *any* gain-of-function research? What requests from Wuhan for DTRA or DARPA funds were denied? Certainly, the Wuhan request to use DARPA funds to insert a furin cleavage site into a coronavirus is pertinent to an investigation.

The Deep State

The great COVID cover-up began in China. No one should be surprised that a totalitarian government would seek to hide any responsibility for a worldwide pandemic. But it was mind-jarring to witness the cover-up that took place in our own country, supposedly the land of the free. Fauci and his yes-men might have gotten away with it if a federal judge hadn't ordered their emails released, revealing that virtually all of Fauci's colleagues initially believed that COVID originated with a lab leak. The emails showed in real time these very same scientists publicly disavowing the lab-leak theory while privately concluding that in all likelihood the virus did leak from the Wuhan lab.[21]

To those who disdain the moniker "deep state," they fail to understand the nature of the epithet. It's not an accusation of evil men sitting in the dark, rubbing their hands together with glee and plotting to devastate the world by releasing a super-virus. The truth is much more mundane. George Carlin put it well when he said, "You don't need a formal conspiracy when interests converge."[22] Why are eight federal agencies resisting my records releases? Why are so many in league that "deep state" describes it well?

It's precisely that their interests converge. Any agency that funded the gain-of-function research in Wuhan or in the United States or anywhere in the world now denies that the research was gain of function and fights tenaciously to keep any record that they funded this dangerous research from the public eye. So fierce is their will that they have refused to divulge records even when I enlisted twenty-five fellow senators to sign the records requests. The deep state is simply an alignment of interests among bureaucrats throughout the federal government to cover up any responsibility for funding research that, in all likelihood, led to a lab leak that killed millions.

CHAPTER 27

Glimpses of Sanity as the Information Embargo
Begins to Crack

David Relman, a Stanford University microbiologist and one of
the authors of regulatory reform for gain-of-function research,
commented on the DOE's new conclusions: "Kudos to those who are
willing to set aside their preconceptions and objectively re-examine
what we know and don't know about Covid origins.... My plea is that
we not accept an incomplete answer or give up because of political
expediency."[1]

The *Wall Street Journal* story that revealed the DOE's new conclusion on COVID's origin reminded readers that "U.S. State Department
cables written in 2018 and internal Chinese documents show that there
were persistent concerns about China's biosafety procedures, which
have been cited by proponents of the lab-leak hypothesis."

The report also reminded skeptics that "the three researchers from the Wuhan Institute of Virology became sick enough [to be hospitalized] in November 2019," months before the Chinese admitted any infections had occurred.[2]

A day after the *Wall Street Journal* revealed the DOE's new conclusion that COVID "likely" leaked from a Wuhan lab, FBI director Christopher Wray announced that the FBI also concluded that the virus leaked from the lab in Wuhan.[3] For some unintelligible reason, the fact that the FBI had made this conclusion was classified until Wray made this announcement. Though it took nearly two years for the FBI to admit it, the announcement seemed to be an acknowledgment that it was now suddenly acceptable for Democrats to allow an investigation.

Perhaps it was the Chinese balloon incursion or the fearmongering against all things China that allowed Wray to find his voice. Wray further commented that the Chinese government, at every turn, was attempting to "thwart and obfuscate" investigations into the origins of COVID.[4]

Wray's public confirmation of the FBI's COVID origin's conclusion pried loose a rare comment from Chuck Schumer (D-NY) on the subject: "The bottom line is we've got to get to the bottom of this...the Biden administration is committed to it. They have all kinds of people looking at it, and we'll wait to see their results."[5]

What a joke! They have done nothing but stonewall, obfuscate, censor, and lie for nearly three years—but now suddenly we're supposed to believe the Biden administration and Democrats are committed to getting to the bottom of this.

The Truth Emerges

In late February of 2023, when the *Wall Street Journal* revealed that the DOE now acknowledged that COVID likely leaked from a Wuhan lab, Elon Musk tweeted to his 130 million followers that Fauci had indeed funded the Wuhan lab and, yes, they had been doing dangerous gain-of-function research.

Musk's tweet was in response to a montage video of my exchanges with Fauci where Fauci repeatedly and pointedly denied funding any "gain-of-function" research.

The video that Musk linked to was titled "Dr. Anthony Fauci funded gain-of-function research at the Wuhan lab, lied to Congress about it, and now both the FBI & the Department of Energy have concluded that the coronavirus originated at the Wuhan lab. Does that mean Dr. Anthony Fauci funded the development of COVID-19?" In response, Musk tweeted, "He did it through a pass-through organization (EcoHealth)."[6]

Musk was confirming that I was correct when I challenged Anthony Fauci in committee and Fauci had angrily and vehemently denied funding any gain-of-function research. When I asked Fauci again at a subsequent hearing, "Dr. Fauci, knowing that it is a crime to lie to Congress, do you wish to retract your statement . . . that the NIH has never funded gain of function research in Wuhan?" Fauci, in a transparent attempt to change the subject, abruptly pivoted to the shrill accusation that I was somehow responsible for death threats against him.[7]

The Mainstream Media's Partisan Interference and Denial

And how did the media respond to these exchanges? How did they respond to Fauci's dissembling? Consider the headlines from some popular media outlets when I dared to reveal that the NIH had indeed funded coronavirus research at the Wuhan lab.

Vanity Fair's headline in July of 2021 blared, "Anthony Fauci Once Again Forced to Basically Call Rand Paul a Sniveling Moron."[8] And yet two months later, this headline: "In Major Shift, NIH Admits

Funding Risky Virus Research in Wuhan." The article starts with the obligatory smear: "You didn't have to be a Democrat to be fed up with all the xenophobic finger-pointing and outright disinformation, coming mainly from the right, up to and including the claim that COVID-19 was a bioweapon cooked up in a lab."[9]

The reader must continue until the bottom of the second paragraph, however, to read, "Based on new information disclosed by the National Institutes of Health, however, Paul might have been onto something."

Ya think?

I don't want an apology for the silly name-calling. I do want our media to stop acting as if everything is a partisan game and stop vilifying and lying about anyone they perceive to be on "the other side."

Indeed, my entire questioning of Fauci's funding of gain-of-function research was consistently framed as an "attack" on Dr. Fauci and not a quest for the truth.

"Fauci Says Senator Paul's Attacks 'Kindle The Crazies' Who Have Threatened His Life"—NBC News, January 11, 2022[10]

"U.S. Sen Rand Paul Driving Violent Threats against Me, Fauci Says"—Reuters, January 11, 2022[11]

"Fauci Accuses Senator Rand Paul of Fueling Threats against Him in the Latest Exchange"—*New York Times*, January 11, 2022[12]

"Fauci Exposes Rand Paul for Fundraising off Covid Lies"—*Rolling Stone*, January 11, 2022[13]

"'If Anybody Is Lying Here, It Is You': Fauci Turns Tables On Inquisitor Rand Paul"—*The Guardian*, July 20, 2021[14]

"Rand Paul Abandons His Hippocratic Oath to Play Politics during a Pandemic"—*The Nation*, January 19, 2022[15]

"Anthony Fauci Basically Calls Rand Paul a Shameless Moron to His Face"—*Vanity Fair*, September 23, 2020[16]

The "Rand Paul attacks Fauci" narrative was replayed daily on all of the mainstream networks. CNN's Brianna Keilar called me "ass" on air for simply questioning the COVID narrative.[17] Gail King of NBC giggled and fawned during the Fauci interview, asking such hard-hitting questions as "Does your whole body tense up when you have to talk to Rand Paul?"[18]

I'll give you another example of the shameful and truly embarrassing level of today's journalists' inability to report the truth, much less uncover it. The day after one of my hearings with Fauci, I was aggressively questioned by a young Kentucky reporter who demanded to know how I felt to be the cause of "Dr. Fauci receiving death threats based on your 'attacks.'"

I looked at the reporter and asked, "And what was my question to Dr. Fauci that caused him to blame me for such things?" The reporter stared blankly back at me. He had no idea. He was simply told to stupidly parrot the narrative that I was somehow "attacking" Fauci. There was no interest in the real news, the source of COVID-19, and the fact that the U.S. government might have funded it.

The reporter had not even watched the hearing.

Pockets of Sanity Remain

This is the sad state of the media and so many of our media outlets, which is why true journalists like Matt Taibbi and Glenn Greenwald, who seek to uncover the truth regardless of whom it benefits or harms, are moving to independent forums like Substack.

It is indeed ironic that fears that the internet would foster unreliable news and supplant the trusted legacy media are now replaced with hope that the internet exists to counter the intellectually lazy and biased mainstream media. Thank God for outlets like Substack for allowing inconvenient and unbiased truth to exist, at least for now.

On May 18, 2021, the famously wrong *Washington Post* fact-checker Glenn Kessler awarded me two Pinocchios for revealing the

NIH funding of coronavirus research in Wuhan, while erroneously reporting that the "balance of the scientific evidence strongly supports the conclusion that the new coronavirus emerged from nature."[19] Wrong again, *Washington Post.*

Glenn Kessler has repeatedly been corrected by Twitter's Community Notes for his inaccurate statements. Community Notes enables Twitter (now called X) users to add context and notes in real time to false claims, such as when Kessler awarded three Pinocchios to a report that New York district attorney Alvin Bragg was being backed by billionaire left-wing donor George Soros. The Community Notes correction of Kessler's false "fact-check" stated, "Soros donated $1 million to the Color of Change PAC, the largest individual donation it received in the 2022 election cycle, days after it endorsed Bragg for district attorney and pledged more than $1 million in spending to support his candidacy."[20]

One would think that Kessler would have been chastened by the thousands of tweets correcting his blatant misinformation, but no, he blasted back with insults, calling those who corrected him "twitter trolls."[21]

Elon Musk responded with a tweet: "Only thing on fire are Kessler's pants."[22]

It's great that Twitter—or X—is a place for free speech again. With so much misinformation coming from formerly reliable media outlets, Twitter has become a forum for fact-checking the fact-checkers.

Mask Sanity Begins to Dawn

On February 21, 2023, Bret Stephens of the *New York Times* admitted, for the whole left-wing world to see, that masks don't work.[23] A remarkable eight-day stretch, indeed! First, the DOE and FBI publicly state their conclusions that COVID originated in a lab in Wuhan and then the *New York Times*, the citadel of left-wing misinformation, was admitting that masks don't work, much to the chagrin of virtue-signaling celebrities and Democrats with "Wear a damn mask!" in their social media profiles.

My time in the YouTube penalty box for saying "masks don't work" was even more savored now as a badge of honor.

Stephens wrote, "The most rigorous and comprehensive analysis of scientific studies conducted on the efficacy of masks for reducing the spread of respiratory illnesses—including Covid-19—was published late last month. Its conclusions, said Tom Jefferson, the Oxford epidemiologist who is its lead author, were unambiguous."

Jefferson went on to say, "'There is just no evidence that they'"— masks—"make any difference. Full stop.'"

But surely Jefferson's analysis is only about inferior cloth masks, not the high-quality N-95s? Jefferson responded: "Makes no difference—none of it."

Jefferson was asked about the CDC studies showing that masks prevented transmission of COVID: "They were convinced by nonrandomized studies, flawed observational studies."

As Stephens explained, "These observations don't come from just anywhere. Jefferson and 11 colleagues conducted the study for Cochrane, a British nonprofit that is widely considered the gold standard for its reviews of health care data."[24]

Of course, there was no correction to previous *New York Times* misinformation headlines such as this beauty on November 6, 2020: "On Masks and Clinical Trials, Rand Paul's Tweeting Is Just Plain Wrong." That article came with the equally absurd subhead: "Scientists know masks limit the coronavirus's spread, but it's impossible for randomized trials to prove that."[25] You can't make this stuff up (although apparently you can if you are the *New York Times*).

Columnist Bret Stephens in his February 21, 2023, article titled "The Mask Mandates Did Nothing. Will Any Lessons Be Learned?"

detailed the Cochrane study, which was "based on 78 randomized controlled trials, six of them during the Covid pandemic, with a total of 610,872 participants in multiple countries. And they track what has been widely observed in the United States: States with mask mandates fared no better against Covid than those without."

Stephens, known for not pulling punches, concluded of the Cochrane study, "When it comes to the *population*-level benefits of masking, the verdict is in: Mask mandates were a bust. Those skeptics who were furiously mocked as cranks and occasionally censored as 'misinformers' for opposing mandates were right."[26]

As one of those voices that was censored and derided by the so-called "scientific consensus," I take particular pride in at least one voice from the mothership of acceptable thought acknowledging that I was right and the "experts" were wrong. Though I'm not holding my breath for a formal apology.

After all the *New York Times* publishes Paul Krugman, who wrote an op-ed on July 27, 2020, titled "The Cult of Selfishness Is Killing America," where he excoriated "the right" for refusing to mandate mask-wearing, which he falsely claimed would protect others and therefore was "the kind of thing America's right just hates, hates to hear." He went on to attack me and other "right-wingers" who "make a point of behaving irresponsibly."[27]

Who exactly was politicizing COVID again?

No corrections or apologies have been issued from Paul Krugman for his ad hominem attacks and misinformation, but then again this is the guy who famously predicted that "By 2005 or so, it will become clear that the internet's impact on the economy has been no greater than the fax machine's."[28] Paul, let me know if you'd like to fax me an apology!

CHAPTER 28

Trust Collapses for Institutions and Experts

Much ink has been spilled about vaccine hesitancy and loss of trust in public health. Most of what has been written simply blames the dissenters rather than analyze the problem. Stephens, though, gets it. He writes, "The C.D.C.'s increasingly mindless adherence to its masking guidance is none of those things. It isn't merely undermining the trust it requires to operate as an effective public institution. It is turning itself into an unwitting accomplice to the genuine enemies of reason and science—conspiracy theorists and quack-cure peddlers—by so badly representing the values and practices that science is supposed to exemplify."

Stephens is right when he concludes, "This is the mentality that once believed that China provided a highly successful model for pandemic response."[1]

In an eight-day period of head-turning admissions on COVID's origins and masking's failures, Ben Shapiro of the Daily Wire wrote, "First, it was supposedly a conspiracy theory. Then, it was banned. Finally, it was true."[2]

But how and why did it take years for any kind of serious investigation of COVID's origins to occur? Shapiro explains it, as I have, as a sort of variant of Trump Derangement Syndrome. Liberals avoided, at all costs, discussing the "lab-leak" theory because, as Nate Silver admitted, "The Bad People thought the lab leak might be true, therefore as journalists we couldn't be expected to actually evaluate the evidence for it."[3]

Shapiro explains the phenomenon:

> A huge number of people have decided that there [is] a cadre of people who are so vile that any opinion they touch is immediately toxified beyond investigation. Claims are not to be evaluated on their own merits; instead, we can simply determine whether a claim ought to be supported based on those who posit it. This helps to explain why political crossover has become nearly impossible: We're not judging the claims of our opponents; we're judging *each* other. And this means that we can discard any argument simply by dint of the fact that we don't like the person offering it.[4]

That in a nutshell explains our contemporary political climate. The truth no longer matters. In fact, the truth is simply what your tribal spokesman declares, and objective standards of evaluating the truth are, in today's environment, illegitimate.

Shapiro sums up how intelligent debate has been upended during the pandemic: "Whether it was ignoring the actual evidence regarding masks and mask mandates, the evidence regarding post-vaccination transmissibility or the evidence regarding the lab leak theory, experts decided that the *wrong people* had to be ignored."[5] Now that the facts are irrefutable and we know that "the experts" were wrong, their credibility lies in ruins, and the public's trust in public health is at an all-time low.

Will Government Documents Ever See the Light of Day?

In March 2023, the Senate and House voted unanimously to declassify all documents related to COVID and the Wuhan lab.[6] I was ecstatic, at least for a moment, until I realized that the deep state would still simply withhold the unclassified documents. I had for more than a year been trying to get unredacted, unclassified documents from HHS, NIH, and the Defense Department concerning COVID and Wuhan applications for U.S. tax dollars and been stonewalled at every turn. I had gone repeatedly to four different Democrat committee chairmen with no success. Now we had a unanimous vote to declassify the documents. And yet the realist in me knew that the fight was not over, that the bureaucracy would still resist exposing information on the COVID cover-up. Was it because they feared that the revelation of COVID's origin would hurt our relations with China? Or was it the fear that Americans would discover that the deep state had indeed funded this incredibly dangerous gain-of-function research in China?

Yet even amidst this progress, the Biden administration announced that it continued to support gain-of-function research to "help prevent future pandemics," despite presenting no evidence that gain-of-function research had ever helped prevent a pandemic.[7]

Pushing Onward

I met with the Chinese chargé d'affaires in the spring of 2023. The ambassador had been recalled or retired, and Xu Xueyuan was the second in command until a new ambassador arrived. During our discussion, it was apparent that she was aware that I had argued against inflaming the language of the Taiwan Relations Act. Senators Rubio, Risch, and Menendez collaborated to harangue and condemn the People's Liberation Army by filling the 1970s language with bombastic rhetoric. The Chinese chargé d'affaires was, I think, favorably disposed to listening to me because of my desire at that moment not to stir controversy with Taiwan.

I took advantage of her favorable impression to ask her pointedly if China might consider improving relations with the United States by "discovering" new evidence that COVID-19 might have leaked from the Wuhan lab. I positioned my question as "not an attack on China" but rather a concern that similar research in twelve institutions in the United States also threatened accidental release of a pathogen causing a pandemic. She smiled opaquely and inscrutably. The meeting ended without any illusion the Chinese would cooperate in the COVID investigation.[8]

Meanwhile, the Biden administration signed an agreement with the WHO to subvert our national autonomy and make us answerable to international health edicts. The U.S. ambassador to the WHO announced that America was committed to obeying a new international "Pandemic Accord."[9] There was no mention of any request for congressional approval before this binding treaty was announced as concluded and in place. So much for democracy.

Believe me, they will have me and many others to deal with if they try to enforce this agreement.

According to Scott Atlas, M.D., a former senior advisor to President Trump, the "signers of the Pandemic Accord clearly relinquish critical autonomy to the WHO. Most ominous is that the WHO defines 'public health emergency' on its own terms—giving it full leeway to determine the fundamental justification for public restrictions." Atlas asks, "Why should any sovereign nation allow a third party to legally define and impose such a critical state?"[10]

The Pandemic Accord also disturbingly restricts American intellectual property and lays the ground for price controls on medicine. And to make sure the public understands how woke they are at the WHO, the accord uses the word "equity" at least ten times.[11] Good to know that during the next pandemic Americans will not only be subject to domestic petty tyrants but the international variety as well.

Blinken Stonewalls

A month or so after Wendy Sherman informed the world that she had no idea that the State Department was funding coronavirus research in China, I got a chance to ask Secretary of State Antony Blinken the same question.

This was our exchange:

> **Senator Paul:** On September 12 and November 7 of last year, I sent letters to the State Department asking for records about coronavirus research that had been funded by the State Department. The State Department refused to comply.
>
> When Assistant Secretary Sherman came, I asked her the same question. She did not seem to be aware that you had been funding coronavirus research, but you are. And I got the "I will get back to you" line.
>
> A couple of weeks later, I met personally with you at the State Department and asked you the same question: Will you not divulge to us the records of the State Department's support for coronavirus research, particularly in China? You assured me you would help.

We communicated several times over the phone with another assistant secretary of state who finally sent us a letter and said, "No, we are not going to give you anything."

So that is where we stand, and it is—my question is, what is the State Department hiding? Why will you not give these records to the American people?"

Secretary Blinken: Senator, thank you, and yes, I appreciated you raising this when we saw each other a month or so ago. And my understanding is that our teams have been working to find accommodation. There is long-standing—

Senator Paul: We got a refusal, a blanket refusal, no, they are not going to give us the records.

Secretary Blinken: We cannot directly provide the unredacted—

Senator Paul: Sure, you can.

Secretary Blinken: —unredacted cables. We have a long-standing practice with this committee about how we do—

Senator Paul: You are refusing—you are refusing to release them, not that you cannot.

Secretary Blinken: No, but I think—

Senator Paul: There is a difference between "can" and "may." You won't do it. But you can do it.

Secretary Blinken: My hope is that we can find a way forward that answers your concerns so that you get the information that you are looking for. My understanding is that our team has been working on that, and I commit to continue to do that so we can get you the—

Senator Paul: We are talking about unclassified material. Most of this is unclassified. And so, we just had a unanimous vote in the Senate and in the House, and President Biden just signed a bill saying he is going to declassify stuff.

But if you declassify it and you still hide it from the American people, that's a problem. I mean, we spend all of this time lambasting authoritarians for lack of transparency—we have these silly networks on TV that are aligned with the Democrat Party saying democracy is under attack.

Do you think transparency has something to do with democracy? You are refusing to give records on research—money that went for research. We want to read the research grant proposals.

We want to read what the people in Wuhan sent back to the State Department saying they did. Which viruses did they create? Because the thing is, it sounds all great. We are going to identify all the viruses of the world.

But part of what they do is they take a virus they found two hundred feet down in a cave, and they mix it with another virus to create a virus that doesn't exist in nature because they say that is how we are going to further identify it.

There is a big debate that should be had whether that is safe, to take a virus from a hundred feet down a bat cave twelve hours south of Wuhan and take it to a city of ten million, and yet you will not help us investigate this. You refuse, and it makes—it is reminiscent of the countries we criticize for lack of transparency, and yet you sit there and say you are still going to continue to refuse.

Secretary Blinken: Senator, I think there are very important debates that certainly go beyond my knowledge and expertise, for example, on gain of function, that I know there is a vigorous debate about whether the risk outweighs the reward. I do not have the expertise to know that and—

Senator Paul: But how do we have oversight or investigate it if you will not give us the record?

Secretary Blinken: So, we—so the program that in this instance USAID was involved in was not engaged in gain of function—

Senator Paul: That is a debate—

Secretary Blinken: But—

Senator Paul: —and that is your opinion. We would like to see the records.

Secretary Blinken: So—

Senator Paul: Fauci says there was no gain of function in Wuhan, and nobody believes him anymore.

Secretary Blinken: You know, again, there is a, I think, an important debate about this. As I recall, during the Obama administration, there was actually a moratorium put on—

Senator Paul: I know, but it isn't the debate. I do not want to have that debate with you. I only want to have the records.

Secretary Blinken: Again, I believe that we can find a way to get you the information that you are looking for—

Senator Paul: All right. But the last response we have from you is no. So, the American public needs to know. I have asked many, many times.

I have asked you in person. This is the second time in person. I have talked to two assistant secretaries of state, and the writing we get back from you is "no." Not "maybe." Not "we'll work with you." It is "no." So that is where we are now.

Secretary Blinken: So, Senator—no, and it is not—it is not no, just to be clear. We did reach back out to your team just as recently as this week to offer to provide all of that information in briefing form, which is to say—

Senator Paul: Which means you get to read it and interpret it and spin it, and we get to hear your spin. We do not want to hear your spin. We want to look at the—we are talking about—

Secretary Blinken: We are not in—we are not in—we are not in the business—

Senator Paul: We are talking about grant proposals—you act as if we are talking about the secrets of the Manhattan Project. We are talking about grant proposals, and we are talking about grant updates where someone has to write in and say, oh, we did this experiment, this experiment, and we got this result. That is what we are talking about.

Same thing from NIH. Same thing from HHS. Everybody is hiding it. And it is not even really something to protect the Biden administration. Most of this stuff happened in the previous administration. But I don't get it.

Why circle the wagons? Maybe there is nothing to see here. But then it makes the whole world think you are hiding something if you will not give it to us—

Secretary Blinken: Again, this goes—

Senator Paul: —so just give it to us. It is a bunch of bureaucratic paper that we are looking to sift through to see if there are any clues, because one of the biggest clues we have that they did this is they asked DARPA—and we only know this through a whistleblower—they asked DARPA for money to take a coronavirus and put a furin cleavage site in it to make it more infectious. And, lo and behold, that is what COVID-19 is.

It looks just like what they said they wanted to create with our money, and we turned them down. That does not mean they did not do the research. We are looking for research like that that they were performing.

We are looking for something that may be in their notes that hasn't been public, that has not been sifted through. But what we feel is that people at State Department and at NIH and HHS are conflicted. Why? Because if you funded research that somehow is linked to the pandemic or leakage of that, that does not look so good for the people who funded it.

So we see this as a circling of the wagons and a conflict of interest that maybe there are people within the State Department who funded research who are worried that it might be linked to the pandemic.

We can't just accept your spin on it because people there may be self-interested, the people who funded the program. We are just asking to look at the data. But so far it has been no. We have had a few phone calls. Well, we do not want your spin on it. We want to look at the documents ourselves.
Secretary Blinken: We are not providing spin. As I said, I believe we can provide the information you are looking for. We have long-standing practices and procedures in terms of actually providing documents and cables with this committee that we are not prepared to change. But in terms of getting you the information you are looking for—
Senator Paul: The only cables we have that are of value we got leaked to us, or actually they were declassified by the Trump administration. Those cables from our State Department folks in Wuhan were amazing. [They warned us that unsafe lab practices in Wuhan threatened the possibility of an accident or lab leak.] I do not fault anybody for [glossing over the cables at the time]. I am sure there are thousands of cables. But in 2018 or '17, they were sending cables back saying, "Holy you know what, they are over

here working without gloves in unsafe conditions in a BSL-2 that should be a BSL-4," not a very safe condition, and that is why some of our intelligence people have leaned towards [the pandemic originating in] a lab.[12]

Why would you not want to help us? Why would everybody not *want* to help us?

Secretary Blinken: I have seen those cables. You are right. They have come out, and I think what they said, at least as I read them, was that there were concerns based on State Department officials visiting the lab. There were not a number of sufficiently trained—

Senator Paul: Right. But we only know those because someone had the gumption to declassify them. And I will end with this because I know my time is up.

Mr. Chairman, it takes one signature. He will give all this stuff to me tomorrow if you will sign a document, because he says he won't sign it unless the chairman of a committee does it, and he is hiding behind some ruse. There is no law saying this. He could do it if he wants. But he is hiding behind some opinion that his own administration makes the rules to say they won't give it to Congress. But if you will help me, we can get the information tomorrow. Everything he is saying he will not give me he will give me, tomorrow if you will sign a letter.

The Chairman: I appreciate—the Senator's time has expired—but I appreciate your concern. I understand that my committee counsel has spoken to your counsel this past Monday and your counsel followed up with us today, and we are in pursuit of trying to see how you can be accommodated, and I look forward to making that happen.

Senator Paul: Thank you.[13]

Government Mandates and Immoral Profiteering

Meanwhile, in the Health and Labor Committee, Bernie Sanders was feeling his oats and dragging in every capitalist he could grab to chastise them for the audacity of creating wealth.

He threatened to subpoena the CEO of Moderna, Stéphane Bancel, who finally, under duress, came in "voluntarily." My beef with Bancel was not that he earned too much money but that he earned it on the back of government mandates that, especially for children, ignored important science.

Here is our exchange:

> **Senator Paul:** Mr. Bancel, Moderna recently paid the NIH $400 million. Do you believe it creates a conflict of interest for the government employees who are making money now off of the vaccine to also be dictating the policy about how many times we have to take the vaccine?
>
> **Mr. Bancel:** Good morning, Senator. Indeed, we recently made, before Christmas last year, a $400 million payment to the NIH for an old patent that they had developed not related to COVID, but useful in the development of a COVID vaccine, to pay them for their work. It is for the U.S. government to assess how that money should be—
>
> **Senator Paul:** Do you think it creates a conflict of interest for the same people deciding the policy of how often we have to take the vaccine to also be making money the more times we take the vaccine, yes or no?
>
> **Mr. Bancel:** This is for the government to decide, Senator.[14]

This opening exchange set the tone for the remainder. It was clear that Bancel's plan was simply to filibuster and blather on and evade any real answers. I turned to the side effects of Moderna's vaccine in children.

Senator Paul: You have no opinion on whether or not it creates a conflict of interest. Is there a higher incidence of myocarditis among adolescent males sixteen to twenty-four after taking your vaccine?

Mr. Bancel: So, thank you for the question, Senator. First, let me say we care deeply about safety, and we are working closely with the CDC and the FDA—

Senator Paul: It is pretty much a yes or no. Is there a higher incidence of myocarditis among boys, sixteen to twenty-four, after they take your vaccine?

Mr. Bancel: The data have shown actually—I have seen, sorry, from the CDC actually—have shown that there is less myocarditis for people to get the vaccine versus who get COVID infection.

Senator Paul: You are saying that for ages sixteen to twenty-four, among males who take the COVID vaccine, their risk of myocarditis is less than people who get the disease?

Mr. Bancel: That is my understanding, Senator.

Senator Paul: That is not true. And I would like to enter into the record six peer-reviewed papers, from the journal *Vaccine*, the *Annals of Medicine* that say the complete opposite of what you say. I also spoke with your president just last week, and he readily acknowledged in private that, yes, there is an increased risk of myocarditis.[15]

In fact, a recent peer-reviewed article in *Circulation* shows a link between free spike antigens produced by the mRNA COVID vaccines and… myocarditis.[16] I continued pushing Bancel:

Senator Paul: The fact that you can't [admit the linkage between Moderna's vaccine and myocarditis] in public is quite disturbing. Do you think it is scientifically sound to mandate three vaccines for adolescent boys?

Mr. Bancel: This is for the public health leaders to decide, Senator.

Senator Paul: You have been advocating for it. You have been interviewed, and you have been advocating for boosters. Do you know when the myocarditis is most common among these adolescent boys? After the second dose. When I spoke with Moderna's president, he readily acknowledged in private, yes, that maybe there ought to be a discussion whether we ought to have one vaccine versus two versus three. If 90 percent of the myocarditis comes after the second dose, why don't we have a rational discussion about one? Marty Makary, a physician from Johns Hopkins, has said exactly the same thing. It has been discussed. And yet we have this ridiculous notion from the CDC. So, the CDC says, and I will ask you this question, let's start it as a question.

Your sixteen-year-old has had COVID. Your sixteen-year-old gets better and now has recovered from COVID. You vaccinate them and they get myocarditis. Are you going to give them two more vaccines, your child, give them two more vaccines?

Mr. Bancel: I am not a clinician. I would have to discuss[....]

Senator Paul: [. . .] So, the CDC recommends this, and, you know, you are obviously someone who is self-interested in the outcome here—but the CDC says that if your fifteen-, sixteen-year-old, gets COVID, recovers, takes a vaccine and gets myocarditis, is hospitalized with elevated heart enzymes, and is very sick—the CDC says, as soon as he gets better, vaccinate him again. Do you know how many American parents think that that is a rational, reasonable thing to do? Do you know how many countries don't do this for children?

Sweden doesn't offer the vaccine for kids under twelve unless they are at risk for severe disease. And I agree with that. I am not saying never on any of this. I think it is a very reasonable position to say kids at risk or who have some diseases, that there may be a reason for vaccinating some children.

Finland doesn't recommend it for under age twelve, and Norway also. England as well. France, Poland, Germany, Switzerland all vaccinate twelve and up. So, we have got half the world who have looked at these studies.

There is a study in Israel of thousands of patients, and yet you sit here and act as if you have never heard of myocarditis and you don't think it is an increased risk for young adolescent males when all of the studies who isolate out people by age have found that, yes, there is an increased risk after taking your vaccine. Pfizer, too, but worse with Moderna.[17]

Even the WHO concluded in the spring of 2023 that COVID vaccines are not needed in healthy children.[18]

In response to Bernie Sanders's harangue about raising the price of the vaccine, Bancel opined that the volume of sales was declining as the severity of COVID declined. I agreed with Bancel on that point:

You are right, you are going to make less money [a strong incentive for Bancel to argue that the CDC mandate the vaccine for schools—and the CDC has now added the COVID vaccine to their schedules]. They are going to try to force all the kids in America to do this through school. But guess what? Parents aren't going to do it. They have seen that COVID is not deadly in children. And you are right, it has become less deadly over time.

Your market is going down, so you aren't going to make as much money. I am all for you making money in an honest way, but I don't like the idea that the people making the decisions in government are also receiving money and are now conflicted in their interest.[19]

Forging Ahead with the Fight for Truth

While I continued my daily quest for U.S. government records that might help my investigation into the origins of COVID, the Senate finally passed legislation to end the pandemic emergency first ordered by Donald Trump in 2020 and continued unabated under the Biden administration.

In the fall of 2022, the Senate voted in a bipartisan manner to end the pandemic. President Biden vetoed the repeal. Now, in the last days of March 2023, the Senate again voted to end the pandemic emergency, and this time the Biden administration announced the president would not veto the bill.[20] Hallelujah! At least the usurpation of power under emergency presidential order was coming to an end.

And yet the vaccine mandates continue, particularly in the hospital setting. Even though the CDC now admits that the vaccines have little efficacy for the current variants of COVID. One study found that both the Pfizer and Moderna vaccines had lost any effectiveness at all after a month and might even make vaccinated people more likely to succumb to an Omicron infection.[21]

Nevertheless, hospitals and many universities continued to blindly require three or four COVID vaccines. The story of Nicole Saphier, M.D., illustrates the monstrously unscientific methodology of these mandates. Dr. Saphier, a well-known radiologist and director of breast imaging at Memorial Sloan Kettering Cancer Center and a Fox News contributor, wrote in the *Wall Street Journal*: "When the

Covid vaccines became available two years ago, my rheumatologist, dermatologist and primary-care physician all worried that the shot might trigger an inflammatory response that would exacerbate an existing autoimmune disease. I spoke with a member of the Pfizer scientific team, who suggested that with my autoimmune history I should consider a lesser dose of the vaccine. That wasn't an option at the pharmacies and hospitals that administered the shot, so I reluctantly received the full doses."

Within two weeks of her second vaccine, Dr. Saphier developed nodular scleritis (a painful inflammation of the eyes) and "chest pain from pericarditis." She was understandably leery of getting a third vaccine. But her hospital refused to let her make her own medical decision and demanded either a third vaccine or weekly COVID test, which she still is forced to submit to in 2023 when virtually the entire planet has either vaccine- or infection-induced immunity to COVID. (She has also had COVID.)[22]

When will the scientific illiteracy end?

Pushing for Sanity

In between the continuous COVID misinformation coming from the government, there are occasional glimpses of sanity. Even the notoriously unscientific CDC director Rochelle Walensky admitted that the viral load was indistinguishable between the vaccinated and the unvaccinated and the vaccines no longer prevent infection. Nevertheless, the CDC continues to mandate and push states to add mandatory COVID vaccines to the school schedule.[23]

What should have been readily apparent to all—that COVID vaccine mandates shouldn't be dictated by anyone who stands to gain monetarily—is still not understood or accepted. Now that the NIH had begun receiving hundreds of millions of dollars in royalties from

Moderna's COVID vaccine, no one in their right mind should consider the NIH capable of making unbiased policy concerning vaccine mandates. For nearly four decades, Anthony Fauci controlled this spigot to billions of research dollars. And as his tenure wore on, he became essentially the czar of healthcare mandates and policy.

Stanford's Jay Bhattacharya, M.D., Ph.D., and Harvard's Martin Kulldorff, Ph.D., describe the inherent problems of this arrangement: "If we want scientists to speak freely in the future, we should avoid having the same people in charge of public health policy and medical research funding."[24]

To date, the NIH refuses to divulge if any of the scientists on the vaccine-approval committees receive royalties from the vaccine manufacturers. But now the problem has grown exponentially worse. Instead of just being concerned with the eighteen hundred scientists who received $193 million in royalties, we now must grapple with the entire agency getting *$400 million* from Moderna. Now any NIH scientist who also sits on a vaccine-approval board is conflicted by the allure of all those millions padding the pockets of the NIH ready to be distributed to thousands of scientists.

Adding insult to injury, NIH grant recipients often haven't revealed "publicly traded equity interests from foreign entities."

Justice Department investigations have revealed that the Chinese government has thousands of foreign scientists on its payroll. The *Wall Street Journal* reports that a "U.S. intelligence report assessed that China had recruited 2,629 scientific experts from the U.S. through its flagship 'Thousand Talents Plan.'"[25]

Pushing for the Records and Reforms

During the spring of 2023, I continued my relentless pursuit of government records on the origins of COVID-19. The revelations that the FBI and the Department of Energy both concluded that the virus leaked from a lab in Wuhan put some added weight behind my thirty letters to eight different agencies. A whistleblower gave us a direct phone number to the FBI agent in charge of the COVID origins investigation. After multiple failures to get the head of the FBI's Weapons of Mass Destruction to respond, I tried cold-calling the agent directly. He didn't return the call, but within hours we received an email from FBI headquarters justifying its denial of information because "[t]he President's decision to declassify" some of the COVID information is "complicating matters…" The email went on to inform me in no uncertain terms that "it is unlikely we will put a line agent in front of a member of congress anytime soon."[26] So, in other words, go pound sand. Is it any wonder the American people want the deep state to be reined in? Is it any surprise that trust in government agencies like the FBI is at a historic low?

As my investigation of COVID-19 origins continued in the spring of 2023, there were signs of Democrat resistance finally weakening. Under duress, Gary Peters (D-MI) had begun to selectively cosign records requests while continuing to stymie any real bipartisan investigation into COVID's origins. He has verbally agreed to consider a gain-of-function reform bill.

Patient Zero Identified

Then in June of 2023, the smokescreen of obfuscation and denial finally began to dissipate. Three years after the pandemic began, Michael Shellenberger, Matt Taibbi, and Alex Gutentag at Public and Racket News revealed to the public that the first individual infected by COVID-19 was none other than Ben Hu, a gain-of-function researcher and colleague of Dr. Shi Zhengli at the Wuhan Institute of Virology.[27]

In other words, "patient zero" was a scientist who worked at the Wuhan Institute of Virology and contracted COVID-19 months before the public became aware of the pandemic. Hu was Dr. Shi's lead investigator and hands-on experimenter creating new viruses not found in nature.

As Shellenberger and the others reported, "Sources within the US government say that three of the earliest people to become infected with SARS-CoV-2 were Ben Hu, Yu Ping, and Yan Zhu. All were members of the Wuhan lab suspected to have leaked the pandemic virus."

The source also maintains that these three researchers were working with coronaviruses genetically similar to COVID-19. Shellenberger and colleagues further report that their source was 100 percent certain of the "identities of the three WIV scientists who developed symptoms consistent with COVID-19 in the fall of 2019...."

Alina Chan, the coauthor of *Viral*, describes Ben Hu as "essentially the next Shi Zhengli.... If I had to guess who would be doing this risky virus research and most at risk of getting accidentally infected, it would be him."[28]

If ever there was a smoking gun, this announcement is it. The public had known since January of 2021 that three researchers at the Wuhan Virology Institute became sick with a COVID-like illness in the fall of 2019 well before the pandemic was recognized.

But their names were never released. Why? Perhaps the powers that be worried that if "patient zero" were known to be a gain-of-function researcher at the Wuhan Institute of Virology, then Congress might ask who in the U.S. government made the decision to fund the research that led to an accident that killed millions of people worldwide.

Why did Anthony Fauci direct funds to this lab for more than a decade?

How long had the State Department known the names of the researchers that first became ill? Why did they hide it from my investigation? When I got wind of this new knowledge, I fired off a letter to

Secretary of State Antony Blinken demanding that he either confirm or deny this new revelation.

I cornered the Democrat chairman of the Intelligence Committee Mark Warner when he boarded the Capitol subway to his office building. He was polite and gave lip service to exploring this new revelation, but to date he has refused to help the investigation get records from the Biden administration.[29]

Jamie Metzl, who once sat on the World Health Organization's human genome committee, explains the significance of this new information: "It's a game changer if it can be proven that Hu got sick with COVID-19 before anyone else."[30]

Ben Hu is well known as Dr. Shi's main understudy. Hu has coauthored several papers on creating chimeric coronaviruses with Shi and others. Hu is also infamous for videos showing his unsafe handling of potential pathogens in the field and in the lab.[31]

By January 2021, the entire world knew that three researchers at WIV had been infected with a COVID-like illness in the fall of 2019. Did Dr. Fauci know earlier? Why did Fauci continue to beat the drum for a "natural" origin for COVID even after it became public that the researchers had fallen ill? Was Fauci privy to the actual name of the researcher that now is believed to be "patient zero"?

Fauci's diversionary tactics to this day have discouraged a full discussion of any meaningful reform or regulation of "gain-of-function" research.

Fauci Knew about Gain-of-Function Research All Along

Finally, in the summer of 2023, any lingering doubt of Anthony Fauci's deception was laid to rest. In a 2020 email, in his own words, Fauci refuted his repeated claim that NIH had never ever funded gain-of-function research in Wuhan. In fact, his refutation came in early 2020 in an email to an assistant at NIAID. Fauci wrote,

They [consulted virologists] were concerned about the fact that upon viewing the sequences of several isolates of [COVID], there were mutations in the virus that would be most unusual to have evolved naturally in the bats and that there was a suspicion that this mutation was intentionally inserted. The suspicion was heightened by the fact that scientists in Wuhan University are known to have been working on gain of function experiments to determine the molecular mechanisms associated with bat viruses adapting to human infections, and the outbreak originated in Wuhan.[32]

In this same tranche of documents obtained by the House Select Subcommittee on COVID, we also discover that the Fauci apologist and virologist Kristian Andersen acknowledged early on that the scientists in Wuhan were conducting gain-of-function research. Andersen further noted that the scientists in Wuhan were performing ". . . SARS GOF [gain-of-function] studies," and that "they created a reverse genetics system for their bat virus on a whim."[33]

In taking a deeper look at the material, keen-eyed observers found more Slack messages that were even more astounding. Andersen wrote, "[T]he lab escape version of this is so friggin' likely to have happened because they were already doing this type of work and the molecular data is fully consistent with that scenario."[34]

Later on the Slack channel, the "Proximal Orgin" coauthor Robert Garry commented, "It's not crackpot to suggest this could have happened, given the Gain of Function research we know is happening." And finally in a February 11 email, Ian Lipkin, another "Proximal Origin" coauthor, wrote of the "possibility of inadvertent release...at the institute in Wuhan. Given the scale of bat CoV research pursued there and the site of emergence of first human cases we have a nightmare of circumstantial evidence to assess."[35]

And while Andersen was publicly working with Fauci to debunk and ridicule the lab-leak theory, he stated privately, "The main issue is that accidental escape is in fact highly likely—it's not some fringe theory."[36]

Yes, Anthony Fauci had lied to the American public about funding the dangerous research that may have led to the pandemic. Lying under oath during sworn congressional testimony is a felony. The email confirms Fauci knew over a year before he came to my committee to testify that gain-of-function research had occurred in Wuhan.

I immediately updated my criminal referral with this information and requested the attorney general begin proceedings against Fauci, though it is unlikely that Merrick Garland—one of the most partisan attorney generals to ever hold office—will ever lift a finger to administer justice to Anthony Fauci.

Gain-of-Function Research Marches On

Yet the scientific community continues to push the envelope on dangerous research. Boston University created a novel virus not found in nature by combining the spike protein from the incredibly infectious Omicron COVID-19 variant with the original "wild" variant from early 2020. Realize what this experiment's goal was—to create a virus that combines the lethality of the original COVID-19 with the enhanced infectivity of the Omicron variant. Is that not a death wish for civilization?

The Boston University researchers found that the new virus killed 80 percent of mice versus the original virus that killed 100 percent of the mice. So, at first blush, you might think the scientists have created a virus less dangerous than the original. You would be wrong. The newly created virus might be slightly less lethal but would be exponentially more transmissible—a deadly combination.[37]

How would Fauci reply? He has never retracted his 2012 conclusion that the risks of gain-of-function research are worth the information gained.

The Biden administration's official view is not far removed from Fauci's dogged defense of gain-of-function research. In the spring of 2023, Biden's National Security Council spokesman John Kirby was still responding in the affirmative to the question of whether "gain-of-function research is prudent," noting that Biden "believes that it's important to help prevent future pandemics...."[38]

For every step forward, a great deal of resistance to reform still exists.

CHAPTER 29

Conclusion

The Public Rebels

In April of 2020, Martin Kulldorff, Harvard professor of medicine and one of the world's most respected biostatisticians and epidemiologists, wrote an article called "COVID-19 Counter Measures Should Be Age Specific" and posted it on his LinkedIn page. In the article, he stated, "Among COVID-19-exposed individuals, people in their 70s have roughly twice the mortality of those in their 60s, 10 times the mortality of those in their 50s, 40 times that of those in their 40s, 100 times that of those in 30s, 300 times that of those in their 20s, and a mortality that is more than 3000 times higher than for children. Since COVID-19 operates in a highly age specific manner, mandated counter measures must also be age specific. If not, lives will be unnecessarily lost."[1]

Why did one of the most respected scientists in the world have to resort to publishing on his LinkedIn page? Why would no medical journal publish his work? He was censored for the crime of questioning the lockdown edicts—despite the fact that his statistics were correct. His work threatened the consensus that schools must be closed, society must be shut down, that COVID threatened civilization as we know it.

In other words, his work threatened the control being seized across the country by Democrat governors.

In addition to the elderly, the obese were more at risk due to the increased inflammatory response in the body. Yet since it was deemed politically incorrect to speak the truth, our public health officials did not stress diet and exercise during the pandemic. Instead, they closed the gyms. They put DO NOT ENTER tape around outdoor walking trails and playgrounds. They took the hoops off of basketball goals and poured giant dump trucks full of sand into skate parks.

A young man paddleboarding alone off the coast of California was followed by the Los Angeles County Sherrif's Department, hauled in, and cited for breaking COVID lockdown rules.[2]

It was utter madness. And yet the George Floyd protests, and the riots and looting they spawned, were encouraged and supported by everyone from Michigan governor Gretchen Whitmer to Kamala Harris. Harris went on social media to encourage people to contribute to bail funds for the rioters, one of whom was promptly bailed out and later went on to commit murder. Vice President Harris was never criticized.[3] As Dr. Aaron Kheriaty reminds us in his excellent book *The New Abnormal*, "thousands of public health 'experts' rushed to sign a statement declaring racism a public health emergency during the BLM protests of 2020."[4] So, according to these experts, the public health emergency of "racism" was a valid exception to the COVID public emergency lockdowns.

Children—at statistically zero risk for COVID—were denied fresh air, exercise, outdoor play, and most important, school. They were marooned in front of screens at home. Thousands of kids from strug-gling homes or with neglectful parents lost all structure and completely fell off the grid. Rich kids like California governor Gavin Newsom's four children were quickly back in person at their $60,000-a-year pri-vate Country Day School.[5] They had access to private clubs for outdoor play, tennis, golf, and swimming. And yet Newsom shut down public schools, parks, and playgrounds as being "too dangerous" for the rest of the children in his state.

California had some of the most draconian lockdowns in the country, with public school children denied in-person education for nearly a year and a half.

The teachers' unions nationwide opposed keeping the schools open. An internet watchdog group, Guerilla Momz, caught the head of a California teachers' union, Matt Meyer, on camera dropping his child off at school, even though Meyer was spearheading a fight to enforce the local public school lockdown.

Guerilla Momz presented the video with this message: "Meet Matt Meyer. White man with dreads and president of the local teachers' union. He's been saying it is unsafe for *your kid* to be back at school, all the while dropping his kid off at private school."[6]

Stanford professor of medicine Jay Bhattacharya, one of the heroes of COVID for his brave stand against the anti-science madness, was relentlessly censored and shadow-banned on Twitter by government demand.[7] Bhattacharya tweeted, "Gov. @GavinNewsom kept my kids out of their public schools for nearly a year and a half with no good scientific or epidemiological justification. His record on education is the worst in the country."[8] Even when they did finally return to school, California required kids to wear masks through March of 2022, well after it was shown that masks did nothing to mitigate the spread.

While Gavin and his wife dined at French Laundry (with California "healthcare" lobbyists—oh, the irony!) and spent thousands on wine, mom-and-pop restaurants in his state were shuttered by his edicts.[9] Of course, it was too dangerous for the common folk to eat out or send their kids to school. The list of Governor Newsom's hypocrisies is long, but unfortunately, he was not alone in his zeal to deny civil liberties in the name of "safety," with Governor Gretchen "Gardening is Verboten" Whitmer and my own governor, Andy Beshear, coming in right behind him.

As the pandemic wore on, an unnameable unease was growing. Despite the unrelenting fearmongering from the media and government, with daily death counts inflated to include anyone who tested positive—even if they died in a car accident—the truth began to come out. People could see for themselves who was at risk for severe disease, with over 99 percent of people under seventy recovering from illness similar to a moderate-to-bad flu.[10]

The unease was not fear of impending death or sickness but of discomfort from prolonged quarantine and loss of freedom. The elites continued to revel in levying pronouncements and edicts, but the common man began to rebel. A spontaneous convoy of truckers clogged the streets of Ottawa, honking their horns at the Byzantine COVID rules hurled at them by Trudeau's heavy hand. The government responded with anti-riot soldiers and sent bank police to freeze the truckers' accounts. Taking over their money and livelihoods wasn't enough. The authoritarian Trudeau demanded that private crowd-funding sources deny the truckers access to fundraising from private citizens to feed their families and pay their rent. The truckers had to be broken completely. They had to comply.[11] Where was free speech in the supposedly "free" world?

After the first months of the pandemic, when I had finished nearly three weeks of quarantine for my asymptomatic COVID-19 infection, I was back to flying twice a week to Washington. As I walked through mostly empty airports, something unusual started happening. I was used to getting reactions like a request for a selfie, a "thumbs up," or occasionally a scowl, but now people were quietly approaching me to whisper, "Keep it up." "Don't let Fauci's lies go unanswered." "We're behind you."

It wasn't exactly "Who is John Galt?" but it was a sort of secret nod of the head and hushed encouragement. At first it was quiet, almost as if they were afraid of being reported. After all, look what happened to the truckers. But as the months turned into years, people became bolder, to the point that I was hearing "Keep going after Fauci, Rand!" yelled at me wherever I went. After twelve years in public office, I had never felt such a spontaneous public response from people from all walks of life, encouraging and exhorting me: "Don't stop grilling Fauci! Don't give up. We want the truth."

I was approached by business people in suits and ties, restaurant servers, college kids, retired tourists in T-shirts, baggage handlers, pilots and flight attendants, people of all ages, races, and genders. TSA agents and flight attendants passed notes of encouragement to me. I had my guard up at first, given that some federal union employees are not often friendly to Republicans, but on this issue we agreed: Americans were being locked down, masked, and denied our civil liberties by people that were lying to us. The American people were tired of busybodies and boors. Their patience was growing thin. The American streak of independence and rebellion was percolating as the government's lies were becoming ever more apparent. And people wanted me to know they appreciated my fight for the truth.

Fauci: "I Sleep Fine"

In April of 2023, Fauci's Teflon coating began showing signs of permeability. David Wallace-Wells of the *New York Times* published a lengthy interview with Anthony Fauci that actually asked a few probing questions. The most revealing part of the interview occurred when Wallace-Wells asked Dr. Fauci this:

> I'm not suggesting that the work described in that particular EcoHealth grant led to the pandemic. But we know that there was a lot of other work being done in Wuhan. And if I were you, and I was going to sleep every night thinking that there was even some very small chance that the virus came from a laboratory doing the kinds of research that I had helped promote and fund over the last few decades, I think that might weigh on me a bit, even if I was absolutely sure I had done everything I had done with the best intentions.
>
> **Fauci:** Now you're saying things that are a little bit troublesome to me. That I need to go to bed tonight worrying that N.I.H.-funded research was responsible for pandemic origins.
>
> **Wallace-Wells:** I'm not saying you need to do anything. I'm putting myself in your shoes and telling you what I think it would mean to me to really believe there's a chance, even a very small one, that this pandemic was the result of a lab leak.
>
> **Fauci:** Well, I sleep fine. I sleep fine. And remember, this work was done in order to be able to help prepare us for the next outbreak.[12]

Fauci's Wake-Up Call

Fauci says he sleeps fine. He's unconcerned that he has any culpability regarding the origin of the COVID pandemic. However, Dr. Shi admitted that she had trouble sleeping at first, concerned that the pandemic might have begun in her lab. In all likelihood, Fauci is lying—lying to himself, or the public, maybe both. His hubris and ego may not allow him to question his own role and responsibility, even at 3:00 in the morning.

And yet the human conscience gnaws at anyone capable of remorse. Outwardly, Fauci may insist, "I sleep fine," but the truth is that most capable scientists believe there is a measurable possibility that the COVID pandemic began in a lab in Wuhan. These scientists are the canary in the coal mine, and the real question should be to these objective scientists: Do they sleep well knowing that Dr. Fauci and his decades of appointees seem not to have learned any lesson, nor gained any insight into the dangers of gain-of-function research? If millions of deaths in a worldwide pandemic are not enough, what will be?

Some worry that the deception, the cover-up, and the elaborate escape from responsibility will succeed and Fauci, the Wuhan lab, and Peter Daszak will somehow avoid culpability.

As the media laps up the Fauci platitudes and dissembling, those seeking truth should also note that most experts, as well as a majority of Americans, believe that COVID-19 did, indeed, escape from the Wuhan lab.[13] Fauci's once unmatched approval numbers have fallen below 50 percent.[14] His pontifications from on high are now examined in the light of day. His conflicts of interest have been exposed.

Most of the public now scrutinizes Fauci in light of his support and funding for the dangerous research that likely caused the pandemic and can clearly see that he lied to the American people.[15] When I called him on it, most Democrats refused to hold him accountable. Their intransigence makes it more difficult to pass legislation to prevent another lab leak.

A high-ranking former CDC official told me in confidence that he believes the next leak will be worse, with a fatality rate ranging from 5 percent to as high as 50 percent.[16] And yet with that sword of Damocles hanging above us, the Democrats holding the reins of power continue to stonewall the investigation and have slow-walked any serious oversight or regulation of gain-of-function research.

I find it ironic that Democrats, who advocate for government regulation of every aspect of business, refuse to do the oversight necessary to protect people from the next lab-manipulated virus that could result in untold human suffering and death. Democrats demand worthless and harmful mandates like forced masking and lockdowns, but when asked to do the vital job of regulating lab experiments on deadly viruses that could kill millions, they suddenly have no interest!

Such is the cult of Tony Fauci.

But it is not just about one man. It is the profound danger of putting blind belief in "the experts," with the rest of us taking no responsibility for questioning, for transparency, or for oversight of the very experiments being funded by the American people. Experiments that could kill them.

The GOP-led House investigation promises to make public the evidence. We will bring the perpetrators to justice.

The public largely now knows that Fauci is no philosopher-king, dispassionate and beyond conflict. The public now knows that his personal wealth nearly doubled under the pandemic restrictions,[17] and that he continues to seek to conceal his royalties as well as those of his government-funded scientist buddies.

What is it that made Fauci such a lightning rod? It wasn't just that he funded dangerous research in Wuhan that likely leaked to create the pandemic—and lied to me about it in a Senate committee. It wasn't just that he lied about masking and flip-flopped on virtually every one of his prognostications. It wasn't just that his edicts defied science and likely cost lives. It wasn't just that he stooped to new lows to attack and smear his scientific critics. The reaction to Anthony Fauci can best be explained if you understand Fauci to be the apotheosis of C. S. Lewis's description of the moral busybody:

Of all tyrannies, a tyranny sincerely exercised for the good of its victims may be the most oppressive.... [T]hose who torment us for our own good will torment us without end for they do so with the approval of their own conscience.[18]

As Fauci wagged his finger at the American public and told us that it was none of our business whether scientists on the vaccine committees received royalties or grants funded by royalties, Americans were justifiably appalled. But time and time again, the left-wing media resurrected his image and allowed him to largely avoid having to answer any difficult questions concerning his conflicts of interest.

Fauci would endlessly aver that he was simply a disinterested public servant doing his job. If he needed to lie to the public about the need to mask or about natural immunity, it was simply a Platonic lie, intended to bring about a greater good. Or so his defenders say.

The Aftermath of Delusion

When the experts pronounced that mass gatherings for "worthy" purposes such as the George Floyd protests were not risky, but gatherings for school and church were dangerous and therefore outlawed, we were told to shut up and comply. We were not allowed to challenge this absurdity, or we would be labeled a racist. The experts told us the virus would not spread when one was screaming into a bullhorn and chanting arm-in-arm for social justice. It also definitely wouldn't spread while looting, setting fires, and attacking police. These gatherings were necessary during the pandemic. As for church? Well, God could wait.

It wasn't just schools, churches, and businesses. Your elderly parents locked down in solitary confinement in an assisted-living condo? They could spend the year lonely and isolated. It was too dangerous to give them any human contact. Your loved one's funeral? That was too risky and not allowed. Grieve alone, the experts said. George Floyd, however, required four massive funerals with thousands of mourners, because again, the virus does not spread when one is singing and chanting for social justice. Don't you know anything?

In the face of such obvious contradictions and lies, Americans were astonishingly compliant. We were told so many absurdities repeatedly by the media that a form of mass manipulation of the American psyche occurred. Remember the famous image of a CNN reporter standing in front of a burning street filled with looters and broken windows while the chyron below him read, "Fiery but Mostly Peaceful Protests"?[19] Nothing to see here! Don't believe your eyes. Don't think too hard. Just listen to the experts. Stay home. We are all in this together! Wear a mask. Watch Netflix. Order from Amazon. Take your Soma.

Above all, do not question. To do so risks social condemnation as a racist, a "denier" of the latest approved belief, an "anti-vaxxer" or "anti-masker." Once branded as such, you could lose not just friends and family members, but your job. Your bank could cancel you. Best to remain silent. Listen to the experts. Believe the science. And as Anthony Fauci famously told you, "I am the Science."

How did Dr. Anthony Fauci, lifelong government bureaucrat, become "The Science"?[20] As Jean Giraudoux is quoted as saying, "The secret of success is sincerity. Once you can fake that you've got it made."[21] Likely, no other government official, elected representatives included, could fake sincerity like Anthony Fauci.

Whether or not the U.S. House of Representatives will indict Fauci for lying to Congress or illegally hiding federal communications using a private email address is unknown at the time of this publication. Will Peter Daszak ultimately be punished for withholding evidence from collaborative work done with Dr. Shi and the Wuhan Institute of Virology?

Will investigators finally uncover, from purposefully lost databases, the real precursor to COVID-19?

History Will Judge

Time will tell. But from what we know of the COVID cover-up, the evidence is clear that Fauci, Shi, and Daszak worked together to obscure and distort the truth. The Chinese government orchestrated its own cover-up. Multiple U.S. government agencies to this day continue to hide evidence that they funded dangerous research in Wuhan. I believe that history will judge them harshly.

In the end, one must imagine Fauci, Shi, and Daszak all believe they got away with it. But still, late at night, even the guilty must become anxious, rerunning the scenarios through their minds, wondering... latching onto lingering doubts...and worrying: Did their actions lead to the largest man-made plague in human history? Are the millions dead the result of their experiments to increase the pathogenicity of deadly viruses? History will judge. But the facts as we now know them paint a sordid tale of dishonesty, misjudgment, and ultimately hubris the likes of which this world has rarely seen.

Acknowledgments

Deception: The Great COVID Cover-Up came to its final form with the expert editing of Tony Daniel and Joshua Monnington—many thanks. The project became a reality with the guidance of Tom Spence and the entire Regnery team, to whom I am grateful. And, of course, the book couldn't have come into being without the insightful, thorough, persistent, and loving attention of my bride—Kelley.

Notes

Preface

1. Cheryl Teh, "Shanghai Is Flying Drones over Districts to Tell Citizens under Lockdown to 'Curb Your Soul's Desire for Freedom' and Comply with COVID-19 Restrictions," Insider, April 7, 2022, https://www.insider.com/shanghai-deploys-drones-robot-dogs-broadcast-covid-19-lockdown-guidelines-2022-4.

2. Yong Xiong and Nectar Gan, "This Chinese Doctor Tried to Save Lives, but Was Silenced. Now He Has Coronavirus," CNN, February 4, 2020, https://www.cnn.com/2020/02/03/asia/coronavirus-doctor-whistle-blower-intl-hnk/index.html.

3. "Facebook's Lab-Leak About-Face" (editorial), *Wall Street Journal*, May 27, 2021, https://www.wsj.com/articles/facebooks-lab-leak-about-face-11622154198.

4. See "Deaths by Select Demographic and Geographic Characteristics," Centers for Disease Control and Prevention, June 21, 2023, https://www.cdc.gov/nchs/nvss/vsrr/covid_weekly/index.htm; "Resident Population of the United States by Sex and Age as of July 1, 2021," Statista, 2022, https://www.statista.com/statistics/241488/population-of-the-us-by-sex-and-age/.

5. James Griffiths, "Wuhan Coronavirus Whistleblower Doctor Dies as Confirmed Cases Top 30,000," CNN, February 7, 2020, https://www.cnn.com/2020/02/06/asia/wuhan-coronavirus-update-intl-hnk/index.html.

6. Parveen Shakir, *Khusbhu* [Fragrance] 2nd ed. (Pakistan: Jahangir Books, 1976), 239.

7. Griffiths, "Wuhan Coronavirus."

8. "Wuhan's Early Covid Cases Are a Mystery. What Is China Hiding?" (editorial), *Washington Post*, November 17, 2022, https://www.washingtonpost.com/opinions/2022/11/17/covid-early-cases-wuhan-china-mystery/.

427

Introduction

1. "Head of NIAID-Funded Galveston Lab Relayed Lab Leak Concerns to Head of Wuhan Institute at Onset of Pandemic," Truth USA, December 6, 2021, https://truthusa.us/news/head-of-niaid-funded-galveston-lab-relayed -lab-leak-concerns-to-head-of-wuhan-institute-at-onset-of-pandemic/; U.S. House Committee on Oversight and Accountability, "COVID Origins Hearing Wrap Up: Facts, Science, Evidence Point to a Wuhan Lab Leak," press release, March 8, 2023, https://oversight.house.gov/release/covid-origins-hearing-wrap-up-facts-science-evidence-point-to-a-wuhan-lab-leak%EF%BF%BC/.

Chapter 1

1. World Health Organization (WHO) (@WHO), "Preliminary investigations conducted by the Chinese authorities have found no clear evidence of human-to-human transmission…," Twitter, January 14, 2020, 6:18 a.m., https://twitter.com/WHO/status/1217043229427761152.

2. Anthony Fauci's approval of gain-of-function will be later noted, as it is a major part of this account's thesis. To evade the Department of Health and Human Services Proposed Research Involving Enhanced Potential Pandemic Pathogens Review Committee (P3CO) required Fauci's permission or acquiescence. Some agree, some disagree, for instance, see Reality Check Team, "Coronavirus: Was US Money Used to Fund Risky Research in China?," BBC, August 2, 2021, https://www.bbc.com/news/57932699. See also, Zachary Stieber, "US Government Suspends Funding to Wuhan Laboratory over Risky Experiments," *Epoch Times*, July 19, 2023, https://www.theepochtimes.com/us-government-suspends-funding-to-wuhan-laboratory-over-risky-experiments_5408425.html; Zachary Stieber, "Fauci Knew Chinese Lab Was Conducting Risky Experiments: Email," *Epoch Times*, July 18, 2023, https://www.theepochtimes.com/fauci-knew-chinese-lab-was-conducting-gain-of-function-experiments-email_5403748.html.

3. Jeremy Farrar and Anjana Ahuja, *Spike: The Virus vs the People; The Inside Story* (London: Profile Books Ltd, 2021), 18.

4. Ibid., 19.

5. Ibid., 25; Derrick Bryson Taylor, "A Timeline of the Coronavirus Pandemic," *New York Times*, March 17, 2021, https://www.nytimes.com/article /coronavirus-timeline.html; Jon Cohen, "Chinese Researchers Reveal Draft Genome of Virus Implicated in Wuhan Pneumonia Outbreak,"

Science, January 11, 2020, https://www.science.org/content/article/chinese
-researchers-reveal-draft-genome-virus-implicated-wuhan-pneumonia
-outbreak.

6. Paul D. Thacker, "Former CDC Director Robert Redfield on Inside Battles
with Anthony Fauci, and Why Classified Information Will Point to a Lab
Accident in Wuhan," The DisInformation Chronicle (Substack), September
15, 2022, https://disinformationchronicle.substack.com/p/former-cdc
-director-robert-redfield.

7. Katherine Eban, "'This Shouldn't Happen': Inside the Virus-Hunting
Nonprofit at the Center of the Lab-Leak Controversy," *Vanity Fair*, March
31, 2022, https://www.vanityfair.com/news/2022/03/the-virus-hunting
-nonprofit-at-the-center-of-the-lab-leak-controversy.

8. Thacker, "Former CDC Director Robert Redfield."

9. Ibid.

10. Ibid.

11. Ibid.

12. "Covid: White House Defends Dr Fauci over Lab Leak Emails," BBC, June
4, 2021, https://www.bbc.com/news/world-us-canada-57352992.

13. Thacker, "Former CDC Director Robert Redfield."

14. Ibid.; Robert Roos, "Fouchier Study Reveals Changes Enabling Airborne
Spread of H5N1," CIDRAP, June 21, 2012, https://www.cidrap.umn.edu
/news-perspective/2012/06/fouchier-study-reveals-changes-enabling
-airborne-spread-h5n1.

15. Eban, "'This Shouldn't Happen.'"

16. Thacker, "Former CDC Director Robert Redfield."

17. Ibid.

18. Eban, "'This Shouldn't Happen'"; Amanda Nieves, "Smoking Gun: WCW
FOIA Investigation Proves NIH Allowed Gain-of-Function Research;
Wuhan Lab Funder Calls It 'Terrific!'," White Coat Waste Project,
November 4, 2021, https://blog.whitecoatwaste.org/2021/11/04/bombshell-
wcw-foia-investigation-proves-nih-ignored-gof-research-wuhan-lab-funder-
calls-it-terrific/.

19. Nathan Robinson, "Why the Chair of the Lancet's COVID-19 Commission
Thinks the US Government Is Preventing a Real Investigation into the
Pandemic," *Current Affairs*, August 2, 2022, https://www.currentaffairs.

org/2022/08/why-the-chair-of-the-lancets-covid-19-commission-thinks-the-us-government-is-preventing-a-real-investigation-into-the-pandemic.

20. Farrar and Ahuja, *Spike*, 54.
21. Ibid., 10.
22. Ibid., 11.
23. Ibid., 56.
24. Ibid., 11.
25. Ibid., 53.
26. Ibid.
27. Thacker, "Former CDC Director Robert Redfield."
28. Ibid.
29. From House Oversight FOIA-obtained material that can be found here: Emily Kopp, "Timeline: The Proximal Origin of SARS-CoV-2," U.S. Right to Know, April 11, 2023, https://usrtk.org/covid-19-origins/timeline-the -proximal-origin-of-sars-cov-2/.
30. Video: "An Update from Federal Officials on Efforts to Combat COVID-19," U.S. Senate Health, Education, Labor and Pensions Committee, May 11, 2021, at 1:13:50, https://www.help.senate.gov/hearings/an-update-from -federal-officials-on-efforts-to-combat-covid-19. Written transcript: U.S. Senate Health, Education, Labor and Pensions Committee, *An Update from Federal Officials on Efforts to Combat COVID-19* (Washington, D.C.: U.S. Government Publishing Office, 2022), https://www.govinfo.gov/ content/pkg/CHRG-117shrg46765/pdf/CHRG-117shrg46765.pdf.
31. Farrar and Ahuja, *Spike*, chapter 2; Kopp, "Timeline: The Proximal Origin of SARS-CoV-2."
32. Kopp, "Timeline: The Proximal Origin of SARS-CoV-2."
33. Farrar and Ahuja, *Spike*, chapter 2.
34. Kopp, "Timeline: The Proximal Origin of SARS-COV-2."
35. Farrar and Ahuja, *Spike*, chapter 2.
36. Ibid., chapter 3; Kopp, "Timeline: The Proximal Origin of SARS-COV-2."
37. Farrar and Ahuja, *Spike*, chapter 2; Kopp, "Timeline: The Proximal Origin of SARS-COV-2."
38. Farrar and Ahuja, *Spike*, chapter 3.
39. Ibid.; Kopp, "Timeline: The Proximal Origin of SARS-COV-2."
40. Kopp, "Timeline: The Proximal Origin of SARS-COV-2."

41. Jon Cohen, "Mining Coronavirus Genomes for Clues to the Outbreak's Origins," *Science*, January 31, 2020, https://www.science.org/content/article/mining-coronavirus-genomes-clues-outbreak-s-origins.

42. Ibid.; "Dr. Richard H. Ebright," Rutgers Waksman Institute of Microbiology, 2021, https://www.waksman.rutgers.edu/ebright/people/dr-richard-h-ebright.

43. Kopp, "Timeline: The Proximal Origin of SARS-COV-2"; Cohen, "Mining Coronavirus Genomes for Clues."

44. Ibid.; Jimmy Tobias, "Evolution of a Theory: Unredacted NIH Emails Show Efforts to Rule Out Lab Origin of Covid," The Intercept, January 19, 2023, https://theintercept.com/2023/01/19/covid-origin-nih-emails/.

45. Kopp, "Timeline: The Proximal Origin of SARS-COV-2"; Tobias, "Evolution of a Theory."

46. James Comer and Jim Jordan to Xavier Becerra, January 11, 2022, appendix 1, DocumentCloud, https://s3.documentcloud.org/documents/21177759/house-oversight-letter-and-email-transcriptions.pdf#page=5.

47. Katie Jerkovich, "'That's a Tactic!': Megyn Kelly's Podcast Gets Heated as She Questions Virologist Dodging COVID Lab Leak Theory Questions," The Daily Wire, November 3, 2022, https://www.dailywire.com/news/thats-a-tactic-megyn-kellys-podcast-gets-heated-as-she-questions-virologist-dodging-covid-lab-leak-theory-questions.

48. Emphases Jordan's. Jim Jordan, "What Did Fauci Know and When? His Emails Point to Panic, Lies, and a Possible Cover-Up," The Federalist, July 14, 2021, https://thefederalist.com/2021/07/14/dr-faucis-emails-tell-the-story-of-panic-lies-and-a-possible-cover-up/.

49. Emphasis Jordan's. Ibid.

50. Emphases and brackets Jordan's. Ibid.

51. Ibid.

52. Rebecca Ballhaus et al., "As Covid Hit, Washington Officials Traded Stocks with Exquisite Timing," *Wall Street Journal*, October 19, 2022, https://www.wsj.com/articles/covid-washington-officials-stocks-trading-markets-stimulus-11666192404.

53. Kopp, "Timeline: The Proximal Origin of SARS-COV-2."

54. Ibid.; Josh Christenson, "US Taxpayers Funded $2M Worth of Research in Wuhan, Government Watchdog Reports," *New York Post*, June 14, 2023, https://nypost.com/2023/06/14/us-taxpayers-funded-2-million-for-research-in-wuhan-report/.

55. Brackets Andersen's. Kopp, "Timeline: The Proximal Origin of SARS-COV-2."

56. Ibid.

57. Kopp, "Timeline: The Proximal Origin of SARS-COV-2"; Eban, "'This Shouldn't Happen'"; Emily Crane, "NIH Admits US Funded Gain-of-Function in Wuhan—despite Fauci's Denials," *New York Post*, October 21, 2021, https://nypost.com/2021/10/21/nih-admits-us-funded-gain-of -function-in-wuhan-despite-faucis-repeated-denials/.

58. Jordan, "What Did Fauci Know and When?"; Richard H. Ebright, "Written Testimony of Richard H. Ebright," Homeland Security and Governmental Affairs, August 3, 2022, page 17, https://www.hsgac.senate. gov/wp-content/uploads/imo/media/doc/Ebright%20Testimony%20 Updated.pdf; Sharon Lerner and Mara Hvistendahl, "NIH Officials Worked with EcoHealth Alliance to Evade Restrictions on Coronavirus Experiments," The Intercept, November 3, 2021, https://theintercept.com /2021/11/03/coronavirus-research-ecohealth-nih-emails/; "Drastic Analysis of the Defuse Documents," Drastic Research, September 20, 2021, https:// drasticresearch.org/2021/09/20/1583/; Andrew Kerr, "EXCLUSIVE: Fauci Staffers Flagged Potential Gain-of-Function Research at Wuhan Lab in 2016, Records Reveal," Daily Caller, November 3, 2021, https://dailycaller. com/2021/11/03/fauci-nih-ecohealth-peter-daszak-gain-of-function-wuhan-covid-19/; Personal conversation with Robert Kadlec, fall 2022; Ed Browne, "Fauci Was 'Untruthful' to Congress about Wuhan Lab Research, New Documents Appear to Show," *Newsweek*, September 9, 2021, https://www. newsweek.com/fauci-untruthful-congress-wuhan-lab-research-documents-show-gain-function-1627351; Zachary Stieber, "Fauci Knew Chinese Lab Was Conducting Risky Experiments: Email," *Epoch Times*, July 18, 2023, https://www.theepochtimes.com/fauci-knew-chinese-lab-was-conducting-gain-of-function-experiments-email_5403748.html.

59. Ebright, "Written Testimony of Richard H. Ebright," 17; Kerr, "EXCLUSIVE: Fauci Staffers Flagged Potential Gain-of-Function Research"; Browne, "Fauci Was 'Untruthful' to Congress"; Stieber, "Fauci Knew Chinese Lab Was Conducting Risky Experiments."

60. Gabe Kaminsky, "Top Virologists Who Changed Tune on COVID-19 Lab Leak Theory Received Millions in NIH Grants," *Washington Examiner*, March 2, 2023, https://www.washingtonexaminer.com/policy/healthcare /covid-lab-leak-virologist-changed-tune-fauci-funding; Cassidy Morrison,

"EXCLUSIVE: Peter Daszak's EcoHealth Alliance Has Received $7Million in US Taxpayer Money for Virus Research since Start of Pandemic—despite Ties to the Wuhan Lab at Center of Covid's Origin," *Daily Mail*, October 3, 2022, https://www.dailymail.co.uk/health/article-11274993/Peter-Daszak -received-6-5MILLION-taxpayer-money-ties-China-revealed.html; Scripps Research, "International Research Alliance Launched to Boost Pandemic Preparedness," news relase, August 27, 2022, https://www.scripps.edu/ news-and-events/press-room/2020/20200827-andersen-WAEIDRC.html.

61. Bess Levin, "Anthony Fauci Once Again Forced to Basically Call Rand Paul a Sniveling Moron," *Vanity Fair*, July 21, 2021, https://www.vanityfair.com /news/2021/07/anthony-fauci-rand-paul-covid-19; Eban, "'This Shouldn't Happen.'"

62. Scripps Research, "International Research Alliance Launched."

63. Farrar and Ahuja, *Spike*, 66.

64. Ibid., chapter 3.

65. Select Subcommittee on the Coronavirus Pandemic Majority Staff, "Memorandum," U.S. House Committee on Oversight and Accountability, March 5, 2023, https://oversight.house.gov/wp-content/uploads/2023/03 /2023.03.05-SSCP-Memo-Re.-New-Evidence.Proximal-Origin.pdf; Miranda Devine, "New Emails Show Dr. Anthony Fauci Commissioned Scientific Paper in Feb. 2020 to Disprove Wuhan Lab Leak Theory," *New York Post*, March 5, 2023, https://nypost.com/2023/03/05/new-emails-show -fauci-commissioned-paper-to-disprove-wuhan-lab-leak-theory/; Kopp, "Timeline: The Proximal Origin of SARS-COV-2."

66. Farrar and Ahuja, *Spike*, 64.

67. Caroline Downey, "Fauci and Collins Dismissed Prominent Scientists Who Endorsed Lab-Leak Theory, Emails Show," Yahoo! News, January 11, 2022, https://news.yahoo.com/fauci-collins-dismissed-prominent-scientists -190207092.html.

68. Kopp, "Timeline: The Proximal Origin of SARS-COV-2."

69. Ibid.

70. Farrar and Ahuja, *Spike*, chapter 3.

71. Emily Kopp, "Paper Critical of 'Lab Leak Theory' Cribbed Ideas from Controversial Gain-of-Function Virologist," U.S. Right to Know, November 14, 2022, https://usrtk.org/covid-19-origins/paper-critical-of-lab-leak- theory-cribbed-ideas-from-controversial-gain-of-function-virologist/.

72. Martin Enserink, "Scientists Brace for Media Storm around Controversial Flu Studies," *Science*, November 23, 2011, https://www.science.org/content/article/scientists-brace-media-storm-around-controversial-flu-studies.

73. Ibid.; Thacker, "Former CDC Director Robert Redfield."

74. Brackets original. Roos, "Fouchier Study Reveals Changes."

75. Ibid.

76. Enserink, "Scientists Brace for Media Storm."

77. Ibid.

78. Anthony Fauci, "Research on Highly Pathogenic H5N1 Influenza Virus: The Way Forward," *mBio* 3, no. 5 (September–October 2012): e00359-12, https://www.ncbi.nlm.nih.gov/pmc/articles/PMC3484390/.

79. Browne, "Fauci Was 'Untruthful' to Congress"; Jocelyn Kaiser, "U.S. Should Expand Rules for Risky Virus Research to More Pathogens, Panel Says," *Science*, January 20, 2023, https://www.science.org/content/article/u-s-should-expand-rules-risky-virus-research-more-pathogens-panel-says.

80. Browne, "Fauci Was 'Untruthful'"; Kaiser, "U.S. Should Expand Rules."

81. Robinson, "Why the Chair of the Lancet's COVID-19 Commission."

82. "Senator Paul Accuses Dr. Fauci of Changing Gain of Function Research Definition on NIH Website," C-SPAN, November 4, 2021, https://www.c-span.org/video/?c4985061/senator-paul-accuses-dr-fauci-changing-gain-function-research-definition-nih-website.

83. Jeff Carlson and Hans Mahncke, "Scientists Who Were Instrumental to Covid-19 'Natural Origin' Narrative Received over $50 Million in NIAID Funding in 2020–21," *Epoch Times*, January 25, 2022, https://www.theepochtimes.com/scientists-who-were-instrumental-to-covid-19-natural-origins-narrative-received-over-50-million-in-niaid-funding-in-2020-2021_4220769.html.

84. Emphasis and ellipsis Jordan's. Jordan, "What Did Fauci Know and When?"

85. Kopp, "Timeline: The Proximal Origin of SARS-CoV-2."

86. Ibid.

87. Eban, "'This Shouldn't Happen.'"

88. Art Moore, "Emails: Fauci, Collins Crushed Lab-Leak Theory to Protect 'Science,' China," WND News Center, January 12, 2022, https://www.wndnewscenter.org/emails-fauci-collins-crushed-lab-leak-theory-to-protect-science-china/.

89. Kopp, "Timeline: The Proximal Origin of SARS-CoV-2."

90. Moore, "Emails: Fauci, Collins Crushed Lab-Leak Theory."

91. Thacker, "Former CDC Director Robert Redfield."

92. Ibid.

93. Kopp, "Timeline: The Proximal Origin of SARS-CoV-2."

94. Cf. Thacker, "Former CDC Director Robert Redfield" and Moore, "Emails: Fauci, Collins Crushed Lab-Leak Theory."

95. Carlson and Mahncke, "Scientists Who Were Instrumental to Covid-19 'Natural Origin' Narrative."

96. Ben Gittleson, "White House Asks Scientists to Investigate Origins of Coronavirus," ABC News, February 6, 2020, https://abcnews.go.com/Politics/white-house-asks-scientists-investigate-origins-coronavirus/story?id=68807304.

97. Sharon Lerner, Mara Hvistendahl, and Maia Hibbett, "NIH Documents Provide New Evidence U.S. Funded Gain-of-Function Research in Wuhan," The Intercept, September 9, 2021, https://theintercept.com/2021/09/09/covid-origins-gain-of-function-research/.

98. Fauci, "Research on Highly Pathogenic H5N1 Influenza Virus."

99. Richard H. Ebright, "Written Testimony," 17; Kerr, "EXCLUSIVE: Fauci Staffers Flagged Potential Gain-of-Function Research at Wuhan Lab"; Lerner and Hvistendahl, "NIH Officials Worked with EcoHealth Alliance"; personal conversation with Robert Kadlec, fall 2022.

100. Lisa Schnirring, "China Releases Genetic Data on New Coronavirus, Now Deadly," CIDRAP, January 11, 2020, https://www.cidrap.umn.edu/news-perspective/2020/01/china-releases-genetic-data-new-coronavirus-now-deadly.

Chapter 2

1. Jeremy Farrar and Anjana Ahuja, *Spike: The Virus vs the People: The Inside Story* (London: Profile Books Ltd, 2021), 64.

2. Paul D. Thacker, "Former CDC Director Robert Redfield on Inside Battles with Anthony Fauci, and Why Classified Information Will Point to a Lab Accident in Wuhan," The DisInformation Chronicle (Substack), September 15, 2022, https://disinformationchronicle.substack.com/p/former-cdc-director-robert-redfield.

3. Emily Kopp, "Timeline: The Proximal Origin of SARS-COV-2," U.S. Right to Know, April 11, 2023, https://usrtk.org/covid-19-origins/timeline-the-proximal-origin-of-sars-cov-2/.

4. Kristian G. Andersen, Andrew Rambaut, W. Ian Lipkin, Edward C. Holmes, and Robert F. Garry, "The Proximal Origin of SARS-COV-2," *Nature Medicine* 26 (2020): 450–52, https://www.nature.com/articles/s41591-020-0820-9#ref-CR19; Select Subcommittee on the Coronavirus Pandemic Majority Staff, "Memorandum," U.S. House Committee on Oversight and Accountability, March 5, 2023, https://oversight.house.gov/wp-content/uploads/2023/03/2023.03.05-SSCP-Memo-Re.-New-Evidence.Proximal-Origin.pdf; Miranda Devine, "New Emails Show Dr. Anthony Fauci Commissioned Scientific Paper in Feb. 2020 to Disprove Wuhan Lab Leak Theory," *New York Post*, March 5, 2023, https://nypost.com/2023/03/05/new-emails-show-fauci-commissioned-paper-to-disprove-wuhan-lab-leak-theory/; Kopp, "Timeline: The Proximal Origin of SARS-COV-2."

5. Farrar and Ahuja, *Spike*, 68.

6. Andersen et al., "Proximal Origin," 450.

7. Ibid., 450.

8. Ibid., 451.

9. Ibid., 451–52.

10. Ibid.

11. Alina Chan and Matt Ridley, *Viral: The Search for the Origin of COVID-19* (New York: HarperCollins, 2021), 261.

12. Steven Quay, "Opening Remarks of Dr. Steven C. Quay, MD, PhD," U.S. House Committee on Oversight and Accountability, June 26, 2021, https://oversight.house.gov/wp-content/uploads/2021/06/Steven-Quay-Prepared-Remarks-26-June-2021-12-230-EST-FINAL.pdf; Matt Palumbo, "Top Scientist Lays Out Case for Wuhan Lab Leak—Warns They May Have an Even Deadlier Virus," The Dan Bongino Show, October 9, 2021, https://bongino.com/top-scientist-lays-out-evidence-for-wuhan-lab-leak-warns-they-may-have-an-even-deadlier-virus.

13. Chan and Ridley, *Viral*, chapter 5.

14. Thacker, "Former CDC Director Robert Redfield."

15. Ridley and Chan, *Viral*, 96.

16. Ibid., 98.

17. Emphasis added. Ibid., 97.
18. Ibid.
19. Ridley and Chan, *Viral*, 96–98; Aylin Woodward, "Chinese CDC Now Says the Wuhan Wet Market Wasn't the Origin of the Virus," Science Alert, May 29, 2020, https://www.sciencealert.com/chinese-cdc-now-says-the -wuhan-wet-market-was-the-site-of-a-super-spreader-event.
20. Andersen et al., "Proximal Origin," 452.
21. Shayla Love, "Once and for All, the New Coronavirus Was Not Made in a Lab," *Vice*, March 20, 2020, https://www.vice.com/en/article/xgqkn4/ the-novel-coronavirus-was-not-made-in-a-lab-nature-medicine-study-confirms.
22. Andersen et al., "Proximal Origin."
23. Caroline Downey, "Fauci and Collins Dismissed Prominent Scientists Who Endorsed Lab-Leak Theory, Emails Show," Yahoo! News, January 11, 2022, https://news.yahoo.com/fauci-collins-dismissed-prominent-scientists -190207092.html.
24. Love, "Once and for All."
25. Ibid.
26. Nicholas Wade, "Origin of Covid—Following the Clues," Medium, May 2, 2021, https://nicholaswade.medium.com/origin-of-covid-following-the-clues-6f03564c038.
27. Ibid.
28. Jean-Paul Chretien and Robert Greg Cutlip, "Critical Analysis of *Andersen et al. The Proximal Origin of SARS-CoV-2*," (working paper), Drastic Research, May 26, 2020, https://drasticresearch.files.wordpress.com/2023 /05/an-argument-against-natural-covid-19-creation-copy-2.pdf; Andersen et al., "Proximal Origin," 450.
29. Chretien and Cutlip, "Critical Analysis of *Andersen et al.*"
30. Trump White House Archived, "4/17/20: Members of the Coronavirus Task Force Hold a Press Briefing," YouTube, April 17, 2020, https://www. youtube.com/watch?v=brbArpX8t6I&t=5912s.
31. Wade, "Origin of Covid."
32. Ibid.
33. Ibid.
34. Ibid.

35. Farrar and Ahuja, *Spike*, 65.
36. First three sets of brackets added, last set of brackets original. James Comer and Jim Jordan to Xavier Beccera, January 11, 2022, DocumentCloud, https://s3.documentcloud.org/documents/21177759/house-oversight-letter -and-email-transcriptions.pdf#page=5.
37. Ridley and Chan, *Viral*, 58.
38. Ibid., 10.
39. Ibid., 166.
40. Andersen et al., "Proximal Origin."
41. Elaine Dewar, *On the Origin of the Deadliest Pandemic in 100 Years: An Investigation* (Windsor, Ontario: Biblioasis, 2021), 306–9.
42. Ridley and Chan, *Viral*, 289.
43. Emily Kopp, "Virologist Who Tried to Discredit the Lab Leak Theory Was Once a 'Partner' to EcoHealth Alliance," U.S. Right to Know, July 1, 2022, https://usrtk.org/covid-19-origins/anti-lab-leak-virologist-ecohealth-alliance -partner/.
44. Ibid.

Chapter 3

1. Charles Calisher, Peter Daszak, and Jeremy Farrar et al., "Statement in Support of the Scientists, Public Health Professionals, and Medical Professionals of China Combatting COVID-19," *The Lancet* 395, no. 10226 (2020): E42–E43, https://www.thelancet.com/journals/lancet/article /PIIS0140-6736(20)30418-9/fulltext.
2. Nicholas Wade, "Origin of Covid—Following the Clues," Medium, May 2, 2021, https://nicholaswade.medium.com/origin-of-covid-following-the-clues-6f03564c038.
3. Elaine Dewar, *On the Origin of the Deadliest Pandemic in 100 Years: An Investigation* (Windsor, Ontario: Biblioasis, 2021), 439.
4. Ibid., 393.
5. Elizabeth Redden, "'An Unacceptable Breach of Trust,'" Inside Higher Ed, October 2, 2018, https://www.insidehighered.com/news/2018/10/03/book -publishers-part-ways-springer-nature-over-concerns-about-censorship -china.
6. Ibid.
7. Ibid.

8. Jerry Dunleavy, "Wuhan Lab Collaborator Recused from *Lancet's* COVID-19 Origins Investigation," *Washington Examiner,* June 21, 2021, https://www.washingtonexaminer.com/news/wuhan-lab-collaborator-peter-daszak-recused-from-lancets-covid-19-origins-investigation.

9. Matt Ridley and Alina Chan, *Viral: The Search for the Origin of COVID-19* (New York: HarperCollins, 2021), 249.

10. Ellipses in the original. Ibid., 290.

11. Wade, "Origin of Covid."

12. Ellispes original. Emily Wang Fujiyama and Sam McNeil, "AP Interview: China Granted WHO Team Full Access in Wuhan," Associated Press, February 5, 2021, https://apnews.com/article/china-granted-who-full-access-wuhan-52dae25c21db7c80c404251e481f88bc.

13. Amy Goodman, "'Pure Baloney': Zoologist Debunks Trump's COVID-19 Origin Theory, Explains Animal-Human Transmission," Democracy Now!, April 16, 2020, https://www.democracynow.org/2020/4/16/peter_daszak_coronavirus.

14. Wade, "Origin of Covid."

15. Ridley and Chan, *Viral,* 148.

16. Rowan Jacobsen, "The Non-Paranoid Person's Guide to Viruses Escaping from Labs," *Mother Jones,* May 14, 2020, https://www.motherjones.com/politics/2020/05/the-non-paranoid-persons-guide-to-viruses-escaping-from-labs/.

17. Wade, "Origin of Covid."

18. Ridley and Chan, *Viral,* 268.

19. "We're Still Missing the Origin Story of This Pandemic. China Is Sitting on the Answers" (editorial), *Washington Post,* February 5, 2021, https://www.washingtonpost.com/opinions/2021/02/05/coronavirus-origins-mystery-china/.

20. Dewar, *On the Origin,* 238.

21. Steven Quay, "Opening Remarks of Dr. Steven C. Quay, MD, PhD," U.S. House Committee on Oversight and Accountability, June 26, 2021, https://oversight.house.gov/wp-content/uploads/2021/06/Steven-Quay-Prepared-Remarks-26-June-2021-12-230-EST-FINAL.pdf.

22. Ridley and Chan, *Viral,* 255.

23. Dominic Dwyer, "I Was on the WHO's Covid Mission to China, Here's What We Found," *The Guardian,* February 22, 2021, https:\\www.

guardian.com\commentisfree\2021\feb\22\i-was-on-the-whos-covid-mission-to-china-heres-what-we-found.

24. Fred Guterl, Naveed Jamali, and Tom O'Connor, "The Controversial Experiments and Wuhan Lab Suspected of Starting the Coronavirus Pandemic," *Newsweek*, May 1, 2020, https://www.newsweek.com/controversial-wuhan-lab-experiments-that-may-have-started-coronavirus-pandemic-1500503.

25. Ridley and Chan, *Viral*, 282.

26. Quay, "Opening Remarks of Dr. Steven C. Quay, MD, PhD."

27. Ibid.

28. Emphasis original. Ibid.

29. Aylin Woodward, "The Chinese CDC Now Says the Coronavirus Didn't Jump to People at the Wuhan Wet Market—Instead, It Was the Site of a Superspreader Event," Insider, May 28, 2020, https://www.businessinsider.com/coronavirus-did-not-jump-wuhan-market-chinese-cdc-says-2020-5.

30. One of multiple examples: Graham Massie, "Covid Definitely Started in 'Wet' Market, Two New Studies Find," *Irish Independent*, February 28, 2022, https://www.independent.ie/world-news/covid-definitely-started-in-wet-market-two-new-studies-find-41392258.html.

31. Ridley and Chan, *Viral*, 267.

32. Sharon Lerner, "Leaked Grant Proposal Details High-Risk Coronavirus Research," The Intercept, September 23, 2021, https://theintercept.com/2021/09/23/coronavirus-research-grant-darpa/.

33. Ibid.

34. Personal phone call.

35. Zachary Stieber, "Fauci Testimony 'Not Credible' in Light of Other Evidence: Lawyers," *Epoch Times*, March 8, 2023, https://www.theepochtimes.com/fauci-testimony-not-credible-in-light-of-other-evidence-lawyers_5108458.html.

36. Ibid.

37. "MERS-CoV Research: Current Status and Future Priorities Meeting," NIH Videocasting, June 24, 2013, https://videocast.nih.gov/watch=12908.

38. Stieber, "Fauci Testimony."

39. David Macdonald, "The Wet Market Sources of Covid-19: Bats and Pangolins Have an Alibi," University of Oxford, June 7, 2021, https://www.ox.ac.uk/news/science-blog/wet-market-sources-covid-19-bats-and

-pangolins-have-alibi; Karen E. Lange, "EXCLUSIVE: What You Need to Know about Wildlife Markets and COVID-19," Humane Society of the United States, June 4, 2020, https://www.humanesociety.org/news/exclusive -what-you-need-know-about-wildlife-markets-and-covid-19.

40. @CAPITOLSHEILA, "He Worked with Wuhan Institute, but Forgot to Tell Congress," BatSh*t Crazy (Substack), April 22, 2022, https://capitolsheila .substack.com/p/he-worked-with-wuhan-institute-but.

41. Emily Kopp, "Timeline: The Proximal Origin of SARS-COV-2," U.S. Right to Know, April 11, 2023, https://usrtk.org/covid-19-origins/timeline-the -proximal-origin-of-sars-cov-2/; Dewar, *On the Origin*, 439.

42. Wade, "Origin of Covid."

43. Ridley and Chan, *Viral*, 95.

44. Ibid., 96.

45. Wade, "Origin of Covid."

46. Ibid.

47. Dewar, *On the Origin*.

48. Wade, "Origin of Covid."

49. Rossana Segreto et al., "Should We Discount the Laboratory Origin of Covid-19?," *Environmental Chemistry Letters* 19 (2021): 2747, https://link .springer.com/article/10.1007/s10311-021-01211-0.

50. Quay, "Opening Remarks of Dr. Steven C. Quay, MD, PhD."

51. Ibid.

52. Emphasis original. Ibid.

53. Ibid.

54. Ibid.

Chapter 4

1. Steven Quay, "Opening Remarks of Dr. Steven C. Quay, MD, PhD," U.S. House Committee on Oversight and Accountability, June 26, 2021, https:// oversight.house.gov/wp-content/uploads/2021/06/Steven-Quay-Prepared -Remarks-26-June-2021-12-230-EST-FINAL.pdf.

2. Emphasis original. Ibid.

3. Emphasis original. Ibid.

4. Ibid.

5. Nicholas Wade, "Origin of Covid—Following the Clues," Medium, May 2, 2021, https://nicholaswade.medium.com/origin-of-covid-following-the-clues-6f03564c038.

6. Quay, "Opening Remarks of Dr. Steven C. Quay, MD, PhD."

7. Wade, "Origin of Covid."

8. Ibid.

9. Quay, "Opening Remarks of Dr. Steven C. Quay, MD, PhD."

10. James Gorman and Carl Zimmer, "Scientist Opens Up about His Early Email to Fauci on Virus Origins," *New York Times*, June 20, 2021, https://www.nytimes.com/2021/06/14/science/covid-lab-leak-fauci-kristian-andersen.html.

11. Jeffrey D. Sachs and Neil L. Harrison, "A Call for an Independent Inquiry into the Origin of the SARS-CoV-2 Virus," *Proceedings of the National Academy of Sciences* 119, no. 21 (2022): e2202769119, https://www.pnas.org/doi/10.1073/pnas.2202769119.

12. Quay, "Opening Remarks of Dr. Steven C. Quay, MD, PhD."

13. Ibid.

14. Ibid.

15. Rossana Segreto et al., "Should We Discount the Laboratory Origin of Covid-19?," *Environmental Chemistry Letters* 19 (2021): 2746, https://link.springer.com/article/10.1007/s10311-021-01211-0.

16. Ibid.

17. Matt Ridley and Alina Chan, *Viral: The Search for the Origin of COVID-19* (New York: HarperCollins, 2021), 210.

18. Sheryl Gay Stolberg, Benjamin Mueller, and Carl Zimmer, "The Origins of the Covid Pandemic: What We Know and Don't Know," *New York Times*, March 17, 2023, https://www.nytimes.com/article/covid-origin-lab-leak-china.html; Han Xia et al., "Biosafety Level 4 Laboratory User Training Program, China," *Emerging Infectious Diseases* 25, no. 5 (2019): e180220, https://wwwnc.cdc.gov/eid/article/25/5/18-0220_article; Miranda Devine, "WHO's COVID 'Investigation' Was Dishonest Chinese Propaganda: Devine," *New York Post*, February 10, 2021, https://nypost.com/2021/02/10/whos-covid-investigation-was-dishonest-chinese-propaganda-devine/.

19. MicrobeTV, "TWiV 940: Eddie Holmes in [sic] on Viral Origins," YouTube, September 28, 2022, https://www.youtube.com/watch?v=5u94foNmpKE. Holmes discusses Andersen's "pulled off a ledge" comment at 31:50.

20. Ibid., after 31:50.

21. This sentence, deleted from the current version of the article, can be accessed via Internet Archive's WayBack Machine: Emily Kopp, "Timeline: The Proximal Origin of SARS-COV-2," U.S. Right to Know, September 14, 2022, https://web.archive.org/web/20221021094313/https://usrtk.org/covid-19-origins/timeline-the-proximal-origin-of-sars-cov-2/.

22. Jeremy Farrar and Anjana Ahuja, *Spike: The Virus vs the People; The Inside Story* (London: Profile Books Ltd, 2021), chapter 2.

23. Charles Rixley, "Charles Rixey Op-Ed: Who Watches the Watchmen? Fauci's 'Noble Lie,' Exposed," What Did You Say?, July 30, 2021, https://whatdidyousay.org/2021/07/30/charles-rixey-op-ed-who-watches-the-watchmen-faucis-noble-lie-exposed/.

24. Personal conversation with Robert Kadlec, fall 2022.

Chapter 5

1. Rowan Scarborough, "The Lancet Chides Wuhan Defender Daszak," *Washington Times*, January 6, 2022, https://www.washingtontimes.com/news/2022/jan/6/the-lancet-chides-wuhan-defender-daszak/.

2. Richard Horton, "Offline: The Origin Story," *The Lancet* 398 (2021): 2136, https://www.thelancet.com/action/showPdf?pii=S0140-6736%2821%2902786-0; "Addendum: Competing Interests and the Origins of SARS-COV-2" (editorial), *The Lancet* 397 (2021): 2449–50, https://www.thelancet.com/pdfs/journals/lancet/PIIS0140-6736(21)01377-5.pdf.

3. Ellipsis original. Joe Davies and Victoria Allen, "Lancet Editor Who Published Letter Slamming Covid Lab Leak Theory as 'Conspiracy' Admits He Knew about Lead Author's Links to Chinese Lab at Centre of Cover-Up for a YEAR before Acknowledging Conflict of Interests," *Daily Mail*, October 3, 2022, https://www.dailymail.co.uk/news/article-10320621/Brit-scientist-took-year-declare-links-Chinese-lab-opposing-Covid-lab-leak-theory.html.

4. Josh Christenson, "US Taxpayers Funded $2M Worth of Research in Wuhan, Government Watchdog Reports," *New York Post*, June 14, 2023, https://nypost.com/2023/06/14/us-taxpayers-funded-2-million-for-research-in-wuhan-report/.

5. Jeffrey D. Sachs et al., "The Lancet COVID-19 Commission," *The Lancet* 396, no. 10249 (2020): 454–55, https://www.thelancet.com/journals/lancet/article/PIIS0140-6736(20)31494-X/fulltext; EcoHealth Alliance,

"EcoHealth Alliance Receives NIH Renewal Grant for Collaborative Research to Understand the Risk of Bat Coronavirus Spillover Emergence," news release, May 8, 2023, https://www.ecohealthalliance.org/2023/05/collaborative-research-to-understand-the-risk-of-bat-coronavirus-spillover-emergence; Christenson, "US Taxpayers Funded $2M Worth of Research in Wuhan."

6. Sachs et al., "The Lancet COVID-19 Commission."

7. Personal conversation with Susan Collins.

8. Phone conversation with Jeffrey Sachs.

9. Personal conversation with Chuck Schumer.

10. Personal conversation with Bernie Sanders.

11. Nathan Robinson, "Why the Chair of the Lancet's COVID-19 Commission Thinks the US Government Is Preventing a Real Investigation into the Pandemic," *Current Affairs*, August 2, 2022, https://www.currentaffairs.org/2022/08/why-the-chair-of-the-lancets-covid-19-commission-thinks-the-us-government-is-preventing-a-real-investigation-into-the-pandemic.

12. Edmund DeMarche, "Daszak 'Recused' from Lancet's COVID-19 Commission," Fox News, June 22, 2021, https://www.foxnews.com/health/daszak-recused-from-lancets-covid-19-commission.

13. Robinson, "Why the Chair of the Lancet's COVID-19."

14. Emphasis original. Ibid.

15. Ibid.

16. Personal recollection of Jeffrey Sachs Zoom presentation, December 2022. See also, Robinson, "Why the Chair of the Lancet's COVID-19."

17. Robinson, "Why the Chair of the Lancet's COVID-19."

18. Ibid.

19. Ibid.

20. Ibid.

21. Bracketed note original. Ibid.

22. Emphasis original. Ibid.

23. Ibid.

24. Nicholson Baker, "The Lab-Leak Hypothesis: For Decades, Scientists Have Been Hot-Wiring Viruses in Hopes of Preventing a Pandemic, Not Causing One. But What Is…?," Intelligencer, January 4, 2021, https://nymag.com/intelligencer/article/coronavirus-lab-escape-theory.html.

25. Robinson, "Why the Chair of the Lancet's COVID-19 Commission."

26. Ibid.

27. Jeffrey D. Sachs and Neil L. Harrison, "A Call for an Independent Inquiry into the Origin of the SARS-CoV-2 Virus," *Proceedings of the National Academy of Sciences* 119, no. 21 (2022): e2202769119, https://www.pnas.org/doi/10.1073/pnas.2202769119.

28. Ibid.

29. "We're Still Missing the Origin Story of This Pandemic. China Is Sitting on the Answers" (editorial), *Washington Post*, February 5, 2021, https://www.washingtonpost.com/opinions/2021/02/05/coronavirus-origins-mystery-china/.

30. Steven Nelson, "NIH Director Confirms Agency Hid Early COVID Genes at Request of Chinese Scientists," *New York Post*, May 11, 2022, https://nypost.com/2022/05/11/nih-director-tabak-confirms-agency-hid-covid-genes-per-chinese/.

31. EcoHealth Alliance, "EcoHealth Alliance Receives NIH Renewal Grant."

32. Jocelyn Kaiser, "NIH Restarts Bat Virus Grant Suspended 3 Years Ago by Trump," *Science*, May 8, 2023, https://www.science.org/content/article/nih-restarts-bat-virus-grant-suspended-3-years-ago-trump.

33. Peter Daszak, "Termination of Our Coronavirus Work by NIH Last Friday" (email), U.S. Right to Know, April 28, 2020, https://usrtk.org/wp-content/uploads/2023/01/Request-20-320.pdf#page=792.

34. Carl Zimmer, "Bat Virus Studies Raise Questions about Laboratory Tinkering," *New York Times*, July 15, 2022, https://www.nytimes.com/2022/07/15/science/bat-coronavirus-laboratory-experiments.html.

35. Lee Brown, "Scientists at Wuhan Lab in COVID Probe Admitted Being Bitten by Bats: Reports," *New York Post*, May 28, 2021, https://nypost.com/2021/05/28/scientists-at-wuhan-lab-filmed-being-bitten-by-bats-report/; Sasha Pezenik, Josh Margolin, Kaitlyn Morris, and Terry Moran, "New Report from Senate Republicans Doubles Down on COVID Lab Leak Theory," ABC News, April 18, 2023, https://abcnews.go.com/Health/new-report-senate-republicans-doubles-covid-lab-leak/story?id=98656740.

36. Hanna Panreck, "Dr. Fauci Claims a Coronavirus Lab Leak Could Still Be Considered a 'Natural Occurrence,'" Fox News, March 12, 2023, https://www.foxnews.com/media/dr-fauci-claims-coronavirus-lab-leak-could-still-be-considered-natural-occurrence.

37. Sachs and Harrison, "Call for an Independent Inquiry."

38. Sharon Lerner, "Jeffrey Sachs Presents Evidence of Possible Lab Origin of Covid-19," The Intercept, May 19, 2022, https://theintercept.com/2022/05 /19/covid-lab-leak-evidence-jeffrey-sachs/.

39. Praveen Anand et al., "SARS-CoV-2 Strategically Mimics Proteolytic Activation of Human ENAC," *eLife* 26, no. 9 (2020): e58603, https:// pubmed.ncbi.nlm.nih.gov/32452762/.

40. Sachs and Harrison, "Call for an Independent Inquiry."

41. Ibid.

42. Ibid.

43. Charles Rixey, "Gaslight of the Gods: The New DARPA Report Raises a Lot of Questions No One Is Asking," Prometheus Shrugged (Substack), January 29, 2022, https://prometheusshrugged.substack.com/p/deusexgaslight.

44. Joseph Murphy, Unclassified DARPA Documents, August 13, 2021, https:// assets.ctfassets.net/syq3snmxclc9/2mVob3c1aDd8CNvVnyei6n/95af7dbfd2 958d4c2b8494048b4889b5/JAG_Docs_pt1_Og_WATERMARK_OVER _Redacted.pdf.

45. Ibid.

46. Ibid.

47. Ibid.

48. Ibid.

49. Ibid.

50. Ibid.

51. Ibid.

52. Ibid.

53. Elaine Dewar, *On the Origin of the Deadliest Pandemic in 100 Years: An Investigation* (Windsor, Ontario: Biblioasis, 2021), 41.

54. Sachs and Harrison, "Call for an Independent Inquiry."

55. Ibid.

56. Ibid.

Chapter 6

1. See, e.g., Paul R. La Monica, "Gilead Sciences Drug Remdesivir May Help Treat Coronavirus Symptoms, according to WHO," CNN, February

25, 2020, https://www.cnn.com/2020/02/24/investing/gilead-sciences-coronavirus-who-remdesivir/index.html.

2. Video: "An Emerging Disease Threat: How the U.S. Is Responding to COVID-19, the Novel Coronavirus," U.S. Senate Committee on Health, Education, Labor and Pensions, March 3, 2020, at 1:26:50, https://www.help.senate.gov/hearings/an-emerging-disease-threat-how-the-us-is-responding-to-covid-19-the-novel-coronavirus; written transcript: U.S. Senate Committee on Health, Education, Labor and Pensions, *An Emerging Disease Threat: How the U.S. Is Responding to COVID–19, the Novel Coronavirus* (Washington, D.C.: U.S. Government Publishing Office, 2021), 31, https://www.govinfo.gov/content/pkg/CHRG-116shrg45217/pdf/CHRG-116shrg45217.pdf. Transcript lightly edited to improve readability.

3. "Emerging Disease Threat," at 1:27:10; U.S. Senate Committee on HELP, *Emerging Disease Threat*, 31–32. Transcript lightly edited to improve readability.

4. Jeremy Page, Betsy McKay, and Drew Hinshaw, "How the WHO's Hunt for Covid's Origins Stumbled in China," *Wall Street Journal*, March 17, 2021, https://www.wsj.com/articles/who-china-hunt-covid-origins-11616004512; Miranda Devine, "WHO's COVID 'Investigation' Was Dishonest Chinese Propaganda: Devine," *New York Post*, February 10, 2021, https://nypost.com/2021/02/10/whos-covid-investigation-was-dishonest-chinese-propaganda-devine/.

5. "Emerging Disease Threat," at 1:28:30; U.S. Senate Committee on HELP, *Emerging Disease Threat*, 32. Transcript lightly edited to improve readability. Brackets indicate slight rewording for written clarity throughout.

6. Alex Berenson, *Pandemia: How Coronavirus Hysteria Took Over Our Government, Rights, and Lives* (Washington, D.C.: Regnery Publishing, 2021), 64.

7. Personal communication with Wyche Coleman.

8. Personal recollection.

9. Personal recollection.

10. Sammi Steele, "Midland Memorial Hospital Says Inhaled Steroid Is No 'Silver Bullet' for COVID-19," NewsWest9, July 7, 2020, https://www.newswest9.com/article/news/local/midland-memorial-hospital-says-inhaled-steroid-is-no-silver-bullet-for-covid-19/513-a30477f5-35fb-41cb-97fb-e8aaad6250b2.

11. Ibid.

12. "COVID-19 Coronavirus Pandemic," Worldometer, July 13, 2023, https://www.worldometers.info/coronavirus; Angelo Maria Pezzullo et al., "Age-Stratified Infection Fatality Rate of COVID-19 in the Non-Elderly Population," *Environmental Research* 216 (2023): 114655, https://www.ncbi.nlm.nih.gov/pmc/articles/PMC9613797/.

13. Mirko Griesel et al., "Inhaled Corticosteroids for the Treatment of COVID-19," *Cochrane Database of Systematic Reviews* 3, no. 3 (2022): CD015125, https://pubmed.ncbi.nlm.nih.gov/35262185/.

14. "Table 5b. Inhaled Corticosteroids: Selected Clinical Data," National Institutes of Health, December 16, 2021, https://www.covid19treatmentguidelines.nih.gov/tables/inhaled-corticosteroids-data/.

15. The RECOVERY Collaborative Group, "Dexamethasone in Hospitalized Patients with Covid-19," *New England Journal of Medicine* 384, no. 8 (2021): 693–704, https://www.nejm.org/doi/full/10.1056/NEJMoa2021436.

16. Sébastien Czernichow et al., "Obesity Doubles Mortality in Patients Hospitalized for Severe Acute Respiratory Syndrome Coronavirus 2 in Paris Hospitals, France: A Cohort Study on 5,795 Patients," *Obesity* 28, no. 12 (2020): 2282–89, https://onlinelibrary.wiley.com/doi/10.1002/oby.23014.

17. Jason Hahn, "City Fills Skatepark with 37 Tons of Sand to Keep Kids and Parents Away amid Coronavirus," *People*, April 17, 2020, https://people.com/human-interest/city-fills-skatepark-with-37-tons-sand-coronavirus/.

18. Hannah Fry, "Paddle Boarder Chased by Boat, Arrested in Malibu after Flouting Coronavirus Closures," *Los Angeles Times*, April 3, 2020, https://www.latimes.com/california/story/2020-04-03/paddle-boarder-arrested-in-malibu-after-flouting-coronavirus-closures.

19. Associated Press, "ACT Test Scores Drop to Their Lowest in 30 Years in a Pandemic Slide," NPR, October 12, 2022, https://www.npr.org/2022/10/12/1128376442/act-test-scores-pandemic.

20. Mackenzie Mays, "Newsom Sends His Children Back to Private School Classrooms in California," *Politico*, October 30, 2020, https://www.politico.com/states/california/story/2020/10/30/newsom-sends-his-children-back-to-school-classrooms-in-california-1332811.

21. Aamer Madhani and Brian Slodysko, "Birx Travels, Family Visits Highlight Pandemic Safety Perils," Associated Press, December 20, 2020, https://apnews.com/article/travel-pandemics-only-on-ap-delaware-thanksgiving-52810c22488fff7e6bb70746bdc9bc61.

22. Mays, "Newsom Sends His Children Back to Private School."

23. Daniel Villarreal, "Texas Judge Orders Jail Sentence for Hair Salon Owner Who Kept Business Open Despite Stay-at-Home Order," *Newsweek*, May 5, 2020, https://www.newsweek.com/texas-judge-orders-jail-sentence-hair-salon-owner-who-kept-business-open-despite-stay-home-order-1502164; "Pelosi Caught Getting Hair Done at Coronavirus-Shuttered SF Salon," Fox News, September 2, 2020, https://www.foxnews.com/us/pelosi-caught-getting-hair-done-at-coronavirus-shuttered-sf-salon; Wilson Wong, "Chicago Mayor Lori Lightfoot Defends Hairstylist Visit amid Coronavirus Outbreak," NBC News, April 11, 2020, https://www.nbcnews.com/news/nbcblk/chicago-mayor-defends-hairstylist-visit-amid-coronavirus-outbreak-n1181546.

24. Nick Sibilla, "Michigan Bans Many Stores from Selling Seeds, Home Gardening Supplies, Calls Them 'Not Necessary,'" *Forbes*, April 16, 2020, https://www.forbes.com/sites/nicksibilla/2020/04/16/michigan-bans-many-stores-from-selling-seeds-home-gardening-supplies-calls-them-not-necessary/?sh=1b1d002a5f80; Poppy Noor, "Michigan Governor's Husband under Fire for Asking to Take His Boat Out during Lockdown," *The Guardian*, May 26, 2020, https://www.theguardian.com/us-news/2020/may/26/gretchen-whitmer-husband-marc-mallory-boat-lockdown.

25. Matthew Brown, "Fact Check: Did Kentucky Order Police to Record the License Plates of Easter Churchgoers?," *USA Today*, April 13, 2020, https://www.usatoday.com/story/news/factcheck/2020/04/13/coronavirus-fact-check-ky-police-recorded-info-easter-churchgoers/2980574001/; Chad Mills, "Here's What Businesses Can Stay Open in Kentucky and Indiana," WDRB.com, December 29, 2021, https://www.wdrb.com/news/heres-what-businesses-can-stay-open-in-kentucky-and-indiana/article_2d171e66-6d6f-11ea-8849-07f232dcb241.html; "Documenting Kentucky's Path to Recovery from the Coronavirus (COVID-19) Pandemic, 2020–2021," Ballotpedia, 2023, https://ballotpedia.org/Documenting_Kentucky%27s_path_to_recovery_from_the_coronavirus_(COVID-19)_pandemic,_2020-2021.

26. Vinay Prasad MD MPH (@VPrasadMDMPH), "Very problematic comment…," Twitter, May 12, 2023, 12:02 a.m., https://twitter.com/VPrasadMDMPH/status/1656872331489452034.

27. Peter A. McCullough et al., "Pathophysiological Basis and Rationale for Early Outpatient Treatment of SARS-CoV-2 (COVID-19) Infection,"

American Journal of Medicine 34, no. 1 (2020): 16–22, https://www
.amjmed.com/article/S0002-9343(20)30673-2/fulltext.

28. University of Oxford, "Genetic Susceptibility to Severe Streptococcal Infections," ClinicalTrials.gov, July 30, 2013, https://clinicaltrials.gov/ct2/show/NCT01911572.

29. Hospices Civils de Lyon, "Genetic Predisposition to Severe Forms of COVID-19 (SARS-CoV2 Infection) (COVIDGEN)," ClinicalTrials.gov, November 25, 2020, https://clinicaltrials.gov/ct2/show/NCT04644146.

30. National Research University Higher School of Economics, "Researchers Reveal Genetic Predisposition to Severe COVID-19," Medical Xpress, February 23, 2021, https://medicalxpress.com/news/2021-02-reveal-genetic-predisposition-severe-covid-.html.

31. Pezzullo et al., "Age-Stratified Infection Fatality Rate"; Kamil Yilmaz et al., "Does Covid-19 in Children Have a Milder Course Than Influenza?," *International Journal of Clinical Practice* 75, no. 9 (2021): e14466, https://pubmed.ncbi.nlm.nih.gov/34107134/.

Chapter 7

1. Scott Morefield, "MSNBC's Nicolle Wallace Says It's 'More Difficult' to Hope Rand Paul Recovers from Coronavirus," Daily Caller, March 24, 2020, https://dailycaller.com/2020/03/24/msnbc-nicolle-wallace-more-difficult-rand-paul-coronavirus/. For Wallace's views on waterboarding, see Elias Isquith, "'I Don't Care What We Did': What Nicolle Wallace's Rant Reveals about America's Torture Problem," *Salon*, December 9, 2014, https://www.salon.com/2014/12/09/i_dont_care_what_we_did_what_nicolle_wallaces_rant_reveals_about_americas_torture_problem/.

2. THE LIBERTY DAILY, "MSNBC's Kasie Hunt: Rand Paul Getting Assaulted 'One of My Favorite Stories,'" YouTube, November 20, 2017, https://www.youtube.com/watch?v=I2tY7lD3TAw.

3. Brandon Gee and Ed O'Keefe, "Sen. Rand Paul's Injuries Far More Severe Than Initially Thought," *Washington Post*, November 5, 2017, https://www.washingtonpost.com/powerpost/sen-rand-paul-recovering-from-injuries-suffered-in-alleged-assault/2017/11/05/6380c78a-c250-11e7-84bc-5e285c7f4512_story.html.

4. Allan Smith, "Rand Paul Becomes First Senator Known to Test Positive for Coronavirus," NBC News, March 22, 2020, https://www.nbcnews.

com/politics/congress/rand-paul-becomes-first-known-senator-test-positive-coronavirus-n1166111.

5. Ibid.

6. Seung Min Kim (@seungminkim), "During the Senate GOP lunch today…," Twitter, March 22, 2020, 2:49 p.m., https://twitter.com/seungminkim/status/1241799144559251456.

7. Rand Paul (@RandPaul), "We want to be clear…," Twitter, March 22, 2020, 4:12 p.m., https://twitter.com/RandPaul/status/1241820090804379654.

8. Matthew Daly, "Sen. Rand Paul Tests Positive for Virus, Forcing Quarantines," PBS, March 22, 2020, https://www.pbs.org/newshour/politics/sen-rand-paul-tests-positive-for-covid-19.

9. Matthew Brown, "Fact Check: Did Kentucky Order Police to Record the License Plates of Easter Churchgoers?," *USA Today*, April 13, 2020, https://www.usatoday.com/story/news/factcheck/2020/04/13/coronavirus-fact-check-ky-police-recorded-info-easter-churchgoers/2980574001/.

10. "Kentucky Gov. Andy Beshear Orders Hair Salons, Spas, Gyms, Theaters to Close by 5 p.m. Wednesday," WDRB.com, March 18, 2020, https://www.wdrb.com/news/kentucky-gov-andy-beshear-orders-hair-salons-spas-gyms-theaters-to-close-by-5-p/article_0ba7c534-6890-11ea-8d6f-3b5a49ed7c62.html; "Travel Restrictions Issued by States in Response to the Coronavirus (COVID-19) Pandemic, 2020–2022," Ballotpedia, 2023, https://ballotpedia.org/Travel_restrictions_issued_by_states_in_response_to_the_coronavirus_(COVID-19)_pandemic,_2020-2022; "Documenting Kentucky's Path to Recovery from the Coronavirus (COVID-19) Pandemic, 2020–2021," Ballotpedia, 2023, https://ballotpedia.org/Documenting_Kentucky%27s_path_to_recovery_from_the_coronavirus_(COVID-19)_pandemic,_2020-2021.

11. Jack Brammer and Karla Ward, "Kentucky Supreme Court: New Laws Limiting Beshear's Emergency Powers Are Valid," *Lexington Herald-Leader*, August 21, 2021, https://www.kentucky.com/news/politics-government/article253645283.html; "Federal Judge Rules against Gov. Beshear's Executive Order Requiring Masks in Schools," WLKY, August 19, 2021, https://www.wlky.com/article/federal-judge-rules-against-gov-beshears-executive-order-requiring-masks-in-schools/37352599#; "Documenting Kentucky's Path to Recovery."

12. Andrew Taylor, "Senate Unanimously Passes Massive Coronavirus Aid Plan," Health News Florida, March 26, 2020, https://health.wusf.usf.

edu/health-news-florida/2020-03-26/senate-unanimously-passes-massive
-coronavirus-aid-plan.

13. Ibid.

14. Personal recollection.

15. Taylor, "Senate Unanimously Passes Massive Coronavirus Aid Plan."

16. Ibid.

17. Sacha Pfeiffer, "IRS Says Its Own Error Sent $1,200 Stimulus Checks to Non-Americans Overseas," NPR, November 30, 2020, https://www.npr.org/2020/11/30/938902523/irs-says-its-own-error-sent-1-200-stimulus-checks-to-non-americans-overseas; Brian Faler, "The IRS Thought It Wasn't Allowed to Withhold Stimulus Checks from the Dead. So It Paid More than 1 Million of Them," *Politico*, June 25, 2020, https://www.politico.com/news/2020/06/25/irs-stimulus-checks-dead-people-339530.

18. Dan Mangan, Robert Frank, and Jessica Golden, "NBA's LA Lakers Got $4.6 Million in Coronavirus Federal Loan Money for Small Business, but Repaid It," CNBC, April 27, 2020, https://www.cnbc.com/2020/04/27/coronavirus-los-angeles-lakers-got-4point6-million-federal-small-business-loan.html.

19. Jim Probasco, "The Paycheck Protection Program and Health Care Enhancement Act," Investopedia, November 30, 2022, https://www.investopedia.com/paycheck-protection-program-and-health-care-enhancement-act-4843094.

20. Anita Campbell, "$341 Million in PPP Fraud So Far, and Counting," Small Business Trends, August 19, 2022, https://smallbiztrends.com/2020/08/ppp-fraud.html.

21. Coronavirus Preparedness and Response Supplemental Appropriations Act, H.R. 6074, 116th Cong. (2020), https://www.congress.gov/bill/116th-congress/house-bill/6074.

22. Will Feuer, "California Announces First Coronavirus Death, Bringing US Fatalities to at Least 11," CNBC, March 5, 2020, https://www.cnbc.com/2020/03/04/california-confirms-first-coronavirus-death-bringing-us-fatalities-to-at-least-11.html.

23. Julie Tsirkin and Dareh Gregorian, "Senate Coronavirus Vote Delayed after Rand Paul Pushes Doomed Amendment," NBC News, March 18, 2020, https://www.nbcnews.com/politics/congress/senate-coronavirus-bill-vote-delayed-after-rand-paul-pushes-doomed-n1162356.

24. Office of Senator Rand Paul, "Dr. Paul Secures Senate Vote on Plan to Pay for Federal Coronavirus Response," press release, March 5, 2020, https://www.paul.senate.gov/news-dr-paul-secures-senate-vote-plan-pay-federal-coronavirus-response/.
25. "All Actions," Coronavirus Preparedness and Response Supplemental Appropriations Act, H.R. 6074, 116th Cong. (2020), https://www.congress.gov/bill/116th-congress/house-bill/6074/all-actions?overview=closed&q=%7B%22roll-call-vote%22%3A%22all%22%7D.
26. Kellie Moss et al., "The Families First Coronavirus Response Act: Summary of Key Provisions," KFF, March 23, 2020, https://www.kff.org/coronavirus-covid-19/issue-brief/the-families-first-coronavirus-response-act-summary-of-key-provisions/; Niv Elis, "Coronavirus Response Bill Estimated to Cost $104 Billion," *The Hill*, March 17, 2020, https://thehill.com/policy/finance/487977-coronavirus-response-bill-estimated-to-cost-104-billion/; Campbell, "$341 Million in PPP Fraud So Far."
27. "All Actions," Families First Coronavirus Response Act, H.R. 6201, 116th Cong. (2020), https://www.congress.gov/bill/116th-congress/house-bill/6201/all-actions?overview=closed&q=%7B%22roll-call-vote%22%3A%22all%22%7D.

Chapter 8

1. "Influenza Vaccine," C-SPAN, October 11, 2004, https://www.c-span.org/video/?183885-2/influenza-vaccine&fbclid=IwAR35Fl4rWcpQEuZS8KQ3jurVbwd88Mh9qPXSbQp1XIj2SBSmiNUG7p92wT8.
2. Darragh Roche, "Fauci Said Masks 'Not Really Effective,' Email Reveals," *Newsweek*, June 2, 2021, https://www.newsweek.com/fauci-said-masks-not-really-effective-keeping-out-virus-email-reveals-1596703.
3. U.S. Senate Committee on Health, Education, Labor and Pensions, *Examining Our COVID-19 Response: An Update from Federal Officials* (Washington, D.C.: U.S. Government Publishing Office, 2022), 38, https://www.govinfo.gov/content/pkg/CHRG-117shrg46755/pdf/CHRG-117shrg46755.pdf. Transcript lightly edited to improve readability.
4. Nikolas Lanum, "Fawning over Fauci: A Look Back at the Media's Praise of the Face of U.S. COVID-19 Response," Fox News, July 19, 2022, https://www.foxnews.com/media/fawning-fauci-look-back-medias-praise-face-us-covid-19-response.

5. Jon Miltimore, "New Danish Study Finds Masks Don't Protect Wearers from COVID Infection," FEE, November 18, 2020, https://fee.org/articles /new-danish-study-finds-masks-don-t-protect-wearers-from-covid-infection/.

6. Gina Kolata, "A New Study Questions Whether Masks Protect Wearers. You Need to Wear Them Anyway," *New York Times*, November 18, 2020, https://www.nytimes.com/2020/11/18/health/coronavirus-masks-denmark .html.

7. Antonio I. Lazzarino, "Rapid Response: Conclusions from the Danish Mask Study," *British Medical Journal* 371 (2020): m4586, https://www. bmj.com/content/371/bmj.m4586/rr-6.

8. Abrar A. Chughtai, Holly Seale, and C. Raina Macintyre, "Effectiveness of Cloth Masks for Protection against Severe Acute Respiratory Syndrome Coronavirus 2," *Emerging Infectious Diseases* 26, no. 10 (2020): e2, https:// doi.org/10.3201/eid2610.200948.

9. Tyler Durden, "Massive Peer-Reviewed Mask Study Shows 'Little to No Difference' in Preventing COVID, Flu Infection," ZeroHedge, February 2, 2023, https://www.zerohedge.com/political/massive-mask-study-shows-little-no-difference-preventing-covid-flu-infection.

10. Damian Guerra and Daniel Guerra, "Mask Mandate and Use Efficacy in State-Level COVID-19 Containment," medRxiv, May 25, 2021, https:// www.semanticscholar.org/paper/Mask-mandate-and-use-efficacy-in-state -level-Guerra-Guerra/06c2052b29f624c13a0fa0a60e13f83553098e74.

11. Paul E. Alexander, "More than 170 Comparative Studies and Articles on Mask Ineffectiveness and Harms," The Brownstone Institute, December 20, 2021, https://brownstone.org/articles/studies-and-articles-on-mask -ineffectiveness-and-harms/.

12. Robby Soave, "CNN's Leana Wen: 'Cloth Masks Are Little More than Facial Decorations,'" *Reason*, December 21, 2021, https://reason.com/2021/12/21/ leana-wen-cloth-mask-facial-decorations-covid-cdc-guidance/; Leana S. Wen, "I'm a Doctor. Here's Why My Kids Won't Wear Masks This School Year," *Washington Post*, August 23, 2022, https://www.washingtonpost .com/opinions/2022/08/23/my-kids-wont-wear-masks-school/.

13. Brianna Keilar (@brikeilarcnn), "I stand by my characterization of Sen. Paul and I'll explain in a moment...." (thread), Twitter, October 22, 2021, 12:58 p.m., https://twitter.com/brikeilarcnn/status/1451593837563060283.

14. Vinay Prasad MD MPH (@VPrasadMDMPH), "12 guards are smarter than even some deans of public health schools...." (thread), Twitter, February 3, 2023, 6:05 p.m., https://twitter.com/VPrasadMDMPH/status /1621646129426489344.

15. Salvador Rizzo, "Rand Paul's False Claim That Masks Don't Work," *Washington Post*, December 2, 2021, https://www.washingtonpost.com/ politics/2021/12/02/rand-pauls-false-claim-that-masks-dont-work/.

16. World Health Organization, *Non-Pharmaceutical Public Health Measures for Mitigating the Risk and Impact of Epidemic and Pandemic Influenza* (Geneva: World Health Organization, 2019), 26, https://apps.who.int/iris/ bitstream/handle/10665/329438/9789241516839-eng.pdf; Jingyi Xiao et al., "Nonpharmaceutical Measures for Pandemic Influenza in Nonhealthcare Settings—Personal Protective and Environmental Measures," *Emerging Infectious Diseases* 26, no. 5 (2020): 967–75, https://doi.org/10.3201/ eid2605.190994.

17. World Health Organization, *Non-Pharmaceutical Public Health Measures*, 26.

18. Jon Miltimore, "Fauci's Mask Flip-Flop, Explained (by Economics)," FEE, June 3, 2021, https://fee.org/articles/fauci-s-mask-flip-flop-explained-by -economics/; Cory Stieg, "Dr. Fauci: Double-Masking Makes 'Common Sense' and Is Likely More Effective," CNBC, January 25, 2021, https:// www.cnbc.com/2021/01/25/dr-fauci-double-mask-during-covid-makes- common-sense-more-effective.html.

19. Olga Perski, David Simons, Robert West, and Susan Michie, "Face Masks to Prevent Community Transmission of Viral Respiratory Infections: A Rapid Evidence Review Using Bayesian Analysis," Qeios, May 1, 2020, https://www.qeios.com/read/1SC5L4.

20. Matt Taibbi, "Twitter, the FBI Subsidiary," The Twitter Files (Substack), April 12, 2023, https://twitterfiles.substack.com/p/twitter-the-fbi- subsidiary; David Molloy, "Zuckerberg Tells Rogan FBI Warning Prompted Biden Laptop Story Censorship," BBC, August 26, 2022, https://www. bbc.com/news/world-us-canada-62688532; Jenin Younes and Aaron Kheriaty, "The White House Covid Censorship Machine," *Wall Street Journal*, January 8, 2023, https://www.wsj.com/articles/white-house- covid-censorship-machine-social-media-facebook-meta-executive-rob- flaherty-free-speech-google-11673203704; Paul D. Thacker (@thackerpd), "1) Twitter Files #FauciPharmaFiles..." (thread), April 20, 2023, 9:09

a.m., https://twitter.com/thackerpd/status/1649037538663727106; Chris Donaldson, "New Twitter Files Drop Brings Long-Promised Hammer to Fauci, with of [sic] Promise 'More to Come!'," BizPac Review, April 21, 2023, https://www.bizpacreview.com/2023/04/21/new-twitter-files-drop-brings-long-promised-hammer-to-fauci-with-of-promise-more-to-come-1352124/; Matt Taibbi, "Stanford, the Virality Project, and the Censorship of 'True Stories,'" The Twitter Files (Substack), April 12, 2023, https://twitterfiles.substack.com/p/stanford-the-virality-project-and.

21. Christopher Brito, "Rand Paul Suspended from YouTube for 7 Days after COVID Mask Claims," CBS News, August 11, 2021, https://www.cbsnews.com/news/rand-paul-suspended-youtube-face-mask/; "YouTube Suspends Rand Paul after Misleading Video on Masks," Associated Press, August 11, 2021, https://apnews.com/article/technology-business-health-coronavirus-pandemic-rand-paul-9e8a970398830ea415f7d1fb68f0a95e.

22. Brito, "Rand Paul Suspended"; Office of Senator Rand Paul, "Dr. Rand Paul Blasts YouTube for Continued Censorship," press release, August 10, 2021, https://www.paul.senate.gov/news-dr-rand-paul-blasts-youtube-continued-censorship/.

23. Gino Spocchia, "Rand Paul Suspended from YouTube Video Full of Covid Lies," The Independent, August 11, 2021; "YouTube Suspends Rand Paul."

24. Daniel Victor, "YouTube Suspends Rand Paul for a Week over a Video Disputing the Effectiveness of Masks," New York Times, August 11, 2021, https://www.nytimes.com/2021/08/11/business/youtube-rand-paul-covid-masks.html.

25. Jackie Borchardt, "'Kind of a Lunatic': Sen. Sherrod Brown Calls Out Sen. Rand Paul for Not Wearing a Mask," Cincinnati Enquirer, May 4, 2021, https://www.cincinnati.com/story/news/politics/2021/05/04/ohio-sen-sherrod-brown-calls-out-kentucky-sen-rand-paul-not-wearing-mask/4944256001/.

26. Ibid.

27. Ibid.

28. jeremytai, "Apple Think Different—Steve Jobs Narrated Version," YouTube, October 6, 2011, https://www.youtube.com/watch?v=GEPhLqwKo6g&t=43s.

29. Saint Augustine, "A Quote by Augustine of Hippo." Goodreads, n.d., https://www.goodreads.com/quotes/798196-the-truth-is-like-a-lion-you-don-t-have-to.

30. B. D. Colen, "Russian Flu Has Arrived in the U.S.," *Washington Post*, January 28, 1978, https://www.washingtonpost.com/archive/politics/1978 /01/28/russian-flu-has-arrived-in-the-us/3d24b12b-5f75-480d-afc4 -f31f1de81113/.

31. Olga Khazan, "The U.S. Is Repeating Its Deadliest Pandemic Mistake," *The Atlantic*, July 6, 2020, https://www.theatlantic.com/health/archive/2020/07 /us-repeating-deadliest-pandemic-mistake-nursing-home-deaths/613855/.

32. "Cyanide for Peace," Brown University Library, n.d., https://library.brown .edu/create/protest6090/cyanide-for-peace/.

33. Carla Herreria Russo, "Rand Paul Says He's Immune to COVID-19 despite Lack of Research," HuffPost, May 5, 2020, https://www.huffpost. com/entry/rand-paul-no-mask-senate-immune_n_5eb1e86bc5b66d3bfcd d1b91.

34. Emmarie Huetteman, "Nurses and Doctors Sick with COVID Feel Pressured to Get Back to Work," KFF Health News, August 12, 2020, https://khn.org /news/nurses-and-doctors-sick-with-covid-feel-pressured-to-get-back-to-work/.

35. "Strategies to Mitigate Healthcare Personnel Staffing Shortages," Centers for Disease Control and Prevention, last updated March 16, 2023, https:// www.cdc.gov/vaccines/covid-19/clinical-considerations/faq.html.

36. Anders Hagstrom, "New York Supreme Court Reinstates All Employees Fired for Being Unvaccinated, Orders Backpay," Fox News, October 25, 2022, https://www.foxnews.com/us/new-york-supreme-court-reinstates-all -employees-fired-being-unvaccinated-orders-backpay.

37. Haley Britzky, "Pentagon Officially Rescinds Covid-19 Vaccine Requirement for Troops," CNN, January 11, 2023, https://www.cnn.com/2023/01/10/ politics/military-covid-vaccine-rescinded/index.html.

38. Jenni Fink, "Will Fired Unvaccinated Employees Get Their Jobs Back after SCOTUS Blocks Biden Mandate?," *Newsweek*, January 14, 2022, https:// www.newsweek.com/will-fired-unvaccinated-employees-get-their-jobs- back-after-scotus-blocks-biden-mandate-1669519.

39. Suzanne Burdick, "New Analysis Shows Studies of COVID Vaccine- Induced Myocarditis Hid Critical Safety Signal," The Defender, January 6, 2023, https://childrenshealthdefense.org/defender/covid-vaccine-induce -myocarditis/.

40. "FAQs for the Interim Clinical Considerations for COVID-19 Vaccination," Centers for Disease Control and Prevention, last updated March 16, 2023, https://www.cdc.gov/vaccines/covid-19/clinical-considerations/faq.html.

41. Personal recollection of staff member.

42. Personal conversation with Tom Carper.

43. Russo, "Rand Paul Says He's Immune to COVID-19."

44. Ibid.

45. Michael Klompas et al., "Universal Masking in Hospitals in the COVID-19 Era," *New England Journal of Medicine* 382, no. 21 (2020): e63, https://www.nejm.org/doi/full/10.1056/NEJMp2006372.

46. Ibid.

47. Perski, Simons, West, and Michie, "Face Masks to Prevent Community Transmission"; World Health Organization, *Non-Pharmaceutical Public Health Measures.*

48. Michael Klompas, Charles A. Morris, and Erica S. Shenoy, "Universal Masking in the Covid-19 Era," *New England Journal of Medicine* 383, no. 2 (2020), e9, https://www.nejm.org/doi/full/10.1056/NEJMc2020836.

49. Russo, "Rand Paul Says He's Immune to COVID-19."

50. Sam Janney, "Politifact and Their So-Called COVID 'Fact-Checker' (with No Medical Experience) Dragged in Brutal Thread," twitchy.com, January 2, 2023, https://twitchy.com/samj-3930/2023/01/02/thread-takes-politifact -and-their-covid-disinformation-fact-checker-apart-tweet-by-brutal-tweet/.

51. Russo, "Rand Paul Says He's Immune to COVID-19."

52. Apoorva Mandavilli, "The C.D.C. Stands by a Decision Not to Require Testing to Leave Isolation," *New York Times*, January 4, 2022, https://www .nytimes.com/2022/01/04/health/cdc-testing-isolation.html.

53. Russo, "Rand Paul Says He's Immune to COVID-19."

54. "102-Year-Old Woman Born during Spanish Flu Pandemic Survives Coronavirus," News4JAX, April 28, 2020, https://www.news4jax. com/health/2020/04/28/102-year-old-woman-born-during-spanish-flu -pandemic-survives-coronavirus/.

55. "90 Years Later, 1918 Flu Lives on in Antibodies, Research," PBS, August 22, 2008, https://www.pbs.org/newshour/science/science-july-dec08 -influenza_08-22.

56. Brackets original. Ibid.

57. Michael Mosley, "The Flu Virus That Nearly Killed Me," BBC, January 25, 2013, https://www.bbc.com/news/magazine-21125713.

58. Office of Attorney General Jeff Landry, "Louisiana, Missouri Release Full Fauci Deposition Transcript," news release, December 5, 2022, https://agjefflandry.com/Article/13094.

59. Ibid.

60. Nina Le Bert et al., "SARS-CoV-2-Specific T Cell Immunity in Cases of COVID-19 and SARS, and Uninfected Controls," *Nature* 584, no. 7821 (2020): 457–62, https://www.nature.com/articles/s41586-020-2550-z.

61. Steve Templeton, "Rev. Cotton Mather and the 18th-Century Battle over Smallpox Inoculation," The Brownstone Institute, November 5, 2021, https://brownstone.org/articles/rev-cotton-mather-and-the-18th-century-battle-over-smallpox-inoculation/.

62. "On This Day in 1721, Dr. Zabdiel Boylston Inoculates His Son against Smallpox," City of Boston, June 26, 2017, https://www.boston.gov/news/day-1721-dr-zabdiel-boylston-inoculates-his-son-against-smallpox.

63. Ellipsis Templeton's. Templeton, "Rev. Cotton Mather."

64. Ibid.

65. "On This Day in 1721."

66. Vanessa Chalmers, "Could Immunity Last 17 Years? Researchers Find SARS Patients Still Have Crucial T Cells," *Daily Mail*, July 16, 2020, https://www.dailymail.co.uk/news/article-8529429/Could-immunity-17-YEARS-Singaporean-researchers-SARS-patients-crucial-T-cells.html.

67. Xiaoqin Guo et al., "Long-Term Persistence of IgG Antibodies in SARS-CoV Infected Healthcare Workers," medRxiv, February 14, 2020, https://www.medrxiv.org/content/10.1101/2020.02.12.20021386v1.

68. Nicoletta Lanese, "Macaque Monkeys Can't Become Reinfected with COVID-19, Small Study Suggests," *Live Science*, March 18, 2020, https://www.livescience.com/monkeys-cannot-get-reinfected-with-coronavirus-study.html.

69. Margery Smelkinson, "Remarks to the Select Subcommittee on the Covid Pandemic," U.S. Committee on Oversight and Accountability, May 2023, https://oversight.house.gov/wp-content/uploads/2023/05/Congressional-testimony-Smelkinson.pdf; Laith J. Abu-Raddad et al., "Assessment of the Risk of Severe Acute Respiratory Syndrome Coronavirus 2 (SARS-CoV-2) Reinfection in an Intense Reexposure Setting," *Clinical Infectious Diseases* 73, no. 7 (2021): e1830–e1840, https://doi.org/10.1093/cid/ciaa1846.

70. Raymond A. Harvey et al., "Association of SARS-CoV-2 Seropositive Antibody Test with Risk of Future Infection," *Journal of the American Medical Association Internal Medicine* 181, no. 5 (2021): 672–79, https://jamanetwork.com/journals/jamainternalmedicine/fullarticle/2776810.

71. Victoria Jane Hall et al., "SARS-CoV-2 Infection Rates of Antibody-Positive Compared with Antibody-Negative Health-Care Workers in England: A Large, Multicentre, Prospective Cohort Study (SIREN)," *The Lancet* 397, no. 10283 (2021): 1459–69, https://www.thelancet.com/journals/lancet/article/PIIS0140-6736(21)00675-9/fulltext.

72. Jackson S. Turner et al., "SARS-CoV-2 Infection Induces Long-Lived Bone Marrow Plasma Cells in Humans," *Nature* 595, no. 7867 (2021): 421–25, https://www.nature.com/articles/s41586-021-03647-4.

73. Marty Makary, "The Power of Natural Immunity," *Wall Street Journal*, June 8, 2021, https://www.wsj.com/articles/the-power-of-natural-immunity-11623171303.

74. Tomás M. León et al., "COVID-19 Cases and Hospitalizations by COVID-19 Vaccination Status and Previous COVID-19 Diagnosis—California and New York, May–November 2021," *Morbidity and Mortality Weekly Report* 71, no.4 (2022): 125–31, http://dx.doi.org/10.15585/mmwr.mm7104e1.

75. Ibid.

76. Russo, "Rand Paul Says He's Immune to COVID-19."

77. Rand Paul (@RandPaul), "The fake news can't stand that some people might not need to submit to the new authoritarianism of the left because they are immune to coronavirus.... ," May 5, 2020, 7:03 p.m., https://twitter.com/RandPaul/status/1257808245130956800.

78. Rand Paul (@RandPaul), "Dr. Fauci: 'We know with infections like this…'" (thread), Twitter, May 5, 2020, 7:03 p.m., https://twitter.com/RandPaul/status/1257808252324249600.

79. Russo, "Rand Paul Says He's Immune to COVID-19."

80. Paul (@RandPaul), "The fake news can't stand that some people might not need to submit to the new authoritarianism." See also, "Concepts of Biology: 17.3 Adaptive Immunity," OpenStax, accessed April 29, 2023, https://openstax.org/books/concepts-biology/pages/17-3-adaptive-immunity.

81. Jessica McDonald, "Paul Misleads on Natural Infection and COVID-19 Vaccines," FactCheck.org, April 19, 2021, https://www.factcheck.org/2020/11/paul-misleads-on-natural-infection-and-covid-19-vaccines/.

82. Rand Paul (@RandPaul), "Great News!–Pfizer Vaccine 90% Effective…," Twitter, November 17, 2020, 2:56 p.m., https://twitter.com/RandPaul/status/1328789051298689027.

83. Rand Paul (@RandPaul), "Why does the left accept immune theory when it comes to vaccines…," Twitter, November 17, 2020, 2:56 p.m., https://twitter.com/RandPaul/status/1328789052565430272.

84. McDonald, "Paul Misleads on Natural Infection and COVID-19 Vaccines."

85. Apoorva Mandavilli, "Coronavirus Reinfections Are Real but Very, Very Rare," *New York Times*, October 13, 2020, https://www.nytimes.com/2020/10/13/health/coronavirus-reinfection.html.

86. Yinjun Mao et al., "Reinfection Rates among Patients Previously Infected by SARS-CoV-2: Systematic Review and Meta-Analysis," *Chinese Medical Journal* 135, no. 2 (2021): 145–52, https://pubmed.ncbi.nlm.nih.gov/34908003/.

87. Brackets original. McDonald, "Paul Misleads on Natural Infection and COVID-19 Vaccines."

88. Ibid.

89. Rand Paul (@RandPaul), "More Great News on Immunity for People Who've Survived Covid….," Twitter, November 18, 2020, 8:38 a.m., https://twitter.com/RandPaul/status/1329056442310078471.

90. Apoorva Mandavilli, "Immunity to the Coronavirus May Last Years, New Data Hint," *New York Times*, November 17, 2020, https://www.nytimes.com/2020/11/17/health/coronavirus-immunity.html.

91. Ibid.

92. McDonald, "Paul Misleads on Natural Infection and COVID-19 Vaccines."

93. Victoria Knight, "Explaining What Rand Paul Said about Vaccines for People Who Had COVID-19," PolitiFact, June 17, 2021, https://www.politifact.com/article/2021/jun/17/explaining-what-rand-paul-said-about-vaccines-peop/.

94. Ibid.

95. León et al., "COVID-19 Cases and Hospitalizations."

96. Knight, "Explaining What Rand Paul Said about Vaccines."

97. See also, Jennifer Dan et al, "Immunological Memory to SARS-CoV-2 Assessed for up to 8 Months after Infection," *Science* 371, no. 6529 (2021): eabf4063, https://www.science.org/doi/10.1126/science.abf4063.

98. Florian Kramer, "Correlates of Protection from SARS-CoV-2 Infection," *The Lancet* 397, no. 10283 (2021): 1421–23, https://www.thelancet.com/journals/lancet/article/PIIS0140-6736(21)00782-0/fulltext.

99. Venkata Viswanadh Edara et al., "Neutralizing Antibodies against SARS-CoV-2 Variants after Infection and Vaccination," *Journal of the American Medical Association* 325, no. 18 (2021): 1896–98, https://jamanetwork.com/journals/jama/fullarticle/2777898.

100. For Walensky's statements, see Joseph Guzman, "CDC Reverses Statement by Director That Vaccinated People Are No Longer Contagious," *The Hill*, April 2, 2021, https://thehill.com/changing-america/well-being/546234-cdc-reverses-statement-by-director-that-vaccinated-people-are-no/. Op-ed by Rand Paul, "Rand Paul: The Science Proves People with Natural Immunity Should Skip Covid Vaccines," *Courier-Journal*, May 29, 2021, https://www.courier-journal.com/story/opinion/2021/05/27/rand-paul-says-people-natural-covid-immunity-should-skip-vaccine/7468051002/. Portions of this op-ed have been updated to account for the progression of the pandemic since 2021.

101. Marty Makary MD, MPH (@MartyMarkary), "Rochelle Walensky has been known for her kindness and collegiality in academia...." (thread), Twitter, May 5, 2023, 7:02 p.m., https://twitter.com/MartyMakary/status/1654622631998660608.

102. Ibid.

103. Morgan Watkins, "Kelley Paul: Package Sent to Her and Sen. Rand Paul's Home 'Pure Terrorism,'" *Courier-Journal*, May 27, 2021, https://www.courier-journal.com/story/news/politics/rand-paul/2021/05/27/rand-pauls-wife-kelley-says-package-sent-home-pure-terrorism/7465433002/; "Sen. Rand Paul, Wife Kelley on Death Threat Package Sent to Their Home: 'Pure Terrorism,'" Fox Business, May 27, 2021, at 1:10, https://www.foxbusiness.com/video/6256252715001. Account of events lightly edited to improve readability.

104. Dennis Perkins, "Supervillain Richard Marx Breaks into *The Late Show* Feed to Mock Rand Paul's Twitter Accusations," AV Club, May 26, 2021, https://www.avclub.com/supervillain-richard-marx-breaks-into-the-late-show-fee-1846971051.

105. "Sen. Rand Paul, Wife Kelley on Death Threat Package," at 3:05.

106. Kelley Paul, "My Husband, Rand Paul, and Our Family Have Suffered Intimidation and Threats," CNN, October 6, 2018, https://www.cnn.com /2018/10/03/opinions/rand-paul-suffer-intimidation-and-threats-kelley-paul/index.html; Bobby Shipman, "Bette Midler Tweets an Apparent Call for More Harm to Rand Paul. And Twitter Wasn't Having It," *Courier-Journal*, February 10, 2018, https://www.courier-journal.com/story/news/ politics/2018/02/10/bette-midler-tweets-rand-paul-attack/325701002/.

107. Jake Epstein, "Rand Paul Calls Out Nancy Pelosi's Daughter as He Wishes Her Husband a 'Speedy Recovery' from the Early Morning-Attack That Left Him Hospitalized," Insider, October 28, 2022, https://www. businessinsider.com/rand-paul-calls-out-nancy-pelosi-daughter-wishes-husband-well-2022-10.

108. Perkins, "Supervillain Richard Marx Breaks into *The Late Show* Feed."

109. Looks like Marx deleted his vile tweet at some later point, but plenty of people saw it: Jim Treacher, "Stephen Colbert Was 'Right Here Waiting' to Laugh Up a Violent Threat against Sen. Rand Paul," PJ Media, May 26, 2021, https://pjmedia.com/culture/jim-treacher/2021/05/26/stephen-colbert -and-some-80s-singer-yuk-it-up-about-death-threats-against-rand-paul -n1449775.

110. Perkins, "Supervillain Richard Marx Breaks into *The Late Show* Feed."

111. Rebecca Downs, "Tweet from 'C-List Celebrity' Inciting Violence against Rand Paul Taken Down," Townhall, May 26, 2021, https://townhall.com/ tipsheet/rebeccadowns/2021/05/26/twitter-takes-down-tweet-from-richard -marx-to-do-with-rand-paul-n2590025; Epstein, "Rand Paul Calls Out Nancy Pelosi's Daughter."

112. "Sen. Rand Paul, Wife Kelley on Death Threat Package," at 4:30.

113. Jared S. Hopkins and Stephanie Armour, "Pfizer's Covid-19 Vaccine for Kids Isn't Working Well against Omicron So Far, Delaying FDA Review," *Wall Street Journal*, February 18, 2022, https://www.wsj.com/articles/ lower-omicron-efficacy-delayed-fda-review-on-pfizer-shot-in-kids-under -5-11645192800.

114. Centers for Disease Control and Prevention, "CDC Strengthens Recommendations and Expands Eligibility for COVID-19 Booster Shots," news release, May 19, 2022, https://www.cdc.gov/media/releases/2022/ s0519-covid-booster-acip.html; Sarah Oliver, "Updates to the Evidence to Recommendation Framework: Pfizer-BioNTech COVID-19 Booster in

Children Aged 5–11 Years," Centers for Disease Control and Prevention, May 19, 2022, https://www.cdc.gov/vaccines/acip/meetings/downloads/slides-2022-05-19/06-COVID-Oliver-508.pdf#page=46.

115. U.S. Senate HELP Committee, *Examining Our COVID-19 Response*, 38. Transcript lightly edited to improve readability.

116. Noah Weiland and Sharon LaFraniere, "Two Top F.D.A. Vaccine Regulators Are Set to Depart during a Crucial Period," *New York Times*, September 22, 2021, https://www.nytimes.com/2021/08/31/us/politics/fda-vaccine-regulators-booster-shots.html.

117. Philip Krause, Marion F. Gruber, and Paul A. Offit, "We Don't Need Universal Booster Shots. We Need to Reach the Unvaccinated," *Washington Post*, December 3, 2021, https://www.washingtonpost.com/outlook/2021/11/29/booster-shots-universal-opinion/.

118. Ronny Reyes, "Top Doctors Refuse to Give Their Own Kids a Third Shot as Studies Find Chances of Vaccinated Boys between 12 and 17 Being Hospitalized Are 0.3 out of 100,000," *Daily Mail*, January 27, 2022, https://www.dailymail.co.uk/news/article-10448853/Top-doctors-refuse-kids-shot-myocarditis-concerns.html.

119. "Sen. Rand Paul Rips Fauci over Contradictory Statements about COVID," Fox News, November 12, 2020, at 2:35, https://www.foxnews.com/video/6209513256001.

120. Ibid.

121. McDonald, "Paul Misleads on Natural Infection and COVID-19 Vaccines."

122. Rand Paul (@RandPaul), "Great news! Cleveland clinic study…" (thread), Twitter, June 8, 2021, 11:14 a.m., https://twitter.com/RandPaul/status/1402282844576260096; Nabin K. Shrestha et al., "Necessity of Coronavirus Disease 2019 (COVID-19) Vaccination in Persons Who Have Already Had COVID-19," *Clinical Infectious Diseases* 75, no. 1 (2022) e662–e671, https://academic.oup.com/cid/article/75/1/e662/6507165.

123. Rand Paul (@RandPaul), "Thus, Recovered COVID-19 Patients Are Likely to Better Defend…" (thread), Twitter, June 8, 2021, 12:27 p.m., https://twitter.com/RandPaul/status/1402301326084775939.

124. Shrestha et al., "Necessity of Coronavirus Disease 2019 (COVID-19) Vaccination."

125. Knight, "Explaining What Rand Paul Said about Vaccines."

126. Ellipsis original. Ibid.

127. Ibid.
128. Ibid.

Chapter 9

1. "COVID-19 Coronavirus Pandemic," Worldometer, July 13, 2023, https://www.worldometers.info/coronavirus.
2. Rand Paul, speech in U.S. Senate, C-SPAN, April 21, 2020, at 48:00, https://www.c-span.org/video/?471366-1/senate-session#!. Transcript lightly edited to improve readability. Brackets indicate slight rewording for written clarity throughout.
3. Mitch McConnell, speech in U.S. Senate, C-SPAN, April 21, 2020, at 2:00, https://www.c-span.org/video/?471366-1/senate-session#!.
4. Mike Lee, speech in U.S. Senate, C-SPAN, April 21, 2020, at 23:30, https://www.c-span.org/video/?471366-1/senate-session#!.
5. Paul, speech in U.S. Senate, at 1:06:40.
6. "H.R. 266: Paycheck Protection Program and Health Care Enhancement Act——House Vote #104——Apr 23, 2020," GovTrack.us, April 23, 2020, https://www.govtrack.us/congress/votes/116-2020/h104.
7. Zachary Evans, "Researcher Tied to Wuhan Lab Thanked Fauci for Dismissing Lab-Leak Theory," *National Review*, June 2, 2021, https://www.nationalreview.com/news/researcher-tied-to-wuhan-lab-thanked-fauci-for-dismissing-lab-leak-theory/.

Chapter 10

1. Video: "COVID-19: Safely Getting Back to Work and Back to School," U.S. Senate Committee on Health, Education, Labor and Pensions, May 12, 2020, at 142:50, https://www.help.senate.gov/hearings/covid-19-safely-getting-back-to-work-and-back-to-school; written transcript: U.S. Senate Committee on Health, Education, Labor, and Pensions, *COVID-19: Safely Getting Back to Work and Back to School* (Washington, D.C.: U.S. Government Printing Office, 2022), 38, https://www.govinfo.gov/content/pkg/CHRG-116shrg45219/pdf/CHRG-116shrg45219.pdf. Transcript lightly edited to improve readability.
2. Michelle A. Waltenburg et al., "Update: COVID-19 among Workers in Meat and Poultry Processing Facilities United States, April–May 2020," *Morbidity and Mortality Weekly Report* 69, no. 27 (2020): 887–92, https://www.cdc.gov/mmwr/volumes/69/wr/mm6927e2.htm.

3. U.S. House of Representatives Select Subcommittee on the Coronavirus Crisis, "Memorandum," U.S. Congress, October 27, 2021, https://web .archive.org/web/20211031061120/https://coronavirus.house.gov/sites /democrats.coronavirus.house.gov/files/2021.10.27%20Meatpacking %20Report.Final_.pdf; Tim A. Bruckner et al., "Estimated Seroprevalence of SARS-CoV-2 Antibodies among Adults in Orange County, California," *Scientific Reports* 11, no. 1 (2021): 3081, https://www.nature.com/articles /s41598-021-82662-x.

4. Jeffrey Klausner and Noah Kojima, "Op-Ed: Quit Ignoring Natural Covid Immunity," MedpageToday, May 28, 2021, https://www.medpagetoday .com/infectiousdisease/covid19/92836.

5. Original transcription: "I think that is important because—in all likelihood is a good way of putting it. The vast majority of these people have immunity, instead of saying there is no evidence. You know, the WHO kind of fed into this by saying no evidence of immunity. And, in reality, there is every evidence stacking up. In fact, a lot of the different studies have shown that it is very unlikely that you get it again in the short term."

6. "COVID-19: Safely Getting Back to Work and Back to School," at 144:15, U.S. Senate HELP Committee, *COVID-19: Safely Getting Back to Work and Back to School*, 39. Transcript lightly edited to improve readability. Brackets indicate slight rewording for written clarity throughout.

7. Stephen Adams, "Professor Who Predicted 500,000 Britons Could Die from Coronavirus Prompted Boris Johnson to Order Lockdown Accused of Having 'Patchy Record of Modelling Pandemics,'" *Daily Mail*, March 28, 2020, https://www.dailymail.co.uk/news/article-8164121/Professor -predicted-500-000-Britons-die-coronavirus-accused-having-patchy-record .html.

8. "COVID-19: Safely Getting Back to Work and Back to School," at 147:20, U.S. Senate HELP Committee, *COVID-19: Safely Getting Back to Work and Back to School*, 39–40. Transcript lightly edited to improve readability.

9. Steerpike, "Six Questions That Neil Ferguson Should Be Asked," *The Spectator*, September 15, 2022, https://www.spectator.co.uk/article/six -questions-that-neil-ferguson-should-be-asked/.

10. Ibid.

11. Heather Stewart, "Neil Ferguson: UK Coronavirus Adviser Resigns after Breaking Lockdown Rules," *The Guardian*, May 5, 2020, https://www

.theguardian.com/uk-news/2020/may/05/uk-coronavirus-adviser-prof-neil
-ferguson-resigns-after-breaking-lockdown-rules.

12. Jacob Sullum, "Gavin Newsom's French Laundry Outing Crystallizes the
Arrogance of COVID-19 Dictators," *Reason*, November 19, 2020, https://
reason.com/2020/11/19/gavin-newsoms-french-laundry-outing-crystallizes
-the-arrogance-of-the-covid-19-dictators/.

13. Nick Sibilla, "Michigan Bans Many Stores from Selling Seeds, Home
Gardening Supplies, Calls Them 'Not Necessary,'" *Forbes*, April 16,
2020, https://www.forbes.com/sites/nicksibilla/2020/04/16/michigan-
bans-many-stores-from-selling-seeds-home-gardening-supplies-calls-them-
not-necessary/?sh=46793dd65f80; Poppy Noor, "Michigan Governor's
Husband under Fire for Asking to Take His Boat Out during Lockdown,"
The Guardian, May 26, 2020, https://www.theguardian.com/us-news/2020
/may/26/gretchen-whitmer-husband-marc-mallory-boat-lockdown.

14. Stewart, "Neil Ferguson."

15. Alistair Haimes, "Lockdown and the R-Number: Is Neil Ferguson Right?,"
The Spectator, June 10, 2022, https://www.spectator.co.uk/article/did-late
-lockdown-double-covid-s-death-toll-fact-checking-neil-ferguson/.

16. John Fund, "'Professor Lockdown' Modeler Resigns in Disgrace," *National
Review*, May 18, 2020, https://www.nationalreview.com/corner/professor
-lockdown-modeler-resigns-in-disgrace/.

17. "Sweden: Coronavirus Deaths," Worldometer, September 1, 2021, accessed
via the Internet Archive's WayBack Machine, https://web.archive.org/
web/20210901074258/https://www.worldometers.info/coronavirus/
country/sweden/.

18. Kevin D. Dayaratna, "Failures of an Influential COVID-19 Model Used to
Justify Lockdowns," The Heritage Foundation, May 18, 2020, https://www
.heritage.org/public-health/commentary/failures-influential-covid-19-model
-used-justify-lockdowns.

19. Ibid.

20. Ibid.

21. Kyle Farrell, "JHB Erupts at 'Completely Wrong' Neil Ferguson Modelling,"
Express, August 3, 2021, https://www.express.co.uk/news/politics/1471469
/neil-ferguson-covid-cases-modelling-forecast-angry-uk-projection-
daily-deaths-news-vn.

22. Ibid.

23. See, e.g., Carlos Garcia, "Architect of Lockdown Policy Admits Sweden Achieved Similar Outcomes without Lockdown," Blaze Media, June 2, 2020, https://www.theblaze.com/news/neil-ferguson-lockdowns-sweden -outcome; Phillip W. Magness, "The Failure of Imperial College Modeling Is Far Worse Than We Knew," American Institute for Economic Research, April 22, 2021, https://www.aier.org/article/the-failure-of-imperial-college -modeling-is-far-worse-than-we-knew/; Anna Mikhailova, Christopher Hope, Louisa Wells, and Michael Gillard, "How Neil Ferguson, the Architect of Lockdown, Was Brought Down by Failing to Obey His Own Rules," *The Telegraph*, May 5, 2020, https://www.telegraph.co.uk/news /2020/05/05/neil-ferguson-architect-lockdown-brought-failing-obey-rules/.

24. See Shannon Brownlee and Jeanne Lenzer, "What Sweden Got Right about COVID," *Washington Monthly*, April 20, 2022, https://washingtonmonthly .com/2022/04/19/what-sweden-got-right-about-covid/.

25. "COVID-19: Safely Getting Back to Work and Back to School," at 147:45; U.S. Senate HELP Committee, *COVID-19: Safely Getting Back to Work and Back to School*, 40. Transcript lightly edited to improve readability.

26. See Emma Colton, "Here Are Fauci's Biggest Flip-Flops and Backtracks amid the Coronavirus Pandemic," *Washington Examiner*, December 1, 2020, https://www.washingtonexaminer.com/news/here-are-faucis-biggest- flip-flops-and-backtracks-amid-the-coronavirus-pandemic.

27. Nicole Mlynaryk, "Kawasaki Disease Rates Dropped during COVID-19 Pandemic," *UC San Diego Today*, June 17, 2022, https://today.ucsd.edu /story/kawasaki-disease-rates-dropped-during-covid-19-pandemic.

28. Carly Vandergriendt, "Kawasaki Disease and the Coronavirus: What's the Connection?," Healthline, April 8, 2022, https://www.healthline.com/health /infection/kawasaki-disease-coronavirus#covid-19-connection.

Chapter 11

1. Video: "COVID-19: Update on Progress toward Safely Getting Back to Work and Back to School," U.S. Senate Committee on Health, Education, Labor and Pensions, June 30, 2020, at 1:29:40, https://www.help.senate.gov /hearings/covid-19-update-on-progress-toward-safely-getting-back-to-work -and-back-to-school; written transcript: U.S. Senate Committee on Health, Education, Labor and Pensions, *COVID-19: Update on Progress toward Safely Getting Back to Work and Back to School* (Washington, D.C.: U.S. Government Printing Office, 2022), 40, https://www.govinfo.gov/content/

pkg/CHRG-116shrg45224/pdf/CHRG-116shrg45224.pdf. Transcript lightly edited to improve readability.

2. Outbreak News Today, "Sweden Report: Teachers Do Not Have a Higher Risk of Being Infected with COVID-19," press release, November 14, 2020, http://outbreaknewstoday.com/sweden-report-teachers-do-not-have-a-higher-risk-of-being-infected-with-covid-19-49944/; Jonas F. Ludvigsson, "Open Schools, Covid-19, and Child and Teacher Morbidity in Sweden," *New England Journal of Medicine* 384, no. 7 (2021): 669–71, https://www.nejm.org/doi/full/10.1056/NEJMc2026670.

3. Anya Kamenetz, "What Parents Can Learn from Child Care Centers That Stayed Open during Lockdowns," NPR, June 24, 2020, https://www.npr.org/2020/06/24/882316641/what-parents-can-learn-from-child-care-centers-that-stayed-open-during-lockdowns.

4. "COVID-19: Update on Progress," at 1:31:30; U.S. Senate Committee on HELP, *COVID-19: Update on Progress*, 40–41. Transcript lightly edited to improve readability. Brackets indicate slight rewording for written clarity throughout.

5. Rafi Eis, "How Eisenhower Predicted Fauci," *Newsweek*, February 13, 2022, https://www.newsweek.com/how-eisenhower-predicted-fauci-opinion-1677267.

6. "COVID-19: Update on Progress," at 1:34:00; U.S. Senate Committee on HELP, *COVID-19: Update on Progress*, 41–42. Transcript lightly edited to improve readability.

7. Jordan Schachtel, "Dr. Flip Flop: A Timeline of Fauci's School Re-Opening Positions," The Dossier (Substack), November 30, 2020, https://www.dossier.today/p/dr-flip-flop-a-timeline-of-faucis?mc_cid=be3cf18f20&mc_eid=a14492f8ea.

8. Ibid.
9. Ibid.
10. Ibid.
11. Ibid.
12. Ibid.
13. Ibid.
14. Ibid.

15. "COVID-19: Update on Progress," at 1:36:15; U.S. Senate Committee on HELP, *COVID-19: Update on Progress*, 42. Transcript lightly edited to improve readability.

16. Ryan Homler, "Dr. Anthony Fauci Advises MLB to Avoid Playing Baseball into October," NBC Sports Washington, June 18, 2020, https://www.nbcsportswashington.com/mlb/dr-anthony-fauci-advises-mlb-to-avoid-playing-baseball-into-october/311658/.

17. "COVID-19: Update on Progress," at 1:37:10; U.S. Senate Committee on HELP, *COVID-19: Update on Progress*, 42. Transcript lightly edited to improve readability.

Chapter 12

1. "United States," Worldometer, accessed April 29, 2023, https://www.worldometers.info/coronavirus/country/us/. The September 2020 number is available via the Internet Archive's WayBack Machine: "United States," Worldometer, September 23, 2020, https://web.archive.org/web/20200923085958/https://www.worldometers.info/coronavirus/country/us/.

2. Ibid.

3. Jon Miltimore, "Sweden Now Has a Lower COVID-19 Death Rate Than the US. Here's Why It Matters," FEE, September 4, 2020, https://fee.org/articles/sweden-now-has-a-lower-covid-19-death-rate-than-the-us-here-s-why-it-matters/.

4. Video: "COVID-19: An Update on the Federal Response," U.S. Senate Committee on Health, Education, Labor and Pensions, September 23, 2020, at 1:44:25, https://www.help.senate.gov/hearings/covid-19-an-update-on-the-federal-response. Transcript: U.S. Senate Committee on Health, Education, Labor and Pensions, *COVID-19: An Update on the Federal Response* (Washington, D.C.: U.S. Government Printing Office, 2022), 47–49, https://www.govinfo.gov/content/pkg/CHRG-116shrg45228/pdf/CHRG-116shrg45228.pdf. Transcript lightly edited to improve readability. Brackets indicate slight rewording for written clarity throughout.

5. Robert E. Sealy and Julia L. Hurwitz, "Cross-Reactive Immune Responses toward the Common Cold Human Coronaviruses and Severe Acute Respiratory Syndrome Coronavirus 2 (SARS-CoV-2): Mini-Review and a Murine Study," *Microorganisms* 9, no. 8 (2021): 1643, https://pubmed.ncbi.nlm.nih.gov/34442723/.

6. Khalid Shrwani et al., "Detection of Serum Cross-Reactive Antibodies and Memory Response to SARS-CoV-2 in Prepandemic and Post-COVID-19 Convalescent Samples," *Journal of Infectious Diseases* 224, no. 8 (2021): 1305, https://pubmed.ncbi.nlm.nih.gov/34161567/.

Chapter 13

1. "United States," Worldometer, accessed April 29, 2023, https://www.worldometers.info/coronavirus/country/us/. For numbers as of November 30, 2020, see the the Internet Archive's WayBack Machine: "United States," Worldometer, November 30, 2020, https://web.archive.org/web/20201130221453/https://www.worldometers.info/coronavirus/country/us/

2. Emma Colton, "Rand Paul Questions Election Results: 'Your Government Sent 1.1 Million Dead People Stimulus Checks,'" *Washington Examiner*, November 9, 2020, https://www.washingtonexaminer.com/news/rand-paul-questions-election-results-your-government-sent-1-1-million-dead-people-stimulus-checks.

3. Vivek Saxena, "Rand Paul Pushes Parler after Tweet 'Our Govt Sent 1.1 Million Dead People Stimulus Checks…' Gets Flagged," BizPac Review, November 11, 2020, https://www.bizpacreview.com/2020/11/11/rand-paul-pushes-parler-after-tweet-our-govt-sent-1-1-million-dead-people-stimulus-checks-gets-flagged-995252/.

4. Ibid.

5. Rich Gardella and Dartunorro Clark, "Dead Wrong: Feds Sent $1.4B in Stimulus Checks to over a Million Deceased," NBC News, June 25, 2020, https://www.nbcnews.com/politics/politics-news/dead-wrong-feds-sent-1-4b-stimulus-checks-over-million-n1232070.

6. U.S. Attorney's Office, Eastern District of Pennsylvania, "Philadelphia Man Charged with Stealing Nearly $1 Million in PPP Funds," press release, June 15, 2021, https://www.justice.gov/usao-edpa/pr/philadelphia-man-charged-stealing-nearly-1-million-ppp-funds; U.S. Attorney's Office, Eastern District of Pennsylvania, "Philadelphia Man Sentenced to 6 ½ Years in Prison for Stealing Nearly $1 Million in PPP Funds," press release, https://www.justice.gov/usao-edpa/pr/philadelphia-man-sentenced-6-years-prison-stealing-nearly-1-million-ppp-funds.

7. "Maryland Man Charged for Stealing over $3.5m in PPP Funds," CBS New Baltimore, September 27, 2021, https://www.cbsnews.com/baltimore/news /maryland-man-charged-for-stealing-over-3-5m-in-ppp-funds/.

8. Reuters, "U.S. Has Charged 57 People in PPP Fraud Cases, Justice Department Says," CNBC, September 10, 2020, https://www.cnbc. com/2020/09/10/us-has-charged-57-people-in-ppp-fraud-cases-justice -department-says.html.

9. Nina Golgowski, "7 Charged with Stealing Millions in COVID Aid, Using It to Buy Lamborghini, Porsche," HuffPost, November 18, 2020, https://www.huffpost.com/entry/7-charged-in-alleged-ppp-scam _n_5fb51c92c5b664958c7c7e23.

10. James Arkin and Andrew Desiderio, "Trump's Attacks on Senate Republicans Complicate His Georgia Message," *Politico*, January 1, 2021, https://www.politico.com/news/2021/01/01/trump-republican-attacks -georgia-453381.

11. Joseph Curl, "Rand Paul Gives Viral Speech on Senate Floor Railing against Covid Bill," The Daily Wire, December 22, 2020, https:// www.dailywire.com/news/rand-paul-gives-viral-speech-on-senate-floor- railing-against-covid-bill.

12. Ibid.

13. Gabriella Muñoz, "Rand Paul Blasts Senate GOP as New 'Bernie Bros' for the Large Cost of Latest COVID Package," *Washington Times*, July 21, 2020, https://www.washingtontimes.com/news/2020/jul/21/rand-paul- blasts-senate-gop-new-bernie-bros-large-/.

14. Ebony Bowden, "Rand Paul Blasts Congress for Adding to US Debt with COVID Relief Bill," *New York Post*, December 22, 2020, https://nypost .com/2020/12/22/rand-paul-blasts-covid-19-relief-bill-over-growing-deficit/.

15. Rand Paul, "Debt Is Not a Sustainable Policy Decision," *The Hill*, December 21, 2020, https://thehill.com/blogs/congress-blog/economy-budget/531173 -debt-is-not-a-sustainable-policy-decision/.

16. Curl, "Rand Paul Gives Viral Speech."

17. Jon Miltimore, "New Study Reveals That Stay-at-Home Orders Backfired. Here's Why," FEE, May 4, 2021, https://fee.org/articles/new-study -reveals-that-stay-at-home-orders-backfired-heres-why/.

18. Curl, "Rand Paul Gives Viral Speech."

19. Brittany Bernstein, "Why Six Senate Republicans Voted against the COVID Relief Bill," *National Review*, December 23, 2020, https://www.nationalreview.com/news/why-six-senate-republicans-voted-against-the-covid-relief-bill/.

20. Emily Czachor, "Republican Rand Paul Criticizes GOP for Adding to National Debt, Says 'They Are Ruining the Country,'" *Newsweek*, July 21, 2020, https://www.newsweek.com/republican-rand-paul-criticizes-gop-adding-national-debt-says-they-are-ruining-country-1519509.

21. Victor Garcia, "Sen. Rand Paul Blasts GOP Colleagues, Says They Should 'Apologize' to Obama for Past Spending Complaints," Fox News, August 5, 2020, https://www.foxnews.com/media/rand-paul-blasts-gop-colleagues-coronavirus-spending; Summer Lin, "Fellow Republicans Owe Obama an Apology for Complaints about Spending, Rand Paul Says," *Lexington Herald-Leader*, August 6, 2020, https://www.kentucky.com/news/politics-government/article244764442.html.

22. "Fact Sheet: Activity at the Wuhan Institute of Virology," U.S. Department of State, January 15, 2021, https://2017-2021.state.gov/fact-sheet-activity-at-the-wuhan-institute-of-virology/index.html.

23. Brackets and ellipsis original. Emily Jacobs, "Pompeo Slams 'Naïve' Fauci for Defending China from COVID Origin Probe," *New York Post*, June 4, 2021, https://nypost.com/2021/06/04/pompeo-slams-fauci-for-defending-china-from-covid-origin-probe/.

24. Ronn Blitzer, "Pompeo: COVID-19 Leaked from Wuhan Lab," Fox News, June 14, 2021, https://www.foxnews.com/politics/pompeo-covid-leaked-wuhan-lab.

25. Tyler Olson, "Pompeo Says It's 'Outrageous' US Officials, including Fauci, Dismissed Lab Leak Theory," Fox News, November 11, 2021, https://www.foxnews.com/politics/pompeo-outrageous-fauci-lab-leak-theory.

26. David Rutz, "CNN Dismisses Redfield Theory Coronavirus Came from Wuhan Lab as 'Controversial' and 'without Evidence,'" Fox News, March 26, 2021, https://www.foxnews.com/media/cnn-redfield-theory-coronavirus-wuhan-lab-evidence.

Chapter 14
1. "United States," Worldometer, May 1, 2021, https://web.archive.org/web/20210501001542/https://www.worldometers.info/coronavirus/country/us/.

2. Original transcription of this paragraph: "You can't get it again. There is almost—there is virtually o percent chance you are going to get it. And yet you are telling people that have had the vaccine, who have immunity—you are defying everything we know about immunity by telling people to wear masks who have been vaccinated. Instead, you should be saying there is no science to say we are going to have a problem from the large number of people to vaccinate. You want to get rid of vaccine hesitancy? Tell them they can quit wearing their their mask after they get the vaccine. You want people to get the vaccine? Give them a reward instead of telling them the nanny state is going to be there for three more years and you got to wear a mask forever. People don't want to hear it. There is no science behind it."

3. Video: "Examining Our COVID-19 Response: An Update from Federal Officials," U.S. Senate Committee on Health, Education, Labor and Pensions, March 18, 2021, at 1:17:45, https://www.help.senate.gov/hearings /examining-our-covid-19-response-an-update-from-federal-officials; written transcript: U.S. Senate Committee on Health, Education, Labor and Pensions, *Examining Our COVID-19 Response: An Update from Federal Officials* (Washington, D.C.: U.S. Government Publishing Office, 2022), 37–40, https://www.govinfo.gov/content/pkg/CHRG-117shrg46755/pdf/ CHRG-117shrg46755.pdf. Transcript lightly edited to improve readability. Brackets indicate slight rewording for written clarity throughout.

4. Maggie Fox, "Masks Are Not Theater, Fauci Tells Sen. Rand Paul in Hearing Exchange," CNN, March 18, 2021, https://www.cnn.com/2021/03/18/ politics/fauci-paul-masks-theater/index.html

5. Matt Lamb, "*Science* Journal Editor: Agree with Me on Climate Change or Don't Get Published," *Washington Examiner*, March 26, 2023, https://www .washingtonexaminer.com/restoring-america/equality-not-elitism/science -journal-editor-agree-with-me-on-climate-change-or-dont-get-published.

6. Holden Thorp, Science EIC (@hholdenthorp), "In light of @Nature's excellent editorial…" (thread), Twitter, March 21, 2023, 4:40 p.m., https:// archive.is/9xxMR.

7. Ibid.

8. Lamb, "*Science* Journal Editor."

9. Robbi Pickeral, "Holden Thorp Resigns as Chancellor," ESPN, September 17, 2012, https://www.espn.com/college-sports/story/_/id/8390950/north -carolina-tar-heels-chancellor-holden-thorp-resigns-latest-athletic-scandal.

10. H. Holden Thorp, "No Senator, It's Not Theater," *Science*, March 22, 2021, https://www.science.org/content/blog-post/no-senator-s-not-theater.

11. Ibid.

12. Holden Thorp, "Letter in Science Tomorrow" (email thread), May 12–13, 2021, DocumentCloud, https://www.documentcloud.org/documents /23807373-nih_foia_59892_complete_response_redacted.

13. Ibid.

14. Ibid.

15. "How Fauci and Collins Shut Down Covid Debate" (editorial), *Wall Street Journal*, December 21, 2021, https://www.wsj.com/articles/fauci-collins-emails-great-barrington-declaration-covid-pandemic-lockdown -11640129116.

16. Nicholas Wade, "Origin of Covid—Following the Clues," Medium.com, May 2, 2021, https://nicholaswade.medium.com/origin-of-covid-following -the-clues-6f03564c038.

17. David Rutz, "New York Times Health Reporter: Wuhan Lab Leak Coronavirus Theory Has 'Racist Roots,' Isn't 'Plausible,'" Fox News, May 26, 2021, https://www.foxnews.com/media/new-york-times-health-reporter -wuhan-lab-leak-coronavirus-theory-has-racist-roots-isnt-plausible.

18. "An Engineered Doomsday" (editorial), *New York Times*, January 7, 2012, https://www.nytimes.com/2012/01/08/opinion/sunday/an-engineered -doomsday.html.

Chapter 15

1. U.S. House of Representatives Permanent Select Committee on Intelligence: Minority, *Unclassified Summary of the Second Interim Report on the Origins of the COVID-19 Pandemic* (Washington, D.C.: U.S. House of Representatives Permanent Select Committee on Intelligence: Minority, accessed April 30, 2023), https://intelligence.house.gov/uploadedfiles/final _unclass_summary_-_covid_origins_report_.pdf; Josh Christenson, "US Taxpayers Funded $2M Worth of Research in Wuhan, Government Watchdog Reports," *New York Post*, June 14, 2023, https://nypost.com/2023 /06/14/us-taxpayers-funded-2-million-for-research-in-wuhan-report/.

2. Nicholson Baker, "The Lab-Leak Hypothesis: For Decades, Scientists Have Been Hot-Wiring Viruses in Hopes of Preventing a Pandemic, Not Causing One. But What Is…?," Intelligencer, January 4, 2021, https://nymag.com /intelligencer/article/coronavirus-lab-escape-theory.html.

3. Ibid.
4. Video: "An Update from Federal Officials on Efforts to Combat COVID-19," U.S. Senate Health, Education, Labor and Pensions Committee, May 11, 2021, at 1:11:55, https://www.help.senate.gov/hearings/an-update-from -federal-officials-on-efforts-to-combat-covid-19; written transcript: U.S. Senate Health, Education, Labor and Pensions Committee, *An Update from Federal Officials on Efforts to Combat COVID-19* (Washington, D.C.: U.S. Government Publishing Office, 2022), 38–41, https://www.govinfo. gov/content/pkg/CHRG-117shrg46765/pdf/CHRG-117shrg46765.pdf. Transcript lightly edited to improved readability. Brackets indicate slight rewording for written clarity throughout.
5. U.S. Senate HELP Committee, *Update from Federal Officials*, 40. Transcript lightly edited to improve readability.
6. Gabrielle Fonrouge, "Fauci Once Argued for Risky Viral Experiments—Even If They Can Lead to Pandemic," *New York Post*, May 28, 2021, https://nypost.com/2021/05/28/fauci-once-argued-viral-experiments-worth-the-risk-of-pandemic/.
7. Ed Browne, "Fauci Was 'Untruthful' to Congress about Wuhan Lab Research, New Documents Appear to Show," *Newsweek*, September 9, 2021, https://www.newsweek.com/fauci-untruthful-congress-wuhan-lab -research-documents-show-gain-function-1627351; Jocelyn Kaiser, "U.S. Should Expand Rules for Risky Virus Research to More Pathogens, Panel Says," *Science*, January 20, 2023, https://www.science.org/content/article /u-s-should-expand-rules-risky-virus-research-more-pathogens-panel-says; Katherine Eban, "'This Shouldn't Happen': Inside the Virus-Hunting Nonprofit at the Center of the Lab-Leak Controversy," *Vanity Fair*, March 31, 2022, https://www.vanityfair.com/news/2022/03/the-virus-hunting -nonprofit-at-the-center-of-the-lab-leak-controversy.
8. Fonrouge, "Fauci Once Argued for Risky Viral Experiments."
9. Britanny Bernstein, "Fauci Argued Benefits of Gain-of-Function Research Outweighed Pandemic Risk in 2012 Paper," Yahoo! News, May 28, 2021, https://news.yahoo.com/fauci-argued-benefits-gain-function-185934217 .html.
10. Sharon Lerner and Maia Hibbett, "Leaked Grant Proposal Details High-Risk Coronavirus Research" The Intercept, September 23, 2021, https:// theintercept.com/2021/09/23/coronavirus-research-grant-darpa/.

11. Ryan Grim, Katherine Eban, Sharon Lerner, and Mara Hvistendahl, "The Lab-Leak Theory Is Looking Stronger by the Day. Here's What We Know," May 6, 2022, in *Deconstructed*, podcast, https://theintercept.com/2022/05 /06/deconstructed-lab-leak-covid-katherine-eban/.

12. Matt Ridley and Alina Chan, *Viral: The Search for the Origin of COVID-19* (New York: HarperCollins, 2021), 312–13.

13. "Drastic Analysis of the Defuse Documents," Drastic Research, February 6, 2022, https://drasticresearch.org/2021/09/20/1583/.

14. Grim, Eban, Lerner, and Hvistendahl, "The Lab-Leak Theory."

15. Cathy McMorris Rodgers, Brett Guthrie, and H. Morgan Griffith to Francis Collins, March 18, 2021, page 3, CloudFront.net, https://d1dth6e84htgma .cloudfront.net/2021_03_18_Energy_Commerce_Minority_Ltr_to_NIH _COVID_Origins_Investigation_w_Attch_beff845b57.pdf?updated_ at=2022-09-13T16:03:57.608Z.

16. Lawrence A. Tabak to Cathy McMorris Rodgers, May 21, 2021, "Tabak Letter to McMorris Rodgers on NIH Grants, *Washington Post*, May 25, 2021, https://www.washingtonpost.com/context/tabak-letter-to-mcmorris -rodgers-on-nih-grants/16cb2639-e9d7-4658-bce8-e944d899dda1/.

17. Ibid.

18. Oversight Committee (@GOPoversight), "July 28th NIH says 'no NIAID funding was approved for Gain of Function Research at the WIV….," Twitter, October 20, 2021, https://twitter.com/GOPoversight/status /1450934193177903105.

19. Lawrence A. Tabak to Cathy McMorris Rodgers.

20. Ibid.; Robert E. Moffit, "Why Are Feds Still Funding EcoHealth Alliance When Its COVID-19 Role Remains Unresolved?," The Heritage Foundation, October 27, 2022, https://www.heritage.org/public-health/ commentary/why-are-feds-still-funding-ecohealth-alliance-when-its-covid-19-role; Jocelyn Kaiser, "NIH Restarts Bat Virus Grant Suspended 3 Years Ago by Trump," *Science*, May 8, 2023, https://www.science.org/content/ article/nih-restarts-bat-virus-grant-suspended-3-years-ago-trump.

Chapter 16

1. Isaac Schorr, "Biosafety Expert Explains Why Fauci's NIH 'Gain-of-Function' Testimony Was 'Demonstrably False,'" *National Review*, May 13, 2021, https://www.nationalreview.com/news/biosafety-expert-explains-why -faucis-nih-gain-of-function-testimony-was-demonstrably-false/.

2. Ibid.

3. Video: "The Path Forward: A Federal Perspective on the COVID-19 Response," U.S. Senate Committee on Health, Education, Labor and Pensions, July 20, 2021, at 50:40, https://www.help.senate.gov/hearings/the -path-forward-a-federal-perspective-on-the-covid-19-response. Transcript lightly edited to improve readability.

4. "We're Still Missing the Origin Story of This Pandemic. China Is Sitting on the Answers," (editorial), *Washington Post*, February 5, 2021, https://www .washingtonpost.com/opinions/2021/02/05/coronavirus-origins-mystery -china/.

5. Amanda Nieves, "Smoking Gun: WCW FOIA Investigation Proves NIH Allowed Gain-of-Function Research; Wuhan Lab Funder Calls It 'Terrific!,'" White Coat Waste Project, November 4, 2021, https://blog. whitecoatwaste.org/2021/11/04/bombshell-wcw-foia-investigation-proves-nih-ignored-gof-research-wuhan-lab-funder-calls-it-terrific/.

6. Jerry Dunleavy, "Rand Paul Sends Criminal Referral to DOJ Saying Fauci Lied about Gain-of-Function Research Funding," *Washington Examiner*, July 24, 2021, https://www.washingtonexaminer.com/news/rand-paul-sends-criminal-referral-doj-fauci-lied-gain-of-function-research.

7. Ben Hu et al., "Discovery of a Rich Gene Pool of Bat SARS-Related Coronaviruses Provides New Insights into the Origin of SARS Coronavirus," *PLoS Pathogens* 13, no. 11 (2017): 1006698, https://pubmed.ncbi.nlm.nih .gov/29190287/.

8. Rand Paul to Merrick Garland, July 21, 2021, DocumentCloud, https:// s3.documentcloud.org/documents/21014466/rand-paul-letter-to-doj.pdf.

9. "Revisiting Gain of Function Research: What the Pandemic Taught Us and Where Do We Go from Here," Homeland Security and Government Affairs, August 3, 2022, https://www.hsgac.senate.gov/ subcommittees/etso/hearings/revisiting-gain-of-function-research-what-the-pandemic-taught-us-and-where-do-we-go-from-here/; Andrew Kerr, "EXCLUSIVE: Fauci Staffers Flagged Potential Gain-of-Function Research at Wuhan Lab in 2016, Records Reveal," Daily Caller, November 3, 2021, https://dailycaller.com/2021/11/03/fauci -nih-ecohealth-peter-daszak-gain-of-function-wuhan-covid-19/.

10. Gabe Kaminsky, "WaPo Corrects Story from Last February Claiming COVID Lab Leak Theory Was 'Debunked,'" The Federalist, June 1, 2021,

https://thefederalist.com/2021/06/01/wapo-quietly-edits-story-from-last
-february-claiming-covid-lab-leak-theory-was-debunked/.

11. Ibid.

12. Kerr, "EXCLUSIVE: Fauci Staffers Flagged Potential Gain-of-Function Research"; Sharon Lerner and Mara Hvistendahl, "NIH Officials Worked with EcoHealth Alliance to Evade Restrictions on Coronavirus Experiments," The Intercept, November 3, 2021, https://theintercept.com /2021/11/03/coronavirus-research-ecohealth-nih-emails/; Teresa Monroe-Hamilton, "Emails Show NIH, NIAID Were Repeatedly Concerned about 'Gain-Of-Function' Experiments at Wuhan Lab," BizPac, July 18, 2022, https://www.bizpacreview.com/2022/07/18/emails-show-nih-niaid-were-repeatedly-concerned-about-gain-of-function-experiments-at-wuhan-lab-1262955/.

13. Kerr, "EXCLUSIVE: Fauci Staffers Flagged Potential Gain-of-Function Research."

14. Ibid.; Monroe-Hamilton, "Emails Show NIH, NIAID Were Repeatedly Concerned."

15. Kerr, "EXCLUSIVE: Fauci Staffers Flagged Potential Gain-of-Function Research."

16. Katherine Eban, "'This Shouldn't Happen': Inside the Virus-Hunting Nonprofit at the Center of the Lab-Leak Controversy," Vanity Fair, March 31, 2022, https://www.vanityfair.com/news/2022/03/the-virus-hunting -nonprofit-at-the-center-of-the-lab-leak-controversy; "Letter Exchange," Informed Action Consent Network, n.d., https://icandecide.org/wp-content/ uploads/2021/11/Letter-Exchange.pdf.

17. "Revisiting Gain of Function Research," U.S. Senate Committee on Homeland Security and Governmental Affairs.

18. Lerner and Hvistendahl, "NIH Officials Worked with EcoHealth Alliance"; Kerr, "EXCLUSIVE: Fauci Staffers Flagged Potential Gain-of-Function Research"; Monroe-Hamilton, "Emails Show NIH, NIAID Were Repeatedly Concerned."

19. Jerry Dunleavy, "Republicans Argue Fauci Emails Show NIH Funded Gain-of-Function Research at Wuhan Lab," Washington Examiner, July 30, 2021, https://www.washingtonexaminer.com/news/republicans-fauci-emails-nih-funded-gain-of-function-research-wuhan-lab.

20. James Comer and Jim Jordan to Xavier Beccerra, January 11, 2022, in "House Oversight Letter and Email Transcriptions," DocumentCloud,

https://www.documentcloud.org/documents/21177759-house-oversight
-letter-and-email-transcriptions.

21. Lawrence A. Tabak to James Comer, October 20, 2021, DocumentCloud,
https://www.documentcloud.org/documents/21674679-tabak-letter-to
-comer-oct-20-2021.

22. Richard H. Ebright, "Written Testimony of Richard H. Ebright,"
Homeland Security and Governmental Affairs, August 3, 2022, page 14,
https://www.hsgac.senate.gov/wp-content/uploads/imo/media/doc/Ebright
%20Testimony%20Updated.pdf.

23. Lawrence A. Tabak to James Comer, October 20, 2021; Monroe-Hamilton,
"Emails Show NIH, NIAID Were Repeatedly Concerned."

24. Ebright, "Written Testimony of Richard H. Ebright," 16.

25. Ibid.

26. Ibid., 17.

Chapter 17

1. Michael P. Senger, "New Study from Ioannidis: Covid's IFR in 2020 Was
Less than 0.1% for Those under 70, Even Lower than Previously Believed,"
The New Normal (Substack), October 17, 2022, https://michaelpsenger
.substack.com/p/new-study-from-ioannidis-covids-ifr.

2. Jonathan Rothwell and Dan Witters, "U.S. Adults' Estimates of COVID-19
Hospitalization Risk," Gallup, November 29, 2022, https://news.gallup.
com/opinion/gallup/354938/adults-estimates-covid-hospitalization-risk.
aspx.

3. "COVID-19: Democratic Voters Support Harsh Measures against
Unvaccinated," Rasmussen Reports, January 13, 2022, https://www
.rasmussenreports.com/public_content/politics/partner_surveys/
jan_2022/covid_19_democratic_voters_support_harsh_measures_against
_unvaccinated.

4. Rohit, "Novak Djokovic Begins 353rd Week as World No. 1," sportskeeda,
December 29, 2021, https://www.sportskeeda.com/tennis/news-novak
-djokovic-ends-year-spending-353rd-week-world-no-1; Associated Press,
"Novak Djokovic Can't Play in Australian Open after Losing Deportation
Appeal," USA Today, January 16, 2022, https://www.usatoday.com/
story/sports/tennis/aus/2022/01/15/novak-djokovic-loses-appeal-against
-deportation-order-australian-open/6547613001/.

5. James Melville (@JamesMelville), "'Because the principles of decision making on my Body are more important than any title....,'" Twitter, January 10, 2023, 2:39 p.m., https://twitter.com/JamesMelville/status /1612896984041676803.

6. Jordan Dajani, "Aaron Rodgers Explains Decision to Not Get Vaccinated, Calls Out NFL for COVID-19 Protocols," CBS Sports, November 5, 2021, https://www.cbssports.com/nfl/news/aaron-rodgers-explains-decision-to -not-get-vaccinated-calls-out-nfl-for-covid-19-protocols/.

7. Charles Creitz, "NBA's Jonathan Isaac Calls Out Media's 'Blatant Miscarriage of Information' about Vaccine Mandates," Fox News, October 19, 2021, https://www.foxnews.com/media/nbas-jonathan-isaac-calls-out -medias-blatant-miscarriage-of-information-about-vaccine-mandates.

8. "Conservative News Viewers More Accurately Estimate COVID-19 Death Risk," Rasmussen Reports, September 3, 2021, https://www .rasmussenreports.com/public_content/lifestyle/covid_19/conservative_ news_viewers_more_accurately_estimate_covid_19_death_risk.

9. Ibid.

10. Jon Miltimore (@miltimore79), "A new @nberpubs paper shows how US media created a climate of #COVID19 fear.... ," Twitter, December 1, 2020, https://twitter.com/miltimore79/status/1333858435591516165.

11. Bruce Sacerdote, Ranjan Sehgal, and Molly Cook, "Why Is All COVID-19 News Bad News?," (working paper 28110), National Bureau of Economic Research, November 2020, https://www.nber.org/papers/w28110.

12. Leah Barkoukis, "NIH Quietly Edits Section of Website on Gain-of-Function Research," Townhall, October 25, 2021, https://townhall.com/ tipsheet/leahbarkoukis/2021/10/25/nih-quietly-edits-section-of-website-on -gain-of-function-research-n2597968.

13. Kevin M. Esvelt, "Manipulating Viruses and Risking Pandemics Is Too Dangerous. It's Time to Stop," *Washington Post*, October 6, 2021, https:// www.washingtonpost.com/opinions/2021/10/07/manipulating-viruses -risking-pandemics-is-too-dangerous-its-time-stop/.

14. "COVID-19 Coronavirus Pandemic," Worldometer, July 13, 2023, https:// www.worldometers.info/coronavirus/; Michael J. Imperiale and Arturo Casadevall, "Rethinking Gain-of-Function Experiments in the Context of the COVID-19 Pandemic," *mBio* 11, no. 4 (2020): e01868-20, https:// www.ncbi.nlm.nih.gov/pmc/articles/PMC7419723/; Steven Quay, "Written Remarks to Accompany the Testimony of Steven Quay, MD, PhD," U.S.

Senate Committee on Homeland Security and Governmental Affairs, August 3, 2022, pages 4–6, https://www.hsgac.senate.gov/wp-content/ uploads/imo/media/doc/Quay%20Testimony.pdf; Craig W. Day et al., "A New Mouse-Adapted Strain of SARS-CoV as a Lethal Model for Evaluating Antiviral Agents In Vitro and In Vivo," *Virology* 395, no. 2 (2009): 210–22, https://www.ncbi.nlm.nih.gov/pmc/articles/PMC2787736/.

15. Emily Crane, "NIH Admits US Funded Gain-of-Function in Wuhan—despite Fauci's Denials," *New York Post*, October 21, 2021, https://nypost.com/2021/10/21/nih-admits-us-funded-gain-of-function-in-wuhan-despite-faucis-repeated-denials/; Zachary Stieber, "NIH: No Documents Available on Removal of 'Gain-of-Function' Definition from Website," *Epoch Times*, December 9, 2021, https://www.theepochtimes.com/nih-no-documents-available-on-removal-of-gain-of-function-definition-from-website_4147680.html?utm_source=partner&utm_campaign=allsides; Hannah Bleau, "NIH Erases Website's Section on Gain of Function amid Fauci Fallout," Breitbart, October 26, 2021, https://www.breitbart.com/politics/2021/10/26/nih-erases-websites-section-on-gain-of-function-amid-fauci-fallout/; Barkoukis, "NIH Quietly Edits."

16. Crane, "NIH Admits US Funded Gain-of-Function in Wuhan"; Stieber, "NIH: No Documents Available on Removal of 'Gain-of-Function' Definition"; Bleau, "NIH Erases Website's Section on Gain of Function"; Barkoukis, "NIH Quietly Edits."

17. "Next Steps: The Road Ahead for the COVID-19 Response," U.S. Senate Committee on Health, Education, Labor and Pensions, November 4, 2021, at 1:14:45, https://www.help.senate.gov/hearings/next-steps-the-road-ahead-for-the-covid-19-response. Transcript lightly edited to improve readability. Brackets indicate slight rewording for written clarity throughout.

18. Anton Troianovski, "Soviets Once Denied a Deadly Anthrax Lab Leak. U.S. Scientists Backed the Story," *New York Times*, June 20, 2021, https://www.nytimes.com/2021/06/20/world/europe/coronavirus-lab-anthrax.html.

19. Office of Senator Rand Paul, "Dr. Rand Paul Introduces Amendment to Eliminate Dr. Fauci's Position as Director of NIAID," news release, March 14, 2022, https://www.paul.senate.gov/news-dr-rand-paul-introduces-amendment-eliminate-dr-faucis-position-director-niaid/. Announcement adapted for use in this book.

20. Adam Staten, "Dr. Fauci Foe Rand Paul Takes Steps to Eliminate 'Dictator-in-Chief' Job," *Newsweek*, March 15, 2022, https://www.newsweek.com/dr-fauci-foe-rand-paul-takes-steps-eliminate-dictator-chief-job-1688371.

21. Jake Thomas, "Dr. Fauci Hints He May Retire Soon as Rand Paul Works to Get Him Fired," *Newsweek*, March 18, 2022, https://www.newsweek.com/dr-fauci-hints-he-may-retire-soon-rand-paul-works-get-him-fired-1689696.

22. Ashley Rindsberg, "How Dick Cheney Created Anthony Fauci: America's Biodefence Strategy Has Finally Backfired," UnHerd, August 29, 2022, https://unherd.com/2022/08/how-dick-cheney-created-anthony-fauci/.

23. Ibid.

24. Rand Paul, "This Will Be the End to Fauci's NIH as We Know It," Fox News, March 23, 2023, https://www.foxnews.com/opinion/end-faucis-nih. Op-ed adapted and expanded for use in this book.

25. Bess Levin, "Rand Paul Swears There's an Innocent Explanation for Not Disclosing His Wife's COVID Stocks for 16 Months," *Vanity Fair*, August 12, 2021, https://www.vanityfair.com/news/2021/08/rand-paul-wife-gilead-remdesivir-stock.

26. Katherine Eban, "'This Shouldn't Happen': Inside the Virus-Hunting Nonprofit at the Center of the Lab-Leak Controversy," *Vanity Fair*, March 31, 2022, https://www.vanityfair.com/news/2022/03/the-virus-hunting-nonprofit-at-the-center-of-the-lab-leak-controversy.

27. Rand Paul (@RandPaul), "How did EcoHealth Alliance convince Fauci to give them over a $100 million? Well, an invitation to the Cosmos Club AND…" (thread), Twitter, March 31, 2022, 3:45 p.m., https://twitter.com/randpaul/status/1509618008985116678.

28. Matt Taibbi, "Twitter, the FBI Subsidiary," The Twitter Files (Substack), April 12, 2023, https://twitterfiles.substack.com/p/twitter-the-fbi-subsidiary; David Molloy, "Zuckerberg Tells Rogan FBI Warning Prompted Biden Laptop Story Censorship," BBC, August 26, 2022, https://www.bbc.com/news/world-us-canada-62688532; Jenin Younes and Aaron Kheriaty, "The White House Covid Censorship Machine," *Wall Street Journal*, January 8, 2023, https://www.wsj.com/articles/white-house-covid-censorship-machine-social-media-facebook-meta-executive-rob-flaherty-free-speech-google-11673203704; Paul D. Thacker (@thackerpd), "1) Twitter Files #FauciPharmaFiles…" (thread), April 20, 2023, 9:09 a.m., https://twitter.com/thackerpd/status/1649037538663727106; Chris Donaldson, "New Twitter Files Drop Brings Long-Promised Hammer

to Fauci, with of [sic] Promise 'More to Come!'," BizPac Review, April 21, 2023, https://www.bizpacreview.com/2023/04/21/new-twitter-files-drop-brings-long-promised-hammer-to-fauci-with-of-promise-more-to-come-1352124/; Matt Taibbi, "Stanford, the Virality Project, and the Censorship of 'True Stories,'" The Twitter Files (Substack), April 12, 2023, https://twitterfiles.substack.com/p/stanford-the-virality-project-and; Mark Lungariello and Samuel Chamberlain, "White House, Big Tech Colluded to Censor 'Misinformation': Lawsuit," *New York Post*, September 1, 2022, https://nypost.com/2022/09/01/white-house-big-tech-colluded-to-censor-misinformation-lawsuit/; Ken Klippenstein and Lee Fang, "Truth Cops," The Intercept, October 31, 2022, https://theintercept.com/2022/10/31/social-media-disinformation-dhs/.

29. "Jeff Landry Deposed Anthony Fauci Last Week. What Did He Find Out?," The Hayride, November 30, 2022, https://thehayride.com/2022/11/jeff-landry-deposed-anthony-fauci-last-week-what-did-he-find-out/.

30. Ibid.

31. Taibbi, "Twitter, the FBI Subsidiary"; Molloy, "Zuckerberg Tells Rogan FBI Warning"; Younes and Kheriaty, "The White House Covid Censorship Machine"; Thacker (@thackerpd), "1) Twitter Files #FauciPharmaFiles…"; Donaldson, "New Twitter Files Drop"; Taibbi, "Stanford, the Virality Project"; Lungariello and Chamberlain, "White House, Big Tech Colluded"; Klippenstein and Fang, "Truth Cops."

32. "Scott Gottlieb, M.D.," salary.com, 2023, https://www.salary.com/research/executive-compensation/scott-gottlieb-m-d-board-member-of-pfizer-inc.

33. Brett Giroir (@DrGiroir), "It's now clear #COVID19 natural immunity is superior to #vaccine immunity, by ALOT…. ," Twitter, August 28, 2021, 9:49 p.m., https://twitter.com/DrGiroir/status/1431433820054638595.

34. Joseph A. Wulfsohn, "Twitter Files: Pfizer Board Member Dr. Scott Gottlieb Flagged Tweets Questioning Covid Vaccine," Fox News, January 9, 2023, https://www.foxnews.com/media/twitter-files-pfizer-board-member-dr-scott-gottlieb-flagged-tweets-questioning-covid-vaccine.

35. Paul Elias Alexander, "160 Plus Research Studies Affirm Naturally Acquired Immuity to Covid-19: Documented, Linked, and Quoted," The Brownstone Institute, October 17, 2021, https://brownstone.org/articles/research-studies-affirm-naturally-acquired-immunity/.

Chapter 18

1.   Amber Todoroff, "Substack: Case Study: Who Is the #1 Recipient of Third-Party Royalty Payments at NIH?," OpenTheBooks, June 9, 2022, https://www.openthebooks.com/substack-case-study-who-is-the-1-recipient-of-third-party-royalty-payments-at-nih/; Adam Andrzejewski, "Substack Investigation: Fauci's Royalties and the $350 Million Royalty Payment Stream HIDDEN by NIH," OpenTheBooks, May 16, 2022, https://www.openthebooks.com/substack-investigation-faucis-royalties-and-the-350-million-royalty-payment-stream-hidden-by-nih/.

2.   Original transcription: "Well, here's the thing is, why don't you let us know? Why don't you reveal how much you've gotten and from what entities? The NIH refuses. Look, we ask them, we ask them. The NIH, we ask them whether or not, who got it, and how much—they refuse to tell us. They send it redacted. Here's what I want to know—it's not just about you, [it's about] everybody on the vaccine committe. Have any of them ever received money from the people who make vaccines? Can you tell me that? Can you tell me if anybody on the vaccine approval committees ever received any money from the people making the vaccines?"

3.   "An Update on the Ongoing Federal Response to COVID-19: Current Status and Future Planning," U.S. Senate Committee on Health, Education, Labor and Pensions, June 16, 2022, at 1:16:00, https://www.help.senate.gov/hearings/an-update-on-the-ongoing-federal-response-to-covid-19-current-status-and-future-planning. Transcript lightly edited to improve readability. Brackets indicate slight rewording for written clarity throughout.

4.   Robert F. Kennedy Jr., *The Real Anthony Fauci: Bill Gates, Big Pharma, and the Global War on Democracy and Public Health* (New York: Skyhorse Publishing, 2022), 119.

5.   Ibid.

6.   Diana Glebova, "Fauci's Net Worth Nearly Doubled during Pandemic," Yahoo! News, September 30, 2022, https://news.yahoo.com/fauci-net-worth-nearly-doubled-154225312.html.

7.   Rand Paul et al. to Lawrence A. Tabak, June 1, 2022, https://www.ronjohnson.senate.gov/services/files/9AA5C381-911D-4026-8534-5780498A7F46.

8.   D'Angelo Gore, "Some Posts about NIH Royalties Omit Fauci Statement That He Donates His Payments," FactCheck.org, May 20, 2022, https://

www.factcheck.org/2022/05/scicheck-some-posts-about-nih-royalties-omit
-that-fauci-said-he-donates-his-payments/.

9. Adam Andrzejewski, "Substack Investigation: Fauci's Royalties and the $350 Million Royalty Payment Stream HIDDEN by NIH," OpenTheBooks.com, May 16, 2022, https://www.openthebooks.com/substack-investigation-faucis -royalties-and-the-350-million-royalty-payment-stream-hidden-by-nih/.

10. Ibid.

11. Ibid.

12. Benjamin Mueller, "After a Long Delay, Moderna Pays N.I.H. for Covid Vaccine Technique," *New York Times*, February 23, 2023, https://www .nytimes.com/2023/02/23/science/moderna-covid-vaccine-patent-nih.html; Eric Sagonowsky, "Moderna Pays US Government $400M 'Catch-Up Payment' under New COVID-19 Vaccine License," Fierce Pharma, February 24, 2023, https://www.fiercepharma.com/pharma/moderna-pays-us -government-400m-catch-payment-under-new-covid-19-vaccine-license.

13. Mueller, "After a Long Delay, Moderna Pays N.I.H."; Sagonowsky, "Moderna Pays US Government."

14. Personal conversation with Bernie Sanders.

15. Personal conversation with Stephen Hoge.

Chapter 19

1. You can view the clip here: Tom Elliott (@tomselliott), "Fauci, in 2004: 'If she got the flu for 14 days, she's as protected as anybody can be, because the best vaccination is getting infected yourself.…," Twitter, April 1, 2022, 7:18 a.m., https://twitter.com/tomselliott/status/1509852615751962627.

2. Original transcription: "So when you are trying to tell us that kids need a third or a fourth vaccine, are you including the variability or the variable of previous infection in the studies? No, you are not. Because when you have approved vaccines in recent times, and the committees that have approved it for children, don't report anything on hospitalization or death or transmission."

3. Original transcription: "Is it any of the guidelines—any of the guidelines for vaccines—do any of the guidelines for the vaccines from the government include previous infection as something to base your decision on with vaccines? Do any of the guidelines involve previous infection? That's why you're ignoring previous infection, because it doesn't involve any of the guidelines. And furthermore, we've been asking you—and you refuse to

answer—whether anybody on the vaccine committees gets royalties from the pharmaceutical companies."

4. Ronn Blitzer, "Rand Paul Threatens to Investigate Royalties to Fauci, Other Officials, If GOP Takes Senate," Fox News, September 14, 2022, https://www.foxnews.com/politics/rand-paul-threatens-investigate-royalties-fauci-officials-gop-takes-senate.

5. "Stopping the Spread of Monkeypox: Examining the Federal Response," Senate Committee on Health, Education, Labor and Pensions, September 14, 2022, at 1:23:10, https://www.help.senate.gov/hearings/stopping-the-spread-of-monkeypox-examining-the-federal-response. Transcript lightly edited to improve readability. Brackets indicate slight rewording for written clarity throughout.

6. Amber Todoroff, "Substack: Case Study: Who Is the #1 Recipient of Third-Party Royalty Payments at NIH?," OpenTheBooks, June 9, 2022, https://www.openthebooks.com/substack-case-study-who-is-the-1-recipient-of-third-party-royalty-payments-at-nih/; Adam Andrzejewski, "Substack Investigation: Fauci's Royalties and the $350 Million Royalty Payment Stream HIDDEN by NIH," OpenTheBooks, May 16, 2022, https://www.openthebooks.com/substack-investigation-faucis-royalties-and-the-350-million-royalty-payment-stream-hidden-by-nih/.

Chapter 20

1. Video: "Revisiting Gain of Function Research: What the Pandemic Taught Us and Where Do We Go from Here," U.S. Senate Committee on Homeland Security and Governmental Affairs, August 3, 2022, https://www.hsgac.senate.gov/subcommittees/etso/hearings/revisiting-gain-of-function-research-what-the-pandemic-taught-us-and-where-do-we-go-from-here/.

2. Rand Paul, "ETSO Subcommittee Hearing: Revisiting Gain of Function Research: What the Pandemic Taught Us and Where Do We Go From Here? Opening Statement of Ranking Member Paul," U.S. Senate Committee on Homeland Security and Governmental Affairs, August 3, 2022, https://www.hsgac.senate.gov/wp-content/uploads/imo/media/doc/2022-08-03%20Ranking%20Member%20Paul%20Opening%20Statement.pdf. Transcript lightly edited to improve readability.

3. Paolo Barnard, Steven Quay, and Angus Dalgleish, *The Origin of the Virus: The Hidden Truths behind the Microbe That Killed Millions of People* (Bristol, United Kingdom: Clinical Press, 2021).

4. Kevin M. Esvelt, "Manipulating Viruses and Risking Pandemics Is Too Dangerous. It's Time to Stop," *Washington Post*, October 6, 2021, https://www.washingtonpost.com/opinions/2021/10/07/manipulating-viruses-risking-pandemics-is-too-dangerous-its-time-stop/. Reproduced with the author's permission.

5. Ellipsis original. Lori Robertson, "The Wuhan Lab and the Gain-of-Function Disagreement," FactCheck.org, July 1, 2021, https://www.factcheck.org/2021/05/the-wuhan-lab-and-the-gain-of-function-disagreement/.

6. Ibid.

7. Richard Ebright, "Written Testimony of Richard H. Ebright," U.S. Senate Committee on Homeland Security and Governmental Affairs, August 3, 2022, page 3, https://www.hsgac.senate.gov/wp-content/uploads/imo/media/doc/Ebright%20Testimony%20Updated.pdf.

8. Steven Quay, "Written Remarks to Accompany the Testimony of Steven Quay, MD, PhD," U.S. Senate Committee on Homeland Security and Governmental Affairs, August 3, 2022, page 2, https://www.hsgac.senate.gov/wp-content/uploads/imo/media/doc/Quay%20Testimony.pdf.

9. Emphasis original. Ebright, "Written Testimony of Richard H. Ebright," 3.

10. Ibid.

11. Quay, "Written Remarks to Accompany the Testimony of Steven Quay, MD, PhD," 5.

12. Ebright, "Written Testimony of Richard H. Ebright," 4.

13. Ibid., 4–5.

14. Quay, "Written Remarks to Accompany the Testimony of Steven Quay, MD, PhD," 5.

15. Ibid.

16. Ibid., 2–3.

17. Sharri Markson, *What Really Happened in Wuhan: The Cover-Ups, the Conspiracies and the Classified Research* (Sydney, Australia: HarperCollins, 2021), 154–56.

18. Ibid., 159.

19. Ibid., 161.

20. Ebright, "Written Testimony of Richard H. Ebright," 5.

21. Kevin M. Esvelt, "Credible Pandemic Virus Identification Will Trigger the Immediate Proliferation of Agents as Lethal as Nuclear Devices: Testimony

of Professor Kevin M. Esvelt, Massachusetts Institute of Technology," Senate Homeland Security and Governmental Affairs Committee, August 3, 2022, page 2, https://www.hsgac.senate.gov/wp-content/uploads/imo/media/doc/Esvelt%20Testimony.pdf.

22. Josh Rogin, "Opinion | The U.S. Government Is Rushing to Resume Risky Virus Research. Not So Fast," *Washington Post*, October 21, 2021, https://www.washingtonpost.com/opinions/2021/10/21/us-government-is-rushing-resume-risky-virus-research-not-so-fast/; Michael Specter, "In a World of Synthetic Biology, Publishing Virus DNA Sequences May Mean Perishing," STAT, April 6, 2023, https://www.statnews.com/2023/04/06/synthetic-biology-publishing-virus-sequences/.

23. Esvelt, "Credible Pandemic Virus Identification," 2.

24. Ebright, "Written Testimony of Richard H. Ebright," 4.

25. Esvelt, "Credible Pandemic Virus Identification," 2.

26. Ibid.

27. Ebright, "Written Testimony of Richard H. Ebright," 6.

28. "Senator Paul Accuses Dr. Fauci of Changing Gain of Function Research Definition on NIH Website," C-SPAN, November 4, 2021, https://www.c-span.org/video/?c4985061/senator-paul-accuses-dr-fauci-changing-gain-function-research-definition-nih-website.

29. Yella Hewings-Martin, "How Do SARS and MERS Compare with COVID-19?," MedicalNewsToday, April 10, 2020, https://www.medicalnewstoday.com/articles/how-do-sars-and-mers-compare-with-covid-19.

30. Katherine Eban, "'This Shouldn't Happen': Inside the Virus-Hunting Nonprofit at the Center of the Lab-Leak Controversy," *Vanity Fair*, March 31, 2022, https://www.vanityfair.com/news/2022/03/the-virus-hunting-nonprofit-at-the-center-of-the-lab-leak-controversy.

31. Ebright, "Written Testimony of Richard H. Ebright," 12–13.

32. Lawrence A. Tabak to Cathy McMorris Rodgers, May 21, 2021, "Tabak Letter to McMorris Rodgers on NIH Grants," *Washington Post*, May 25, 2021, https://www.washingtonpost.com/context/tabak-letter-to-mcmorris-rodgers-on-nih-grants/16cb2639-e9d7-4658-bce8-e944d899dda1/.

33. Zachary Stieber, "US Government Suspends Funding to Wuhan Laboratory over Risky Experiments," *Epoch Times*, July 19, 2023, https://www.theepochtimes.com/us-government-suspends-funding-to-wuhan-laboratory-over-risky-experiments_5408425.html; EcoHealth Alliance,

"EcoHealth Alliance Receives NIH Renewal Grant for Collaborative Research to Understand the Risk of Bat Coronavirus Spillover Emergence," news release, May 8, 2023, https://www.ecohealthalliance.org/2023/05/collaborative-research-to-understand-the-risk-of-bat-coronavirus-spillover-emergence; Josh Christenson, "US Taxpayers Funded $2M Worth of Research in Wuhan, Government Watchdog Reports," *New York Post*, June 14, 2023, https://nypost.com/2023/06/14/us-taxpayers-funded-2-million-for-research-in-wuhan-report/.

34. "Recommended Policy Guidance for Potential Pandemic Pathogen Care and Oversight," The White House, January 9, 2017, https://obamawhitehouse.archives.gov/blog/2017/01/09/recommended-policy-guidance-potential-pandemic-pathogen-care-and-oversight.

35. U.S. Department of Health and Human Services, "Framework for Guiding Funding Decisions about Proposed Research Involving Enhanced Potential Pandemic Pathogens," Administration for Strategic Preparedness and Response, 2017, https://www.phe.gov/s3/dualuse/Documents/p3co.pdf.

36. Ebright, "Written Testimony of Richard H. Ebright," 7.

37. Ibid., 12.

38. Ibid., 13.

39. Ibid.

40. Ibid.

41. Ibid., 7–8.

Chapter 21

1. Steven Quay, "Written Remarks to Accompany the Testimony of Steven Quay, MD, PhD," U.S. Senate Committee on Homeland Security and Governmental Affairs, August 3, 2022, page 1, https://www.hsgac.senate.gov/wp-content/uploads/imo/media/doc/Quay%20Testimony.pdf.

2. Ibid.

3. Jim Jordan, "What Did Fauci Know and When? His Emails Point to Panic, Lies, and a Possible Cover-Up," The Federalist, July 14, 2021, https://thefederalist.com/2021/07/14/dr-faucis-emails-tell-the-story-of-panic-lies-and-a-possible-cover-up/.

4. Senate HELP Committee Minority Oversight Staff, "Senate HELP Committee Minority Oversight Staff Releases Interim Report Analyzing Origins of COVID-19 Pandemic: The U.S. Senate Committee on Health,

Education, Labor and Pensions," news release, October 27, 2022, https://
www.help.senate.gov/ranking/newsroom/press/senate-help-committee
-minority-oversight-staff-releases-interim-report-analyzing-origins-of-covid
-19-pandemic.

5. Richard Ebright, "Written Testimony of Richard H. Ebright," U.S. Senate
Committee on Homeland Security and Governmental Affairs, August 3,
2022, page 11, https://www.hsgac.senate.gov/wp-content/uploads/imo/
media/doc/Ebright%20Testimony%20Updated.pdf.

6. Ibid.

7. Ibid., 11–12.

8. Quay, "Written Remarks to Accompany the Testimony of Steven Quay,
MD, PhD," 1.

9. Ibid., 1–2.

10. Ibid., 2.

11. Ibid.

12. Ibid.

13. Claire Klobucista, "Will the World Ever Solve the Mystery of COVID-19's
Origin?," Council on Foreign Relations, November 3, 2021, https://www.
cfr.org/backgrounder/will-world-ever-solve-mystery-covid-19s-origin;
Aylin Woodward, "The Chinese CDC Now Says the Coronavirus Didn't
Jump to People at the Wuhan Wet Market—Instead, It Was the Site of a
Superspreader Event," Insider, May 28, 2020, https://www.businessinsider.
com/coronavirus-did-not-jump-wuhan-market-chinese-cdc-says-2020-5.

14. Quay, "Written Remarks to Accompany the Testimony of Steven Quay,
MD, PhD," 2.

15. Ibid.

16. Elaine Dewar, *On the Origin of the Deadliest Pandemic in 100 Years: An
Investigation* (Windsor, Ontario: Biblioasis, 2021), 364.

17. Ibid., 360.

18. Quay, "Written Remarks to Accompany the Testimony of Steven Quay,
MD, PhD," 3.

19. Ibid.

20. Ibid.

21. Ibid.

22. Katherine Eban, "In Major Shift, NIH Admits Funding Risky Virus Research in Wuhan," *Vanity Fair*, October 22, 2021, https://www.vanityfair.com/news/2021/10/nih-admits-funding-risky-virus-research-in-wuhan.

23. Quay, "Written Remarks to Accompany the Testimony of Steven Quay, MD, PhD," 3.

24. Ibid.

25. Ibid.

26. "Open Reading Frame," National Human Genome Research Institute, accessed April 18, 2023, https://www.genome.gov/genetics-glossary/Open-Reading-Frame.

27. Quay, "Written Remarks to Accompany the Testimony of Steven Quay, MD, PhD," 4.

28. Ibid.

29. Yiwen Zang et al., "The ORF8 Protein of SARS-CoV-2 Mediates Immune Evasion through Down-Regulating MHC-I," *Proceedings of the National Academy of Sciences of the United States of America* 118, no. 23 (2021): e2024202118, https://www.pnas.org/doi/10.1073/pnas.2024202118.

30. Xiaosheng Wu et al., "Secreted ORF8 Is a Pathogenic Cause of Severe COVID-19 and Potentially Targetable with Select NLRP3 Inhibitors," bioRxiv, December 3, 2021, https://www.biorxiv.org/content/10.1101/2021.12.02.470978v1.

31. Quay, "Written Remarks to Accompany the Testimony of Steven Quay, MD, PhD," 4.

32. Brackets original. Eban, "In Major Shift, NIH Admits Funding Risky Virus Research in Wuhan."

33. Quay, "Written Remarks to Accompany the Testimony of Steven Quay, MD, PhD," 4–5.

34. Ibid., 6.

Chapter 22

1. Rand Paul (@RandPaul), "Fauci's resignation will not prevent a full-throated investigation into the origins of the pandemic….," Twitter, August 22, 2022, 12:45 p.m., https://twitter.com/RandPaul/status/1561751391332438020.

2. Kevin M. Esvelt, "Credible Pandemic Virus Identification Will Trigger the Immediate Proliferation of Agents as Lethal as Nuclear Devices: Testimony of Professor Kevin M. Esvelt, Massachusetts Institute of Technology,"

Senate Homeland Security and Governmental Affairs Committee, August 3, 2022, page 16, https://www.hsgac.senate.gov/wp-content/uploads/imo/media/doc/Esvelt%20Testimony.pdf.

3. Ibid., 8.

4. Ibid.

5. Ibid., 8–9.

6. Ibid., 9.

7. Ibid., 4.

8. International Gene Synthesis Consortium, 2023, https://genesynthesisconsortium.org/.

9. Esvelt, "Credible Pandemic Virus Identification," 4.

10. Ibid., 4–5.

11. "Synthetic DNA Makers Alerted to Bioterrorism Threats," Homeland Security News Wire, October 22, 2010, https://www.homelandsecurity newswire.com/synthetic-dna-makers-alerted-bioterrorism-threats.

12. Elaine Dewar, *On the Origin of the Deadliest Pandemic in 100 Years: An Investigation* (Windsor, Ontario: Biblioasis, 2021), 230.

13. Esvelt, "Credible Pandemic Virus Identification," 16.

14. Kelsey Piper, "Can We Stop the Next Pandemic by Seeking Out Deadly Viruses in the Wild?," *Vox*, May 7, 2022, https://www.vox.com/future -perfect/2022/5/7/22973296/virus-hunting-discovery-deep-vzn-global -virome-project.

15. Ibid.

16. Esvelt, "Credible Pandemic Virus Identification," 16.

17. Ibid., 6.

18. Ibid., 7, citing Edward C. Holmes, Andrew Rambaut, and Kristian G. Andersen, "Pandemics: Spend on Surveillance, Not Prediction," *Nature* 558, no. 7709 (2018): 180–82, https://pubmed.ncbi.nlm.nih.gov/29880819/.

19. Esvelt, "Credible Pandemic Virus Identification," 7.

20. Sharri Markson, *What Really Happened in Wuhan: The Cover-Ups, the Conspiracies and the Classified Research* (Sydney, Australia: HarperCollins, 2021), 207.

21. Esvelt, "Credible Pandemic Virus Identification," 7.

22. Ibid.

23. Ibid., 8.

Chapter 23

1. Ellipsis Pandolfo's. Chris Pandolfo, "Omnibus Bill Defunds Risky Research Involving 'Pathogens of Pandemic Potential' in Any 'Country of Concern,'" Fox News, December 23, 2022, https://www.foxnews.com/politics/omnibus -bill-defunds-risky-research-involving-pathogens-pandemic-potential -country-concern.

2. Personal conversation with Robert Kadlec.

3. Richard Ebright, "Written Testimony of Richard H. Ebright," U.S. Senate Committee on Homeland Security and Governmental Affairs, August 3, 2022, page 3, https://www.hsgac.senate.gov/wp-content/uploads/imo/ media/doc/Ebright%20Testimony%20Updated.pdf.

4. Barry R. Bloom et al., "Recommendations to Strengthen the US Government's Enhanced Potential Pandemic Pathogen Framework and Dual Use Research of Concern Policies," Center for Health Security, June 29, 2022, page 3, https://centerforhealthsecurity.org/sites/default/files/2023- 02/220629-recstostrengthenusgepppanddurcpolicies.pdf.

5. "From the Starr Referral: Clinton's Grand Jury Testimony, Part 4," *Washington Post*, 1998, https://www.washingtonpost.com/wp-srv/politics /special/clinton/stories/bctesto92198_4.htm.

6. Bloom et al., "Recommendations to Strengthen the US Government's Enhanced Potential Pandemic Pathogen Framework," 2.

7. Ibid.

8. Gabe Kaminsky, "Top Virologists Who Changed Tune on COVID-19 Lab Leak Theory Received Millions in NIH Grants," *Washington Examiner*, March 2, 2023, https://www.washingtonexaminer.com/policy/healthcare /covid-lab-leak-virologist-changed-tune-fauci-funding.

9. Bloom et al., "Recommendations to Strengthen the US Government's Enhanced Potential Pandemic Pathogen Framework," 5.

10. Rand Paul, "S.1973—BASIC Research Act: 115th Congress (2017–2018): Text," Congress.gov, October 17, 2017, https://www.congress.gov/bill/115th -congress/senate-bill/1973/text.

11. Audrey Conklin, "NIH Spent $2.3M Injecting Dogs with Cocaine in Experiment Related to Overdose Research: Report," Fox News, February 2, 2022, https://www.foxnews.com/us/nih-spent-millions-dogs-cocaine; Emma Parry, "Cocaine and Steroid-Fueled Hamster Cage Fights Slammed by Animal Rights Group," *New York Post*, October 26, 2017, https://nypost .com/2017/10/26/cocaine-and-steroid-fueled-hamster-cage-fights-slammed -by-animal-rights-group/.

12. Peter Kasperowicz, "Feds Blow $700K to Find Out What REALLY Happened on the Moon," *Washington Examiner*, October 5, 2016, https://www.washingtonexaminer.com/feds-blow-700k-to-find-out-what-really-happened-on-the-moon.

13. "Senator Rand Paul Introduces Bill to Reform the Federal Grant Review Process," American Geosciences Institute, October 18, 2017, https://www.americangeosciences.org/policy/news-briefs/senator-rand-paul-introduces-bill-to-reform-the-federal-grant-review-process.

14. Rand Paul (@randpaul), "The NSF spent $500,000 on a grant for UC Irvine to research if taking selfies improves happiness and relaxation....," Twitter, May 25, 2021, 12:11 p.m., https://twitter.com/RandPaul/status/1397223864720048141.

15. Rand Paul, *The Festivus Report 2019* (Bowling Green, Kentucky: Rand Paul, 2019), 7–8, https://www.paul.senate.gov/wp-content/uploads/2023/02/Festivus2019WasteReport.pdf.

16. Rand Paul, *2018 Festivus Report* (Bowling Green, Kentucky: Rand Paul, 2018), 7–8, https://www.scribd.com/document/396160193/Chairman-Paul-s-2018-Festivus-Report#from_embed.

17. Julia Barron, "Feds Funded Study Proving Thanos Couldn't Snap His Fingers While Wearing Infinity Gauntlet," ABC 15 News, December 27, 2022, https://wpde.com/news/nation-world/feds-funded-study-proving-thanos-couldnt-snap-his-fingers-while-wearing-infinity-gauntlet.

18. Office of Senator Roger Marshall, "Sen. Marshall Demands NSF and NIH Stop EcoHealth Alliance Grant Funding," news release, October 12, 2022, https://www.marshall.senate.gov/newsroom/press-releases/sen-marshall-demands-nsf-and-nih-stop-ecohealth-alliance-grant-funding/; Jay Landers, "Chips and Science Act Authorizes Billions of Dollars for R&D," American Society of Civil Engineers, August 25, 2022, https://www.asce.org/publications-and-news/civil-engineering-source/civil-engineering-magazine/article/2022/08/chips-and-science-act-authorizes-billions-of-dollars-for-rd.

19. Adam Andrzejewski, "U.S. Senator William Proxmire's Golden Fleece Award Turns 46 Years Old," *Forbes*, June 30, 2021, https://www.forbes.com/sites/adamandrzejewski/2021/06/30/us-senator-william-proxmires-golden-fleece-award-turns-46-years-old/?sh=60df2334283a.

20. Ebright, "Written Testimony of Richard H. Ebright," 10.

21. Steven Quay, "Written Remarks to Accompany the Testimony of Steven Quay, MD, PhD," U.S. Senate Committee on Homeland Security and

Governmental Affairs, August 3, 2022, page 6, https://www.hsgac.senate
.gov/wp-content/uploads/imo/media/doc/Quay%20Testimony.pdf.

22. Ebright, "Written Testimony of Richard H. Ebright," 10.

23. Kevin M. Esvelt, "Credible Pandemic Virus Identification Will Trigger the Immediate Proliferation of Agents as Lethal as Nuclear Devices: Testimony of Professor Kevin M. Esvelt, Massachusetts Institute of Technology," U.S. Senate Homeland Security and Governmental Affairs Committee, August 3, 2022, page 11, https://www.hsgac.senate.gov/wp-content/uploads/imo/media/doc/Esvelt%20Testimony.pdf.

24. Bloom et al., "Recommendations to Strengthen the US Government's Enhanced Potential Pandemic Pathogen Framework," 7.

25. Quay, "Written Remarks to Accompany the Testimony of Steven Quay, MD, PhD," 5–6.

26. Ebright, "Written Testimony of Richard H. Ebright," 10.

27. Esvelt, "Credible Pandemic Virus Identification," 13.

28. Ibid.

29. Bloom et al., "Recommendations to Strengthen the US Government's Enhanced Potential Pandemic Pathogen Framework."

30. Esvelt, "Credible Pandemic Virus Identification," 13.

31. Ibid., 10–11; Quay, "Written Remarks to Accompany the Testimony of Steven Quay, MD, PhD," 6.

32. Esvelt, "Credible Pandemic Virus Identification," 10.

33. Ibid., 9–10.

34. Ibid., 12.

35. Ibid.

36. Ibid.

37. Marko Ateensuu, "Synthetic Biology, Genome Editing, and the Risk of Bioterrorism," *Science and Engineering Ethics* 23, no. 6 (2017): 1541, https://link.springer.com/content/pdf/10.1007/s11948-016-9868-9.pdf.

38. Esvelt, "Credible Pandemic Virus Identification," 13.

39. Ibid., 15.

40. Ryan Cross, "Synthetic Biology Could Enable Bioweapons Development," *Chemical and Engineering News*, June 19, 2018, https://cen.acs.org/biological-chemistry/synthetic-biology/Synthetic-biology-enable-bioweapons-development/96/i26.

41. Ibid.
42. Ibid.
43. Esvelt, "Credible Pandemic Virus Identification," 14.
44. United Press International, "$135 Million Voted by Senate to Fund Flu Immunization," *New York Times*, April 10, 1976, https://www.nytimes.com/1976/04/10/archives/135-million-voted-by-senate-to-fund-flu-immunization.html.
45. Shari Roan, "Swine Flu 'Debacle' of 1976 Is Recalled," *Los Angeles Times*, April 27, 2009, https://www.latimes.com/archives/la-xpm-2009-apr-27-sci-swine-history27-story.html.
46. Victor Cohn, "U.S. Agrees to Pay Those Paralyzed by Swine Flu Shots," *Washington Post*, June 21, 1978, https://www.washingtonpost.com/archive/politics/1978/06/21/us-agrees-to-pay-those-paralyzed-by-swine-flu-shots/26c65a54-e3c9-4e4c-a23f-b8a411b563b3/.
47. K. C. Conway, "Pandemic Insurance," Alabama Real Estate Journal, May 1, 2020, https://acre.culverhouse.ua.edu/2020/05/01/pandemic-insurance/.
48. Rand Paul, "COVID-19 Gain-of-Function Research Too Dangerous for Fauci to Work With China," Fox News, August 15, 2022, https://www.foxnews.com/opinion/covid-gain-function-research-dangerous-fauci-china.
49. Ebright, "Written Testimony of Richard H. Ebright," 3.
50. Paul, "COVID-19 Gain-of-Function Research."
51. Ellipsis original. Ibid.
52. Ibid.

Chapter 24

1. Adam Cancryn and Krista Mahr, "Biden Declared the Pandemic 'Over.' His Covid Team Says It's More Complicated," *Politico*, September 19, 2022, https://www.politico.com/news/2022/09/19/biden-pandemic-over-covid-team-response-00057649.
2. Josh Marcus, "Biden Blames Pollution in Delaware for Him and Others Getting Cancer: The White House Says That President Has Had Several Non-Melanoma Skin Cancers Removed," *The Independent*, July 21, 2022, https://www.independent.co.uk/news/world/americas/us-politics/biden-delaware-cancer-pollution-b2127918.html; Steven Nelson, "Biden Tells US Troops They'll Be in Ukraine in War Gaffe," *New York Post*, March 25,

2022, https://nypost.com/2022/03/25/joe-biden-says-us-troops-will-be-in
-ukraine-in-apparent-gaffe/.

3. Xavier Becerra, "Renewal of Determination That a Public Health
   Emergency Exists," U.S. Department of Health & Human Services, October
   13, 2022, https://aspr.hhs.gov/legal/PHE/Pages/covid19-13Oct2022.aspx.

4. Betsy Klein and Tami Luhby, "Biden Administration Renews COVID-19
   Public Health Emergency," CNN, January 11, 2023, https://www.cnn.com
   /2023/01/11/politics/covid-19-public-health-emergency/.

5. Joseph Patrick, "And Just like That, CNN's COVID-19 'Death Counter'
   Suddenly Disappears," Law Enforcement Today, January 24, 2021, https://
   www.lawenforcementtoday.com/and-just-like-that-cnns-covid-19-death
   -counter-suddenly-disappears/.

6. Katy Stech Ferek, "Senate Votes to End Covid-19 Emergency Declaration,"
   Wall Street Journal, November 16, 2022, https://www.wsj.com/articles/
   senate-votes-to-end-covid-19-emergency-declaration-11668559887.

7. Office of Senator Robert Marshall, "Sen. Marshall Resolution Puts an End
   to COVID State of Emergency," press release, February 15, 2022, https://
   www.marshall.senate.gov/newsroom/press-releases/sen-marshall-resolution
   -puts-an-end-to-covid-state-of-emergency/; National Emergencies Act, 50
   U.S.C. § 202 (1976), https://www.govinfo.gov/content/pkg/HMAN-112/
   pdf/HMAN-112-pg1119.pdf.

8. Office of Senator Robert Marshall, "Sen. Marshall Resolution."

9. Jessica Gresko, "Supreme Court: Trump Can Use Pentagon Funds for
   Border Wall," Associated Press, July 27, 2019, https://apnews.com/article/
   mexico-donald-trump-ap-top-news-courts-supreme-courts-5d893d388c2
   54c7fa83a1570112ae90e.

10. "ArtI.S9.C2.1 Suspension Clause and Writ of Habeas Corpus," in
    *Constitution Annotated: Analysis and Interpretation of the U.S.
    Constitution*, n.d., https://constitution.congress.gov/browse/essay/
    artI-S9-C2-1/ALDE_00001087/.

11. Aaron Kheriaty, *The New Abnormal: The Rise of the Biomedical Security
    State* (Washington, D.C.: Regnery Publishing, 2022), 13.

12. Office of Senator Rand Paul, "Sens. Paul and Wyden Reintroduce the
    REPUBLIC Act to Rein Presidential National Emergency Powers," press
    release, February 26, 2021, https://www.paul.senate.gov/news-sens-paul-and
    -wyden-reintroduce-republic-act-rein-presidential-national-emergency-powers/.

13. Ferek, "Senate Votes to End Covid-19 Emergency Declaration."

14. Mary Ellen McIntire and Niels Lesniewski, "Senate Votes to Overturn COVID-19 National Emergency Order," Roll Call, March 29, 2023, https://rollcall.com/2023/03/29/senate-votes-to-overturn-covid-19-national -emergency-order/.

15. Jonathan Turley, "Pelosi Now Claims That She Was Misled by CIA," Jonathan Turley, May 14, 2009, https://jonathanturley.org/2009/05/14/ pelosi-now-claims-that-she-was-misled-by-cia/; Pam Benson, Kristi Keck, and Deirdre Walsh, "Hoyer Looks to Change Torture Talk Back to 'What Was Done,'" CNN, May 15, 2009, https://www.cnn.com/2009/ POLITICS/05/14/pelosi.waterboarding/index.html.

16. U.S. House of Representatives Permanent Select Committee on Intelligence: Minority, *Unclassified Summary of the Second Interim Report on the Origins of the COVID-19 Pandemic* (Washington, D.C.: U.S. House of Representatives Permanent Select Committee on Intelligence: Minority, 2022), https://intelligence.house.gov/uploadedfiles/final_unclass_summary _-_covid_origins_report_.pdf.

17. Ibid.

18. Andrew Court, "Chinese Scientist 'Filed Patent for a COVID Vaccine before the Virus Was Declared a Global Pandemic and Worked Closely with 'Bat Woman' at Wuhan Institute,'" *Daily Mail*, June 6, 2021, https:// www.dailymail.co.uk/news/article-9658235/Chinese-scientist-filed-patent -COVID-vaccine-virus-declared-global-pandemic.html; "DEAD MEN DON'T TALK: Fauci's NIH Funded Wuhan Military Scientist Who Died Mysteriously after Filing COVID Vaccine Patent," RIELPOLITIK, June 6, 2021, https://rielpolitik.com/2021/06/06/dead-men-dont-talk-faucis-nih -funded-wuhan-military-scientist-who-died-mysteriously-after-filing-covid -vaccine-patent/; Glen Owen, "Did Vaccine Scientist 'Thrown to His Death' Have Proof of Wuhan Lab Leak? Chinese Military Expert Who Filed Patent for Covid Vaccine Barely a Month into Country's First Lockdown Died in Mysterious Circumstances Aged Just 54," *Daily Mail*, June 17, 2023, https://www.dailymail.co.uk/news/article-12205705/Chinese-military- expert-filed-patent-Covid-vaccine-died-mysterious-circumstances.html.

19. Katherine Eban and Jeff Kao, "COVID-19 Origins: Investigating a 'Complex and Grave Situation' inside a Wuhan Lab," *Vanity Fair*, October 28, 2022, https://www.vanityfair.com/news/2022/10/covid-origins-investigation -wuhan-lab.

20. Xi Jin Pig (@KoronaKitaya), "Yusen Zhou's wife, Lanying Du, from Beijing Institute of Microbiology (Academy of Military Medical Science), then worked at @NYBloodCenter," Twitter, October 29, 2022, 9:58 a.m., https://twitter.com/KoronaKitaya/status/1586356915579195392; Sheila (@capitolsheila), "Looks like She was working on SARS1, MERS, spike & vax pre-pandemic & got NIH money when she was at NY Blood Center.... ," Twitter, 8:43 a.m., https://twitter.com/KoronaKitaya/status /1586356915579195392.

21. Lanying Du, interview with Rand Paul's staff.

22. "Peter Hotez, MD, PhD, on His 10 Years of Work on Coronavirus," American Medical Association, February 15, 2021, https://www.ama-assn .org/delivering-care/public-health/peter-hotez-md-phd-his-10-years-work -coronavirus.

23. Emily Kopp, "Vaccine Industry Insider Peter Hotez Helped Fund Wuhan Gain-of-Function Study," The Defender, August 10, 2022, https:// childrenshealthdefense.org/defender/vaccine-industry-peter-hotez-funded -wuhan-gain-of-function-study/.

24. Ibid.

25. Emily DeCiccio, "Dr. Peter Hotez Backs Fauci in His Showdown with Sen. Paul over Masks," CNBC, March 18, 2021, https://www.cnbc.com/2021 /03/18/dr-peter-hotez-backs-fauci-in-his-showdown-with-sen-paul-over -masks.html.

26. Benedette Cuffari, "The Size of SARS-CoV-2 and Its Implications," News Medical Life Sciences, February 15, 2021, https://www.news-medical.net/ health/The-Size-of-SARS-CoV-2-Compared-to-Other-Things.aspx; Bhanu Bhakta Neupane et al., "Optical Microscope Study of Surface Morphology and Filtering Efficiency of Face Masks," PeerJ 7 (2019): e7142, https://www .ncbi.nlm.nih.gov/pmc/articles/PMC6599448/pdf/peerj-07-7142.pdf.

27. U.S. House of Representatives Permanent Select Committee on Intelligence: Minority, *Unclassified Summary*, 14.

28. Ibid., 14.

Chapter 25

1. Karson Yiu, "How a Deadly Apartment Fire Fueled Anti-Zero-COVID Protests across China: ANALYSIS," ABC News, November 27, 2022, https://abcnews.go.com/International/deadly-apartment-fire-fueled-anti- zero-covid-protests/story?id=94045207.

2. Wikipedia, s.v., "*Songbie*," February 20, 2023, https://en.wikipedia.org/wiki /Songbie.

3. Thomas Peter, "In China, Young Women Become Accidental Symbols of Defiance," *Wall Street Journal*, January 25, 2023, https://www.wsj.com/ articles/in-china-young-women-become-accidental-symbols-of-defiance -11674667983.

4. Samuel Osborne, "COVID-19: Australian Riot Police Fire Rubber Bullets at Anti-Lockdown Protesters in Melbourne," Sky News, September 22, 2021, https://news.sky.com/story/covid-19-australian-riot-police-fire-rubber -bullets-at-anti-lockdown-protesters-in-melbourne-12414439.

5. "Inside Australia's Covid Interment Camp," UnHeard, December 2, 2021, https://unherd.com/thepost/inside-australias-covid-internment-camp/.

6. Chantal Da Silva and Associated Press, "Police in the Netherlands Open Fire on Covid Lockdown Protesters as European Nations Reintroduce Restrictions," NBC News, November 20, 2021, https://www.nbcnews. com/news/world/police-netherlands-open-fire-covid-lockdown-protesters -european-nation-rcna6231.

7. Jon Miltimore, "Good Riddance to Jacinda Ardern, New Zealand's Authoritarian in Chief," *Washington Examiner*, January 23, 2023, https:// www.washingtonexaminer.com/opinion/good-riddance-to-jacinda-ardern -new-zealands-authoritarian-in-chief.

8. "Trudeau Vows to Freeze Anti-Mandate Protesters' Bank Accounts," BBC, February 15, 2022, https://www.bbc.com/news/world-us-canada-60383385.

9. Democracy Now!, "'We Can't Trust the Unvaccinated': Dr. Leana Wen on Vaccine Mandates & How to Stop the Delta Variant," YouTube, July 29, 2021, at 4:44, https://www.youtube.com/watch?v=bvtKq79oUX8.

10. Robby Soave, "CNN's Leana Wen: The Unvaccinated Should Not Be Allowed to Leave Their Homes," *Reason*, September 10, 2021, https:// reason.com/2021/09/10/cnn-leana-wen-unvaccinated-travel-outdoor-ban/.

11. Ny Magge, "Don Lemon Argues It's Time to 'Shun' Anti-Vaxxers," Yahoo! News, September 16, 2021, https://news.yahoo.com/don-lemon-argues-time -shun-233600544.html.

12. Ryan Parker, "Howard Stern Says Anti-Vaxxers Should Be Denied Hospital Care Once Infected," *Hollywood Reporter*, September 9, 2021, https:// www.hollywoodreporter.com/news/general-news/howard-stern-covid-anti -vaxxers-denied-care-1235010383/.

13. Ed Mazza, "'You're a Schmuck!': Arnold Schwarzenegger Unloads on Anti-Maskers, Anti-Vaxxers," HuffPost, August 12, 2021, https://www.huffpost.com/entry/arnold-schwarzenegger-mask-mandates_n_6114b90 l5e4b0454ed70a2456.

14. Joseph Biden, "Remarks by President Biden on Fighting the COVID-19 Pandemic," The White House, September 9, 2021, https://www.whitehouse.gov/briefing-room/speeches-remarks/2021/09/09/remarks-by-president-biden-on-fighting-the-covid-19-pandemic-3/.

15. Joe Sonka, "Judge, Quoting from Host of Historical Figures, Argues Andy Beshear Edicts Unconstitutional," *Courier-Journal*, July 21, 2020, https://www.courier-journal.com/story/news/politics/2020/07/21/covid-19-kentucky-judge-argues-andy-beshear-orders-unconstitutional/3287953001/.

16. Christina Carrega, "Kentucky Governor Asks Churches to Close on Easter; Judge Overrules Louisville Mayor's Order to Stop Drive-In Service," ABC News, April 11, 2020, https://abcnews.go.com/US/kentucky-governor-warns-worshipers-congregate-easter-weekend/story?id=70101091.

17. Ibid.

Chapter 26

1. Laura Powell (@LauraPowellEsq), "'We knew about [Infection-Acquired Immunity] since 430 BC... ," Twitter, March 19, 2023, 9:41 p.m., https://twitter.com/LauraPowellEsq/status/1637267941648646145.

2. Matt Taibbi (@mtaibbi), "1.TWITTER FILES #19 The Great Covid-19 Lie Machine..." (thread), Twitter, March 17, 2023, 10:00 a.m., https://twitter.com/mtaibbi/status/1636729166631432195; Michael Shellenberger (@shellenberger), "1. TWITTER FILES: PART 7...," Twitter, December 19, 2022, 11:09 a.m., https://twitter.com/shellenberger/status/1604871630613753856.

3. Taibbi (@mtaibbi), "1.TWITTER FILES #19."

4. Heather Hamilton, "Rand Paul Says He's Confirmed Fauci Has Government-Funded Security Detail amid Alleged Retirement," *Washington Examiner*, July 18, 2023, https://www.washingtonexaminer.com/news/rand-paul-fauci-government-funded-security-detail-retirement.

5. Jack Birle, "Anthony Fauci Charging up to $100k for Speaking Engagements," *Washington Examiner*, February 6, 2023, https://www.washingtonexaminer.com/news/anthony-fauci-charging-100k-for-speaking-engagements.

6. Joseph Murphy, Unclassified DARPA Documents, August 13, 2021, https://
assets.ctfassets.net/syq3snmxclc9/2mVob3c1aDd8CNvVnyei6n/95af7dbfd2
958d4c2b8494048b4889b5/JAG_Docs_pt1_Og_WATERMARK_OVER
_Redacted.pdf.

7. U.S. Department of State, "Fact Sheet: Activity at the Wuhan Institute of
Virology," U.S. Department of State, January 15, 2021, https://2017-2021
.state.gov/fact-sheet-activity-at-the-wuhan-institute-of-virology/index.html.

8. Josh Rogin, "Opinion | State Department Cables Warned of Safety Issues at
Wuhan Lab Studying Bat Coronaviruses," *Washington Post*, April 14, 2020,
https://www.washingtonpost.com/opinions/2020/04/14/state-department
-cables-warned-safety-issues-wuhan-lab-studying-bat-coronaviruses/.

9. "Evaluating U.S.-China Policy in the Era of Strategic Competition," U.S.
Senate Committee on Foreign Relations, February 9, 2023, at 1:39:20,
https://www.foreign.senate.gov/hearings/evaluating-us-china-policy-in-
the-era-of-strategic-competition. Transcript lightly edited to improve
readability. Brackets indicate slight rewording for written clarity throughout.

10. Michael R. Gordon and Warren P. Strobel, "Lab Leak Most Likely Origin
of Covid-19 Pandemic, Energy Department Now Says," *Wall Street Journal*,
February 26, 2023, https://www.wsj.com/articles/covid-origin-china-lab
-leak-807b7b0a.

11. Ibid.; Jared Gans, "FBI Director Says Origin of COVID-19 Pandemic 'Most
Likely' a Lab 'Incident' in Wuhan," *The Hill*, February 28, 2023, https://
Thehill.Com/Policy/National-security/3878243-fbi-director-says-origin-of
-covid-19-pandemic-most-likely-a-lab-incident-in-wuhan/.

12. Michael R. Gordon and Warren P. Strobel, "U.S. Report Found It Plausible
Covid-19 Leaked from Wuhan Lab," *Wall Street Journal*, June 8, 2021,
https://www.wsj.com/articles/u-s-report-concluded-covid-19-may-have
-leaked-from-wuhan-lab-11623106982.

13. Michael Collins and Josh Meyer, "What's the 'Z Division'? A Secret
Team of Scientists Searches for Answers on COVID-19's Origins,"
USA Today, March 1, 2023, https://www.usatoday.com/story/news/
politics/2023/03/01/z-division-secret-team-scientists-investigated-covid-19-
origins/11364009002/.

14. From conversations between DTRA officials, available via Gary Ruskin,
"FOI Documents on Origins of Covid-19, Gain-of-Function Research and
Biolabs," U.S. Right to Know, April 28, 2023, https://usrtk.org/covid-19

-origins/foi-documents-on-origins-of-sars-cov-2-risks-of-gain-of-function
-research-and-biosafety-labs/.

15. Ibid.
16. Ibid.
17. Ibid.
18. Ibid.
19. Ibid.
20. Ibid.
21. Emily Kopp, "Timeline: The Proximal Origin of SARS-CoV-2," U.S. Right
to Know, April 11, 2023, https://usrtk.org/covid-19-origins/timeline-the
-proximal-origin-of-sars-cov-2/; Select Subcommittee on the Coronavirus
Pandemic Majority Staff, "Memorandum," U.S. House Committee on
Oversight and Accountability, March 5, 2023, https://oversight.house.gov/
wp-content/uploads/2023/03/2023.03.05-SSCP-Memo-Re.-New-Evidence
.Proximal-Origin.pdf; Miranda Devine, "New Emails Show Dr. Anthony
Fauci Commissioned Scientific Paper in Feb. 2020 to Disprove Wuhan Lab
Leak Theory," *New York Post*, March 5, 2023, https://nypost.com/2023
/03/05/new-emails-show-fauci-commissioned-paper-to-disprove-wuhan-lab
-leak-theory/.
22. "George Carlin on Conspiracies," Films for Action, May 22, 2014, https://
usrtk.org/covid-19-origins/foi-documents-on-origins-of-sars-cov-2-risks-of
-gain-of-function-research-and-biosafety-labs/.

Chapter 27
1. Michael R.Gordon and Warren P. Strobel, "Lab Leak Most Likely Origin
of Covid-19 Pandemic, Energy Department Now Says," *Wall Street Journal*,
February 28, 2023, https://www.wsj.com/articles/covid-origin-china-lab-leak
-807b7b0a.
2. Ibid.
3. Jared Gans, "FBI Director Says Origin of COVID-19 Pandemic 'Most
Likely' a Lab 'Incident' in Wuhan," *The Hill*, February 28, 2023, https://
Thehill.Com/Policy/National-security/3878243-fbi-director-says-origin-of
-covid-19-pandemic-most-likely-a-lab-incident-in-wuhan/.
4. Ibid.
5. Alison Young, "How Did the Covid Pandemic Begin? We Need to
Investigate All Credible Hypotheses," *The Guardian*, March 2, 2023,

https://www.theguardian.com/commentisfree/2023/mar/02/covid-19-pandemic-origin-answers-political-feud.

6. "BREAKING: Elon Musk Accuses Fauci of Using Pass-Through Organization to Fund Gain-of-Function Research," Trending Politics, February 27, 2023, https://trendingpoliticsnews.com/elon-musk-accuses-fauci-of-funding-gain-of-function-research-in-wuhan-paub/.

7. Andrés R. Martínez, "Fauci Accuses Senator Paul of Fueling Threats against Him in the Latest Exchange," *New York Times*, January 11, 2022, https://www.nytimes.com/2022/01/11/us/politics/rand-paul-fauci-covid.html.

8. Bess Levin, "Anthony Fauci Once Again Forced to Basically Call Rand Paul a Sniveling Moron," *Vanity Fair*, July 21, 2021, https://www.vanityfair.com/news/2021/07/anthony-fauci-rand-paul-covid-19.

9. Katherine Eban, "In Major Shift, NIH Admits Funding Risky Virus Research in Wuhan," *Vanity Fair*, October 22, 2021, https://www.vanityfair.com/news/2021/10/nih-admits-funding-risky-virus-research-in-wuhan.

10. Teaganne Finn, "Fauci Says Sen. Paul's Attacks 'Kindle the Crazies' Who Have Threatened His Life," NBC News, January 11, 2022, https://www.nbcnews.com/politics/congress/fauci-says-sen-paul-s-attacks-kindle-crazies-who-have-n1287299.

11. "U.S. Sen. Rand Paul Driving Violent Threats against Me, Fauci Says," Reuters, January 11, 2022, https://www.reuters.com/world/us/us-sen-rand-paul-driving-violent-threats-against-me-fauci-says-2022-01-11/.

12. Martínez, "Fauci Accuses Senator Paul of Fueling Threats."

13. Ryan Bort, "Fauci Caught on Hot Mic Calling Republican Senator a 'Moron' after Heated Exchange," *Rolling Stone*, January 11, 2022, https://www.rollingstone.com/politics/politics-news/anthony-fauci-rand-paul-covid-fundraising-1282682/; see the original headline via the Internet Archive's Wayback Machine: https://web.archive.org/web/20220111183017/https://www.rollingstone.com/politics/politics-news/anthony-fauci-rand-paul-covid-fundraising-1282682/.

14. David Smith, "'If Anybody Is Lying Here, It Is You': Fauci Turns Tables on Inquisitor Rand Paul," *The Guardian*, July 20, 2021, https://www.theguardian.com/us-news/2021/jul/20/anthony-fauci-rand-paul-coronavirus-research.

15. John Nichols, "Rand Paul Abandons His Hippocratic Oath to Play Politics during a Pandemic," *The Nation*, January 19, 2022, https://www.thenation.com/article/politics/rand-paul-fauci/.

Notes

16. Bess Levin, "Anthony Fauci Basically Calls Rand Paul a Shameless Moron to His Face," *Vanity Fair*, September 23, 2020, https://www.vanityfair.com /news/2020/09/anthony-fauci-rand-paul-coronavirus.

17. Cortney O'Brien, "CNN's Brianna Keilar calls Rand Paul an 'A—' Again for Questioning Fauci," Fox News, May 11, 2021, https://www.foxnews .com/media/cnns-brianna-keilar-calls-rand-paul-ass-questioning-fauci.

18. Ian Hanchett, "CBS' King to Fauci: 'Does Your Body Tense Up' Dealing with Rand Paul?," Breitbart, May 14, 2021, https://www.breitbart.com/clips/2021 /05/14/cbs-king-to-fauci-does-your-body-tense-up-dealing-with-rand-paul/.

19. Glenn Kessler, "Fact-Checking the Paul-Fauci Flap over Wuhan Lab Funding," *Washington Post*, May 18, 2021, https://www.washingtonpost .com/politics/2021/05/18/fact-checking-senator-paul-dr-fauci-flap-over -wuhan-lab-funding/.

20. Glenn Kessler (@GlennKesslerWP), "New #FactChecker -> The incendiary claim that George Soros 'funds' Alvin Brag," Twitter, April 1, 2023, 8:38 a.m., https://twitter.com/GlennKesslerWP/status/1642144423956889600.

21. Christine Rosen, "Four Pinocchios for Glenn Kessler," American Enterprise Institute, April 17, 2023, https://www.aei.org/op-eds/four-pinocchios- for-glenn-kessler/.

22. Elon Musk (@elonmusk), "Only thing on fire are Kessler's pants," Twitter, April 1, 2023, 3:24 p.m., https://twitter.com/elonmusk/status /1642246593087774722?lang=en.

23. Bret Stephens, "The Mask Mandates Did Nothing. Will Any Lessons Be Learned?," *New York Times*, February 21, 2023, https://www.nytimes. com/2023/02/21/opinion/do-mask-mandates-work.html.

24. Ibid.

25. Zeynep Tufekci, "On Masks and Clinical Trials, Rand Paul's Tweeting Is Just Plain Wrong," *New York Times*, November 6, 2020, https://www .nytimes.com/2020/11/06/opinion/sunday/coronavirus-masks.html.

26. Stephens, "Mask Mandates Did Nothing."

27. Paul Krugman, "The Cult of Selfishness Is Killing America," *New York Times*, July 27, 2020, https://www.nytimes.com/2020/07/27/opinion/us -republicans-coronavirus.html.

28. Paul Krugman, "Paul Krugman: The Internet Was an Economic Disappointment," *Pittsburgh Post-Gazette*, April 7, 2023, https://www.post

-gazette.com/opinion/Op-Ed/2023/04/08/paul-krugman-ai-information
-technology-nyt/stories/202304080009.

Chapter 28

1. Bret Stephens, "The Mask Mandates Did Nothing. Will Any Lessons Be Learned?," *New York Times*, February 21, 2023, https://www.nytimes.com/2023/02/21/opinion/do-mask-mandates-work.html.

2. Ben Shapiro, "The Greatest Cover-Up in Human History," Creators Syndicate, March 1, 2023, https://www.creators.com/read/ben-shapiro/03/23/the-greatest-cover-up-in-human-history.

3. Ibid.

4. Ibid.

5. Ibid.

6. Lisa Mascaro, "House Votes to Declassify Info about Origins of COVID-19," Associated Press, March 10, 2023, https://apnews.com/article/covid-origins-china-wuhan-intelligence-7018f8016c7346cfaa8193933ec10063.

7. David Zweig, "Is Gain-of-Function Research a 'Risk Worth Taking'? or 'Insanity'?," The Free Press, March 7, 2023, http://www.thefp.com/p/is-gain-of-function-research-a-risk.

8. Personal conversation with Xu Xueyuan.

9. Betsy McCaughey, "Biden's WHO Pandemic Treaty Would Kill Americans in the Name of 'Equity,'" *New York Post*, March 1, 2023, https://nypost.com/2023/03/01/bidens-who-pandemic-treaty-would-kill-americans-in-for-equity/; U.S. Department of State, "Statement by Ambassador Pamela Hamamoto World Health Organization (WHO) Fourth Meeting of the Intergovernmental Negotiating Body (INB)," news release, February 27, 2023, https://www.state.gov/statement-by-ambassador-hamamoto-who-fourth-meeting-of-the-inb/.

10. Scott W. Atlas, "W.H.O. Do You Trust?," *Newsweek*, March 16, 2023, https://www.newsweek.com/who-do-you-trust-opinion-1787783.

11. Ibid.

12. Josh Rogin, "Opinion | State Department Cables Warned of Safety Issues at Wuhan Lab Studying Bat Coronaviruses," *Washington Post*, April 14, 2020, https://www.washingtonpost.com/opinions/2020/04/14/state-department-cables-warned-safety-issues-wuhan-lab-studying-bat-coronaviruses/.

13. Forbes Breaking News, "JUST IN: Rand Paul Directly Confronts Antony Blinken about COVID-19 Research Funding Records," YouTube, March 22, 2023, https://www.youtube.com/watch?v=7TKiRkmiIkk. Transcript lightly edited to improve readability. Brackets indicate slight rewording for written clarity throughout.

14. "Taxpayers Paid Billions for It: So Why Would Moderna Consider Quadrupling the Price of the COVID Vaccine?," U.S. Senate Committee on Health, Education, Labor and Pensions, March 22, 2023, at 46:05, https://www.help.senate.gov/hearings/taxpayers-paid-billions-for-it-so-why-would-moderna-consider-quadrupling-the-price-of-the-covid-vaccine. Transcript lightly edited to improve readability.

15. Ibid., at 46:58. Transcript lightly edited to improve readability.

16. Lael M. Yonker et al., "Circulating Spike Protein Detected in Post-COVID-19 MRNA Vaccine Myocarditis," *Circulation* 147, no. 11 (2023): 867–76, https://www.ahajournals.org/doi/10.1161/CIRCULATIONAHA.122.061025.

17. "Taxpayers Paid Billions for It," at 48:00. Transcript lightly edited to improve readability. Brackets indicate slight rewording for written clarity throughout.

18. Melissa Rudy, "Covid Vaccines Are Not Needed for Healthy Kids and Teens, Says World Health Organization," Fox News, March 30, 2023, https://www.foxnews.com/health/covid-vaccines-not-needed-healthy-kids-teens-world-health-organization.

19. "Taxpayers Paid Billions for It," at 50:58. Transcript lightly edited to improve readability. Brackets indicate slight rewording for written clarity throughout.

20. Nathaniel Weixel, "Senate Votes to End COVID-19 National Emergency," *The Hill*, March 29, 2023, https://thehill.com/policy/healthcare/3924782-senate-votes-to-end-covid-19-national-emergency/.

21. Christian Holm Hansen et al., "Vaccine Effectiveness against SARS-COV-2 Infection with the Omicron or Delta Variants Following a Two-Dose or Booster BNT162b2 or MRNA-1273 Vaccination Series: A Danish Cohort Study," medRxiv (2021), https://doi.org/10.1101/2021.12.20.21267966.

22. Nicole Saphier, "My Weekly Covid Tests Continue," *Wall Street Journal*, March 29, 2023, https://www.wsj.com/articles/my-weekly-covid-tests-continue-new-jersey-murphy-healthcare-mandate-mask-autoimmune-booster-spread-9fcfce3a.

23. Centers for Disease Control and Prevention, "Statement from CDC Director Rochelle P. Walensky, MD, MPH on Today's MMWR," news release, July 30, 2021, https://www.cdc.gov/media/releases/2021/s0730-mmwr-covid-19 .html; José R. Romero, "CDC Call to Action: Add Routine & COVID-19 Vaccinations to the Back-to-School Checklist," U.S. Department of Health and Human Services, n.d., https://www.cdc.gov/vaccines/hcp/clinical-resources/downloads/safe-return-school.pdf.

24. Jayanta Bhattacharya and Martin Kulldorff, "The Collins and Fauci Attack on Traditional Public Health," The Brownstone Institute, January 3, 2022, https://brownstone.org/articles/the-collins-and-fauci-attack-on-traditional -public-health.

25. Ginger Adams Otis, "NIH Should Strengthen Oversight of Foreign Funding Disclosure, Watchdog Says," *Wall Street Journal*, June 7, 2022, https:// www.wsj.com/articles/nih-should-strengthen-oversight-of-foreign-funding -disclosure-watchdog-says-11654571892.

26. Email correspondence from the FBI.

27. Michael Shellenberger, Matt Taibbi, and Alex Gutentag, "First People Sickened by COVID-19 Were Chinese Scientists at Wuhan Institute of Virology, Say US Government Sources," Public (Substack), June 13, 2023, https://public.substack.com/p/first-people-sickened-by-covid-19.

28. Ibid.

29. Personal conversation with Mark Warner.

30. Shellenberger, Taibbi, and Gutentag, "First People Sickened by COVID-19."

31. Ibid.

32. Select Subcommittee on the Coronavirus Pandemic (@COVIDSelect), "BREAKING: New emails reveal that Dr. Fauci was aware of risky gain-of-function research . . . ," Twitter, July 13, 2023, 5:39 p.m., https://twitter .com/COVIDSelect/status/1679606442414809090.

33. Francisco de Asis (@franciscodeasis), "[#REV0002906 on page 38 of pdf] . . . ," Twitter, July 12, 2023, 5:16 p.m., https://twitter.com/ franciscodeasis/status/1679238202744291329. See also, Francisco de Asis (@franciscodeasis), "Let's go on an Easter egg hunt inside the pdf..." (thread), Twitter, July 11, 2023, https://twitter.com/franciscodeasis/status /1678901425571606528.

34. David Zweig, "Anthony Fauci's Deceptions," The Free Press (Substack), August 7, 2023, https://www.thefp.com/p/anthony-faucis-deceptions.

35.	Ibid.

36.	Francisco de Asis (@franciscodeasis), "Page 19: Drosten here? . . . ," Twitter, July 11, 2023, 6:57 p.m., https://twitter.com/franciscodeasis/status/1678901434341810177/photo/3. See also, Francisco de Asis (@franciscodeasis), "Let's go on an Easter egg hunt inside the pdf . . ." (thread), Twitter, July 11, 2023, 6:57 p.m., https://twitter.com/franciscodeasis/status/1678901425571606528.

37.	Steven Salzberg, "Gain-of-Function Experiments at Boston University Create a Deadly New Covid-19 Virus. Who Thought This Was a Good Idea?," *Forbes*, October 24, 2022, https://www.forbes.com/sites/stevensalzberg/2022/10/24/gain-of-function-experiments-at-boston-university-create-a-deadly-new-covid-19-virus-who-thought-this-was-a-good-idea.

38.	Tim Hains, "RCP's Wegmann to John Kirby: 'Does the President Believe the Reward Outweighs the Risk on Gain-of-Function Research?,'" RealClearPolitics, February 27, 2023, https://www.realclearpolitics.com/video/2023/02/27/rcps_wegmann_to_john_kirby_does_the_president_believe_the_reward_outweighs_the_risk_on_gain-of-function_research.html.

Chapter 29: Conclusion

1.	Martin Kulldorff, "COVID-19 Counter Measures Should Be Age Specific," LinkedIn, April 10, 2020, https://www.linkedin.com/pulse/covid-19-counter-measures-should-age-specific-martin-kulldorff.

2.	Hannah Fry, "Paddle Boarder Chased by Boat, Arrested in Malibu after Flouting Coronavirus Closures," *Los Angeles Times*, April 3, 2020, https://www.latimes.com/california/story/2020-04-03/paddle-boarder-arrested-in-malibu-after-flouting-coronavirus-closures.

3.	Madison Dibble, "Gretchen Whitmer Criticized for Marching Shoulder to Shoulder with Protesters after Months of Social Distancing Orders," *Washington Examiner*, June 5, 2020, https://www.washingtonexaminer.com/news/gretchen-whitmer-criticized-for-marching-shoulder-to-shoulder-with-protesters-after-months-of-social-distancing-orders; Joshua Rhett Miller, "Bail Fund Backed by Kamala Harris Freed Minneapolis Man Charged with Murder," *New York Post*, September 9, 2021, https://nypost.com/2021/09/08/bail-fund-backed-by-kamala-harris-freed-man-charged-with-murder.

4.	Aaron Kheriaty, *The New Abnormal: The Rise of the Biomedical Security State* (Washington, D.C.: Regnery Publishing, 2022), 12.

5. Mackenzie Mays, "Newsom Sends His Children Back to Private School Classrooms in California," *Politico*, October 30, 2020, https://www.politico.com/states/california/story/2020/10/30/newsom-sends-his-children-back-to-school-classrooms-in-california-1332811.

6. Zachary Evans, "Teachers Union Head Taped Sending Child to In-Person Pre-School while Backing School Closures," Yahoo! News, March 1, 2021, https://news.yahoo.com/teachers-union-head-fights-keep-183132140.html; guerillaMomz (@GuerillaMomz), Meet Matt Meyers…," Twitter, February 27, 2021, 8:05 p.m., https://twitter.com/GuerillaMomz/status/1365830556366237702.

7. Justin Hart, "The Twitter Blacklisting of Jay Bhattacharya," *Wall Street Journal*, December 9, 2022, https://www.wsj.com/articles/the-twitter-blacklisting-of-jay-bhattacharya-medical-expert-covid-lockdown-stanford-doctor-shadow-banned-censorship-11670621083; Wesley J. Smith, "Dr. Jay Bhattacharya on the Need for a COVID Response Truth Commission," June 5, 2023, in *Humanize*, podcast, https://overcast.fm/+8rbv2aaEE.

8. Jay Bhattacharya (@DrJBhattacharya), "Gov. @GavinNewsom kept my kids out of their public schools for nearly a year and a half with no good scientific or epidemiological justification…," Twitter, February 19, 2023, 2:35 p.m., https://twitter.com/DrJBhattacharya/status/1627391566313672704.

9. Jeremy B. White, "Newsom Faces Backlash after Attending French Laundry Dinner Party," *Politico*, November 13, 2020, https://www.politico.com/states/california/story/2020/11/13/newsom-faces-backlash-after-attending-french-laundry-dinner-party-1336419.

10. "County Coroner Takes Inaccurate COVID Death Reporting to Governor," Grand Gazette, February 11, 2021, https://grandgazette.net/county-coroner-takes-inaccurate-covid-death-reporting-to-governor/; Andrea Maria Pezzulo et al., "Age-Stratified Infection Fatality Rate of Covid-19 in the Non-Elderly Population," *Environmental Research* 216, no. 3 (2023): 114655, https://www.ncbi.nlm.nih.gov/pmc/articles/PMC9613797/.

11. Aya Elamroussi, Holly Yan, and Amir Vera, "Canadian Authorities Freeze Financial Assets for Those Involved in Ongoing Protests in Ottawa," CNN, February 21, 2022, https://www.cnn.com/2022/02/20/americas/canada-trucker-protest-covid-sunday/index.html.

12. David Wallace-Wells, "Dr. Fauci Looks Back: 'Something Clearly Went Wrong,'" *New York Times*, April 25, 2023, https://www.nytimes.com/interactive/2023/04/24/magazine/dr-fauci-pandemic.html.

13. Alice Miranda Ollstein, "POLITICO-Harvard poll: Most Americans Believe Covid Leaked from Lab," *Politico*, July 9, 2021, https://www. politico.com/news/2021/07/09/poll-covid-wuhan-lab-leak-498847.

14. Casey Harper, "Poll: Majority Say Time Fauci Should Be Removed," The Center Square, January 24, 2022, https://www.thecentersquare.com/national/article_3fd24a10-7d2d-11ec-9661-8364adb79c16.html. An April 2020 poll by Quinnipiac placed Fauci's approval rating at 78 percent: "Fauci, Governors Get Highest Marks for Response to Coronavirus, Quinnipiac University National Poll Finds; Majority Say Trump's Response Not Aggressive Enough," Quinnipiac University Poll, April 8, 2020, https://poll.qu.edu/Poll-Release?releaseid=3753.

15. Harper, "Poll: Majority Say Time Fauci Should Be Removed."

16. Personal conversation.

17. Diana Glebova, "Fauci's Net Worth Nearly Doubled during Pandemic," *National Review*, September 30, 2022, https://www.nationalreview.com/news/faucis-net-worth-nearly-doubled-during-pandemic/.

18. C. S. Lewis, "A Quote from God in the Dock," Goodreads, 2023, https://www.goodreads.com/quotes/526469-of-all-tyrannies-a-tyranny-sincerely-exercised-for-the-good.

19. Khaleda Rahman, "CNN Mocked for Calling Kenosha Riots 'Fiery but Mostly Peaceful Protests,'" *Newsweek*, August 27, 2020, https://www.newsweek.com/cnn-mocked-calling-kenosha-riots-fiery-mostly-peaceful-protests-1527997.

20. Michael Brendan Dougherty, "Anthony Fauci: I Am the Science," *National Review*, November 29, 2021, https://www.nationalreview.com/2021/11/anthony-fauci-i-am-the-science/; Carlie Porterfield, "Dr. Fauci On GOP Criticism: 'Attacks On Me, Quite Frankly, Are Attacks On Science'" *Forbes*, December 10, 2021, https://www.forbes.com/sites/carlieporterfield/2021/06/09/fauci-on-gop-criticism-attacks-on-me-quite-frankly-are-attacks-on-science/?sh=35fafe345429.

21. Jean Giraudoux, "The Secret of Success Is Sincerity. Once You Can Fake That You've Got It Made," Quotes of Famous People, June 3, 2021, https://quotepark.com/quotes/1872806-jean-giraudoux-the-secret-of-success-is-sincerity-once-you-can-f/https://quotepark.com/quotes/1872806-jean-giraudoux-the-secret-of-success-is-sincerity-once-you-can-f/.

Index

Index